T0210186

The Price of Perfection

Recent and Related Titles in Bioethics

Joseph S. Alper, Catherine Ard, Adrienne Asch, Jon Beckwith, Peter Conrad, and Lisa N. Geller, eds. *The Double-Edged Helix: Social Implications of Genetics in a Diverse Society*

Mary Ann Baily and Thomas H. Murray, eds. *Ethics and Newborn Genetic Screening: New Technologies, New Challenges*

Audrey R. Chapman and Mark S. Frankel, eds. *Designing Our Descendants: The Promises and Perils of Genetic Modifications*

Lori P. Knowles and Gregory E. Kaebnick, eds. *Reprogenetics: Law, Policy, and Ethical Issues*

Erik Parens, ed. *Surgically Shaping Children: Technology, Ethics, and the Pursuit of Normality*

Erik Parens, Audrey R. Chapman, and Nancy Press, eds. *Wrestling with Behavioral Genetics: Science, Ethics, and Public Conversation*

Mark A. Rothstein, Thomas H. Murray, Gregory E. Kaebnick, and Mary Anderlik Majumder, eds. *Genetic Ties and the Family: The Impact of Paternity Testing on Parents and Children*

Thomas H. Murray, Consulting Editor in Bioethics

The Price of Perfection

Individualism and Society in the Era of Biomedical Enhancement

MAXWELL J. MEHLMAN

The Johns Hopkins University Press
Baltimore

Printed in the United States of America on acid-free paper
9 8 7 6 5 4 3 2 1

The Johns Hopkins University Press
2715 North Charles Street
Baltimore, Maryland 21218-4363
www.press.jhu.edu

Library of Congress Cataloging-in-Publication Data

Mehlman, Maxwell J.
The price of perfection : individualism and society in the era of biomedical enhancement / Maxwell J. Mehlman.
p. ; cm.
Includes bibliographical references and index.
ISBN-13: 978-0-8018-9263-9 (hardcover : alk. paper)
ISBN-10: 0-8018-9263-5 (hardcover : alk. paper)
1. Medical innovations—Social aspects. 2. Perfection—Moral and ethical aspects. 3. Social medicine. 4. Bioethics. I. Title.
[DNLM: 1. Biomedical Enhancement. 2. Decision Making. 3. Doping in Sports. 4. Social Identification. W 82 M498p 2009]
RA418.5.M4M45 2009
610—dc22 2008037854

A catalog record for this book is available from the British Library.

Research for this book was funded in part by grants from the National Human Genome Research Institute (NIH 1 R01 HG003879-01; NIH RO1 HG01446-05; NIH RO1 HG01446B2; NIH RO1 HG01446-01A1; NIH RO1 HG00683-2) and the National Institute on Aging, National Institutes of Health (NIH 1 R01 AG20916-01).

To Jerry

Contents

The Price of Perfection

Introduction

THANKS TO biomedical enhancement, in six months, you can be transformed. Your eyesight can become 20/5, so that you can see something from 20 feet away as clearly as a person with normal vision sees it at 5 feet. You can increase your muscle mass by 40 percent; improve your cognitive function so that you can remember better, solve harder problems, and cope better with emergencies; elevate your mood; sustain your erection; and surgically reshape your body so completely that even close friends will have trouble recognizing you.

Biomedical enhancement is not new, of course. Large quantities of amphetamines and alcohol were doled out to troops in battle during World War II. Athletes at the turn of the twentieth century ingested them as well, along with narcotics and all sorts of so-called patent preparations. The term *doping* itself comes from the nineteenth-century Afrikaans word *dop,* the name of a potion that Zulu warriors drank in the belief that it would help them vanquish their foes. The cognitive effects of nicotine were discovered five hundred years ago. Caffeine has been around for at least a millennium. Records from the ancient Olympics suggest that the athletes' enhancement of choice was an herbal energy drink. Even Viagra is old hat: the ancient Egyptians brewed an infusion of wild lotus containing a related substance at least a thousand years before Christ.

But modern biomedical enhancements are different. In the first place, some currently available biomedical enhancements produce much greater and more targeted enhancement effects than their predecessors. Steroids actually grow muscles. People who wear overcorrective contact lenses are in effect seeing through low-powered binoculars as a matter of routine. A first-generation drug for Alzheimer disease called Aricept (donepezil) significantly improves the ability of airline pilots to respond to in-flight emergencies in flight simulators, and the effects persist for some time after the pilots discontinue taking the drug.

And this is only the start. In the case of Alzheimer research, for example, the government is spending more than $600 million a year and private companies are conducting research on their own. Promising treatments are being discovered all the time; three new Alzheimer drugs have been marketed since the introduction of Aricept. Some of these new drugs are bound to work better than Aricept in normal subjects, significantly improving cognition with fewer side effects.

More extraordinary developments will emerge from the revolution in human genetics. Gene hunters already have widened their search for mutations beyond those associated with diseases and disabilities and are now seeking genetic factors that influence such positive traits as beauty, height, strength, and intelligence. Once these genes are located, they will generate a cascade of new technologies. Genetic screens will identify a person's genetic endowment for these traits, and parents will learn the genetically based talents of their children. Already, there is a test that allows sports teams and coaches to distinguish a genetic preference for growing slow- or fast-twitch muscles—the difference between having a talent for sprinting rather than for long-distance running. Couples contemplating reproduction soon will be able to test themselves and get a glimpse of the nondisease genes that their offspring would inherit. Parents now test fetuses and preimplantation embryos produced by in vitro fertilization not only to detect genetic diseases and conditions but also to ensure the proper gender. Soon they will be able to select embryos and fetuses on the basis of many other nondisease characteristics.

Recombinant DNA technology has been around since 1975. Splicing foreign DNA into the genomes of bacteria has the effect of programming them to manufacture compounds useful to mankind, such as synthetic hormones. We even have drugs that mimic or block the protein products that the genes encode. The next step also has been taken: we know how to switch a gene on and off, so that it manufactures a hormone only when we tell it to.

The current research frontier already has moved to the next stage, where we begin to reprogram human genes. Ultimately, this might enable us to redesign ourselves to produce a new set of desirable traits. Already researchers have genetically engineered a "smart mouse" as well as a "Methuselah" mouse, which has a lifespan 40 percent longer than average. Human genetic manipulation so far has proved difficult; a few people have died in experiments, and several babies who were thought to have been cured with gene therapy after having been born without a natural immune system nevertheless developed leukemia. But an enormous amount of research is under way. Eventually we will be able safely and reliably to treat genetic illnesses like Huntington disease by rewriting the DNA of the genes that code for them. As we also will have identified the genes that code for nondisease traits, there will be pressure to manipulate them as well.

Beyond this lies the final technological frontier: germline genetic enhancement, making positive changes in the DNA that will be inherited by our descendants. Germline genetic enhancement will take the same enhancements that we have developed with our increasingly sophisticated understanding of human genetics and make them part of our lineages. We could seize the initiative from our genes, a turning point in evolution. Able to reprogram ourselves and our children, we could reprogram humanity.

Many religious leaders think that God objects to this human trajectory, and conservative bioethicists like Francis Fukuyama, Leon Kass, and Michael Sandel complain that, by treading where we were not meant to go, we commit the sin of hubris. Like the medieval Catholic hierarchy that prosecuted Galileo, they want the science to be stopped.

They are joined by a chorus of scientific skeptics. The skeptics point to the complexities of genetics and how little we understand them. Only a few years ago, humans were thought to have about a hundred thousand genes. It turns out that we have less than a third that many, which we figured out when we realized that proteins can come in different shapes as well as chemical compositions. Scientists also point out that genes are only part of the reason for the way we look, how we behave, and what we accomplish; our environment, including the way we are raised, is at least as important. Finally, geneticists note that genes not only code for proteins but also interact with other genes and that most complex human traits, such as beauty or cognition, are likely to be the product of multiple genes at work, and thus not easily manipulated.

These are good arguments. We are indeed genetic babes in the woods, and we therefore must proceed cautiously lest, as the ancient Greeks believed, our *hubris* brings on *nemesis*, or catastrophe. But our efforts to regulate genetic and other enhancements for the good of society so far have been inconsistent and unprincipled. In elite sports, we try to impose a total ban, but it is enforced by a reign of terror and extended to substances that are so safe that a child can purchase them. We do not let adults employ anabolic steroids, yet normal children are given amphetamines to help them do better in school. Outside of sports, we criminalize the use of human growth hormone but pay millions of dollars each year for a military research program whose avowed objective is "sustaining and augmenting human performance" and "enabling new human capabilities." The government forbids doctors from prescribing drugs for nonmedical uses at the same time that the in vitro fertilization and dietary supplement industries are allowed to be virtual free-for-alls.

In any event, no matter how cautious or prohibitive we try to be, the history of science teaches us that genetic engineering and other enhancement technologies will continue to move forward. Given the scientific hurdles, it may take years before we gain the ability to reengineer the human race genetically, but then again, things may move much more quickly than expected. This is thanks to a remarkable historical coincidence, as I pointed out in my previous book, *Wondergenes: Genetic Enhancement and the Future of Society*. We indeed are in the midst of a revolution in science and human genetics, and like most revolutions, it has the capacity to change our way of life radically. But we also are in the grip of another transformation: the computer revolution. A company headed by Craig Venter deciphered the structural components of the human genome in a tenth of the time it took the government by using the largest amount of private supercomputing capacity in the world. Think how much of a difference computerization has made in the world in the last 25 years. Then, to factor in the contribution of genetic science, square it. That's how fast things are moving, just in human genetics. It's as if fire and the wheel had been discovered in the same half-century.

This prompts some important questions. What should society do about the growing sophistication of biomedical enhancement? Should we applaud it or disapprove? If we disapprove, should we invoke the coercive power of the state to stop it? Because we now permit the marketing or use of numerous biomedical enhancements, we would be unlikely to outlaw them altogether. But if only certain uses of biomedical enhancements should be allowed, which ones? Outside of sports, would we tolerate the invasion of privacy and bodily integrity that would be necessary for restrictions to be enforced?

Another challenging set of concerns is raised by the method by which these interventions are distributed. If biomedical enhancements were allowed to be bought and sold in the marketplace with little or no government interference, then we would face a problem of injustice, because those most affluent would enjoy the greatest amount of access. This might be offset by trickle-down benefits to the less affluent, but it also runs a substantial risk of creating a "genobility" that tyrannizes the have-nots. On the other hand, if the government is going to subsidize access, who is eligible? The poor? If so, to how much should they be entitled? Only to certain enhancements? Which ones? What about the problem of infinite regress, because although the poor who receive effective enhancements would no longer rest at the bottom of the socioeconomic ladder, they would be replaced by the group whose socioeconomic status previously had been slightly higher. This new group, being the worst off, would now be entitled to biomedical enhancements, and so on ad infinitum. The only way to avoid injustice seems to be to subsidize an equivalent amount of access for everyone, but such a restriction on individual initiative would require a commitment to communitarianism greater than Americans seem willing to accept.

But even greater challenges await us. Researchers are beginning to fashion chimeras—creatures that contain DNA from different species. They can make artificial genes that facilitate powers that no organism has ever had. These techniques will permit us to rewrite the human genome, or at least, the genome that once was human. Given enough of an opportunity, we could divide not only into separate subspecies but also into different hominids, and these may not be able to reproduce with one another, at least not sexually.

This leaves us asking: Should we stop this? Can we? Were we meant to?

Chapter 1

The Technological Horizon

We can control biomedical enhancement only if we know to what the concept refers. Too broad a definition would sweep up and possibly discourage medical innovation. Too narrow a definition and pernicious enhancements might slip through the net.

According to the dictionary, to enhance is to raise or lift up. A biomedical enhancement, then, is something biomedical that raises a person up by improving performance, appearance, or capability. If only it were that simple. In the first place, what is an improvement? It may be an objectively measured increase, for example, running faster or farther. But what about a more subjective improvement, such as a change in appearance? Suppose a person changes her eye color to an odd variant, say, orange. Is this an improvement? What if other people find it ugly? For the most part, an enhancement is an improvement if the enhanced person thinks it is one. But one of the fundamental questions that will be taken up later in this book is what happens if other people disagree. Do they have the right to interfere?

For the sake of argument, consider a change that most people are likely to regard as an improvement—the ability to read faster without any decrease in comprehension or enjoyment. Oxford professor Julian Savulescu defines *enhancement* as a "change in biology or psychology of a person which increases the chances of leading a good life."[1] So presumably he would regard this type of improvement in reading ability as an enhancement. But what if, before the enhancement, the individual had read at a snail's pace and now manages to keep up with other people? The improvement then would not be so much an enhancement as a remedial step, or, if the person had previously read slowly because of a disorder like dyslexia, a treatment. Remediation and treatment raise interesting issues about how they should be controlled but quite different issues from those raised by enhancements.

Some commentators restrict the notion of enhancement to changes that go beyond what is normal, so that a person whose performance or capabilities stayed within the normal range would not be regarded as enhanced. It is true that a person with below-normal reading ability would be deemed to be enhanced only if they then read faster than normal or at least read significantly better than average. But a person who started out with a reading ability within the range of normality also should be considered enhanced if they can now read faster, even if they remain within a normal range. Above-normal enhancements raise particularly troubling issues discussed later in the book, but it is a mistake to limit the term in this fashion.

But what is "normal"? In some cases, it refers to the frequency with which a trait or capability occurs within a population. A person of normal height, for example, is arbitrarily defined as someone whose height lies within approximately two standard deviations of the population mean. Because approximately 95 percent of a population lies within two standard deviations of the mean (assuming a so-called normal or bell-shaped distribution), about one out of every 20 persons automatically is either abnormally tall or short. In other circumstances, what is considered normal may have no relationship to the distribution of a trait. Instead, the emphasis is on a degree of function that is considered to be a useful baseline, if not an ideal. Normal eyesight is deemed to be 20/20, but only about 35 percent of adults have 20/20 vision without some form of correction.[2] (The 20/20 standard of normality stems from an eye chart created by a nineteenth-century physician; a person with 20/20 vision could read a character on the chart approximately three-eighths of an inch high from 20 feet away.)

What is normal also may vary from place to place and time to time. The average American is taller than the average Japanese, and the average American is taller now than at the beginning of the century. Standards of normality, moreover, might change as the use of enhancements expands; if there were a drug that increased height, for example, the more people who used it, the taller the average height of the population would become. Despite its fluidity, however, the standard of normalcy is critical in appreciating the difference between an enhancement and a therapy.

What if an individual, although starting out below normal, ends up above it? My colleague Eric Juengst cites the example of immunization, which makes people's immune systems better than normal. Because the goal of immunization is to prevent disease, it is not an enhancement; by definition enhancements are not aimed at preventing, treating, or mitigating the effects of a disease or disorder.

But now we have to decide what counts as a disease, and the concept of disease is just as hard to pin down as the notion of normality. Some people regard homosexuality as a disorder rather than a lifestyle choice. Body shapes that were associated with health a hundred years ago are now considered obese. There is a tendency to describe more and more conditions as diseases and more and more interventions as treatments. Cosmetic surgeons maintain, for example, that by enhancing appearance they improve patients' mental health, arguing that their services should be deemed "medical" and, not coincidentally, covered by health insurance. Critics call this "medicalization." They complain that doctors prescribe antidepressants to counteract the ordinary tribulations of daily life rather than to treat depression, and that many male children diagnosed with attention-deficit hyperactive disorder are merely "boys being boys." One group of authors laments that "everyday experiences like insomnia, sadness, twitchy legs and impaired sex drive now become diagnoses: sleep disorder, depression, restless leg syndrome and sexual dysfunction."[3] Many people suffer a mild loss of cognitive function as they age. This has led to a new diagnostic category, "mild cognitive impairment" (MCI), which has been arbitrarily defined as performance on neuropsychological tests that is greater than 1.5 standard deviations from age-associated norms.[4] This instantly makes about 1.75 million people in the United States sufferers of MCI. But do they really suffer from a disorder, or are they simply going through the normal stages of healthy cognitive life, albeit perhaps a little faster than some others? Much depends on the "unit of normality"—a person viewed over a long span of time versus the person at a given moment, for example.

A major controversy surrounds aging itself. Some biogerontologists (biologists who study aging) are adamant that aging is a natural rather than a disease process. Leonard Hayflick argues, for example, that "aging is not a disease, so the concept of seeking a cure for it is tantamount to seeking a cure for embryogenesis or child or adult development."[5] The President's Council on Bioethics maintains that aging is not only natural but also desirable and urges us to "take into account the value inherent in the human life cycle, in the process of aging, and in the knowledge we have of our mortality as we experience it. We should recognize that age-retardation may irreparably distort these and leave us living lives that, whatever else they might become, are in fundamental ways different from—and perhaps less serious or rich than—what we have to this point understood to be truly human."[6] On the other hand, even biogerontologists like Hayflick acknowledge that aging is the greatest risk factor for the leading causes of death and morbidity, and it is often difficult to separate the aging process itself from the deterioration that it causes.[7] If aging is a disease, a pathological process, or even just a state that makes people susceptible to illness, then efforts to combat it should be deemed therapy. But to the members of the President's Council, antiaging interventions are enhancements, and undesirable ones at that.

There also is a third way to conceive of antiaging interventions, one that confounds the treatment/enhancement distinction even further. This is to regard them as preventive measures. Not only does this approach enable antiaging entrepreneurs to finesse the treatment-versus-enhancement controversy, it also confers on them a preferred public policy status, because prevention generally is considered superior to treatment, even to cure, and preventive measures therefore tend to be given high priority in access to scarce government research dollars as well as favorable treatment by the FDA and other health care regulators.

In the end, then, the distinction between therapy and enhancement is not always clear-cut, and there invariably will be borderline cases. A good example is "compensatory enhancement," an intervention that does not treat a disease or condition but instead makes up for it, such as blind people taking cognition-enhancing drugs or, if available, drugs to improve their hearing beyond normal; another example is paraplegics injecting steroids to strengthen their arms. The interventions are enhancement-like in that they improve the person's capabilities without directly affecting the underlying illness or condition, but they are therapeutic-like in that they mitigate the effects of the person's disability.

Finally, what is meant by *biomedical*? The term, while blurry, refers to techniques that employ essentially biological means to alter human characteristics or capacities. There are many other ways of enhancing a person's abilities that are outside the scope of this book, including education, experience, and machines; as with the distinction between enhancement and therapy, it is sometimes difficult to draw the line between biomedical and other types of enhancements. Moreover, the book will cover mechanical prostheses but not implanted computer chips or the enhancement uses of nanotechnology, which, although similar, are the subject of blossoming but largely distinctive ethical and social debates. The types of biomedical enhancements focused on in this book employ techniques familiar to medical researchers and medical professionals. Once public policy has been established for these biomedical enhancements, the same underlying considerations may help formulate policy approaches for other types of enhancements.

So although subject to all of the foregoing reservations and qualifications, we can construct a working definition that says that a biomedical enhancement is a biological intervention that improves normal performance or capability and that is not aimed at preventing, treating, or mitigating the effects of a disease or disorder. Now that we have an idea of what we mean by biomedical enhancement, let's look at the state of the technology.

Enhancing Physical Performance

The cutting edge of efforts to enhance physical performance, not surprisingly, lies within one of the realms in which physical performance garners the greatest social rewards—elite and professional sports. During the nineteenth and early twentieth centuries, athletes' enhancements of choice were stimulants, such as cocaine and amphetamines, and calmatives, such as opium and alcohol. Amphetamines continue to be in vogue. According to John Hoberman, a noted scholar of drug use in sports, professional hockey players take amphetamines to feel more aggressive, which they believe improves their game.[8] Beta blockers, such as propranolol, which slow the heart rate, are modern calmatives. They confer an advantage in sports such as biathlon, where cross-country ski racers must stop suddenly and hold a rifle steady to hit targets.

In the mid-twentieth century, sports enhancement focused on two primary objectives. The first was to increase the number of red blood cells in the circulatory system. Researchers had discovered that the more red blood cells, the more oxygen that gets to the tissues, which improves the athlete's energy and endurance. In 1972, a Swedish sports physician developed what became known as "blood doping"—the use of blood transfusions to increase the number of circulating red blood cells. As sports organizations have become more skilled at detecting banned substances such as erythropoietin (EPO), a naturally occurring substance that stimulates the manufacture of red blood cells in bone marrow, athletes are reported to be reverting to blood doping. The most popular technique is autotransfusion, where athletes remove and store their own blood and then transfuse it back into their bodies before competition. According to a recent British government report, autotransfusion is virtually undetectable.[9]

The next breakthrough came with the development of recombinant DNA manufacturing. This technology enabled drug companies in 1985 to synthesize EPO. Lately, athletes have taken to sleeping in artificial atmospheres in so-called nitrogen tents and houses. These create artificial atmospheres that mimic the effects of sleeping at high altitudes, which stimulates their bodies to produce more red blood cells.

The second major goal of modern performance enhancement in sports has been to grow more muscle tissue. The chief substances of interest have been a class of hormones known as anabolic steroids, which include the male hormone testosterone. Researchers first attempted to isolate testosterone in the 1920s but did not succeed until 1935. At first they concentrated on medical uses, and when steroids first became commercially available in 1956 with the introduction of methandrostenolone (Dianabol), the drug was used to offset the tissue loss suffered by burn victims. But the potential value of anabolic steroids for athletes was obvious. There were rumors in the early 1950s that the Soviet weightlifting team was using testosterone to great effect. Steroids also became popular in track-and-field. Now they are believed to have infiltrated all sports in which additional amounts of muscle would be advantageous. Another recombinant-DNA-manufactured substance is human growth hormone (HGH). Many athletes believe that HGH has anabolic, or tissue-growing, properties and also that it can strengthen and prevent damage to tendons, reduce the likelihood of stress fractures, and speed the healing process after injuries.

Athletes have long experimented with modified diets to give them greater energy and endurance. A prime example is carbohydrate loading, where, to increase levels of glycogen, the storage form of the energizing sugar glucose, athletes follow a special regimen culminating in the consumption of large amounts of carbohydrates before competing. Vitamins and dietary supplements also are widely used. When he was with the Cleveland Browns, football player Jeffrey Faine was reported to swallow 22 specially formulated vitamin and dietary supplement pills every morning, 22 in the afternoon, and another 21 at night, for a total of 23,000 a year.[10] The National Football League even gives a seal of approval that certain supplement products can place on their labels.[11]

Performance enhancement is also at a premium in nonathletic settings. The steadying effect of beta blockers, mentioned earlier in connection with shooting sports, also makes them useful for musicians. The first mention of their use to combat stage fright appeared in a 1976 article in the British medical journal *The Lancet*.[12] In 1987, a survey of the nation's major symphony orchestras found that 25 percent of the musicians used beta blockers, more than two thirds of them obtaining the drugs from acquaintances.[13] Concerns about safety are allayed by the fact that musicians generally take between 5 and 20 milligrams of the drug, and only when they are performing; the drug produces significant side effects only at sustained doses above 700 milligrams per day.[14] Research shows that beta blockers not only reduce stage fright but also improve technical playing ability, and some experts believe that they enable musicians who use them to show how well they can really play.[15] Surgeons also take beta blockers to steady their hands during operations.

Finally, there are enhancements to improve male sexual physical performance. Viagra was first marketed in 1998, and while the FDA only approved it to treat a medical condition, erectile dysfunction, it is also widely used by men with normal erectile functioning to prolong arousal. This has not escaped its manufacturer, Pfizer. In 2004, the FDA required Pfizer to stop airing television commercials in which a voiceover asked viewers to "remember that guy who used to be called 'wild thing,'" and later said "he's back." The FDA felt that this implied that Viagra enabled people to regain youthful levels of sexual interest and performance, a claim that the manufacturer had not submitted any evidence to support.[16]

Enhancing Appearance

In 2006, Americans spent more than $11 billion on more than 11 million cosmetic surgery procedures.[17] Patients seeking a more youthful appearance underwent facelifts, eyelid surgery (bletharoplasty), and tummy tucks. More than 4 million people paid for less-invasive injections of Botox, which the FDA approved in 2002 to remove frown lines between the eyes. Still other people illegally use steroids. Researchers report, for example, that 5 percent of high school girls and 7 percent of middle school girls admit trying steroids at least once, and that two-thirds of users in high school took them not to improve athletic performance but to give themselves a "buff" appearance by controlling their weight and reducing body fat. This led the chair of the American Academy of Pediatrics Sports Medicine Committee to comment that "talking about supplements and steroids needs to start in the third grade."[18]

The most common types of surgical reshaping—nose jobs (rhinoplasty), breast augmentation and reduction, and liposuction for non-morbid obesity—are employed to make parts of the body more attractive. In 2006, the FDA decided there was enough evidence of safety to lift a longstanding ban on silicone breast implants for augmentation. While there is no age restriction on using the implants for reconstruction, the FDA limits cosmetic use to women 22 and older on the grounds that not only do women's breasts continue to develop until that age, but some younger women also may not be mature enough to make informed decisions about the potential risks. This is especially interesting in view of the practice of parents giving their daughters breast implants, including as high school graduation presents. A 2004 article in the *Miami Herald* describes a girl whose parents went along with her decision to have implants when she was 19 as a reward for losing 35 pounds. The implants raised her from a 36AA to a 36C. Her parents assented in part because she paid for the procedure herself, using money she had saved since she was 15 to make a down payment of $2,850, and borrowing the remaining $1,500.[19]

Cosmetic surgery isn't just for women. More than a million men in 2006 had nose reshaping, eyelid surgery, liposuction, hair transplants, and breast reduction. More than a quarter of a million men used Botox injections. Actor Michael Douglas is reported to have had a face-lift, neck wattle prune, tummy tuck, liposuction, and eyelifts. According to one press account, this was connected to his marriage to Catherine Zeta-Jones, who is 25 years younger.[20]

Cosmetic medicine also is an increasingly popular type of practice for physicians. As Natasha Singer reports in the *New York Times*, "Five years ago, cosmetic medicine was primarily the domain of plastic surgeons, facial surgeons and dermatologists—medical school graduates who undergo several years of training in facial skin and its underlying anatomy. But now obstetricians, family practitioners and emergency room physicians are gravitating to the beauty business, lured by lucrative cosmetic treatments that require same-day payments because they are not covered by insurance and by a medical practice without bothersome midnight emergency calls."[21]

Some cosmetic procedures are especially fashionable with certain ethnic groups. Asians request a particular type of double eyelid surgery in which a crease is placed in the upper lid to give the eyes a more "Western" appearance. In the past, Chinese girls were subjected to foot binding in order make them more sexually alluring and to enable them to marry into a higher social class. Bioethicist Carl Elliot explains that "a woman who was homely in every other way could still be considered beautiful if she had small feet. But if she had large feet, her marriage prospects were poor. She would be considered both ugly and common, and would face ridicule for having 'peasant feet.'"[22] In China, where being tall is a premium for certain high-paying jobs, one type of surgery that has become popular is leg-lengthening. The procedure consists of repeatedly sawing through the patient's shin bones and then pulling them apart and fixing them in place with metal pins and braces until the ends of the bone fuse together across the gap. The Chinese government renounced foot binding in the early twentieth century, and banned leg-lengthening surgery in 2006 as unsafe.

Although leg-lengthening surgery in the United States seems confined to dwarfs, there is no question that Americans too favor persons who are tall. A researcher at Harvard Business School noted that "you cannot even think about donating sperm if you're a short man. The average height of a sperm donor is 5-10. The average height of an American male is nowhere near that."[23] The height advantage has led some parents to seek injections of HGH for children who are normal and even tall for their age, in the hopes that their children will grow tall enough to play competitive basketball.[24]

Enhanced appearance is valued not only for the way it makes people feel but also for the social advantages it provides. People who look better do better. They even are treated better as infants. One controversial Canadian study reported that parental use of seatbelts for children increased in direct proportion to the children's attractiveness. "Like lots of animals," one researcher commented, "we tend to parcel out our resources on the basis of value. Maybe we can't always articulate it, but in fact we do. There are a lot of things that make a person more valuable, and physical attractiveness may be one of them."[25]

One venue in which the value of physical beauty is obvious is beauty pageants. Given the hostility of sports to performance enhancements, beauty contests are surprisingly indifferent to contestants' use of cosmetic surgery. After losing previous Miss America pageants as Miss Texas, Debra Sue Moffett had cosmetic enhancement and, competing as Miss California, was crowned Miss America in 1983. The official Miss Universe / Miss USA pageant policy states: "Although Pageant contestants are discouraged from altering their own natural beauty, no restrictions are placed on cosmetic surgery; it would be impossible to enforce such a rule. In fact, since 1990 the Pageant has allowed the use of padding in an effort to discourage participants from permanently altering their bodies for the competition." In 1988, the Miss San Diego pageant (a feeder for the Miss California and Miss America pageants) appointed an "official facial plastic surgery consultant" but eliminated the unpaid position after the press picked up on the story.[26]

Surgical reshaping even has become a spectator sport. Witness the popularity of TV shows like *Nip/Tuck,* a drama set in a south Florida plastic surgery center, and *Extreme Makeover,* in which participants are displayed "before" and "after" undergoing surgical and other forms of cosmetic transformation. The website for *Extreme Makeover* tells viewers for the 2007–2008 season to "expect more emotion, tears and joy as life-long dreams and fairy tale fantasies come true." In 2004, Fox aired a show called *The Swan,* which offered contestants $250,000 of cosmetic surgery and a chance to enter a beauty contest in which one would be crowned "the Ultimate Swan." One French performance artist undergoes a series of cosmetic surgeries which she directs while under local anesthetic.[27]

Plastic surgery is not the only way to enhance appearance. Tattooing is enjoying a surge of popularity, with 1 in 8 Americans getting them, including 40 percent of persons between the ages of 20 and 25.[28] Canadian sociologist Arthur Frank tries to distinguish modern tattooing and body-piercing practices from ritual scarification by claiming that the former are voluntary, personal decisions, while the traditional ones are "a non-negotiable expectation, expressing such matters as a member's gender, family status, and age group (such as having attained puberty)," but this ignores the fact that many tattoos are worn as symbols of gang membership.[29] A more radical approach to body piercing is inserting tiny heart- or crescent-shaped platinum studs into the eyeball. The technique, pioneered in Europe, takes 15 minutes and is performed under local anesthesia.[30]

Enhancing Cognition

Cognition enhancement has an ancient pedigree; after all, Adam and Eve were banished from the Garden of Eden for eating the fruit of the Tree of Knowledge. Caffeine has been in use for more than a thousand years. People flock to Starbucks not only for the cachet and the ambiance, but also for the caffeine: a 16-ounce serving of its regular coffee contains 550 milligrams of caffeine, more than five times the amount in a regular cup of coffee or in a single NoDoz tablet.[31] Some historians credit caffeine with helping to win the Civil War, because the South's supply of coffee beans was severely restricted by the Union naval blockade, while Yankee troops drank huge amounts of coffee, in some cases an "instant" version made from a concentrate, and chewed whole beans on the march if they didn't have time to heat water.[32] Nicotine also promotes cognitive abilities.[33] One study at Duke, for example, found that nicotine patches significantly improved age-associated memory impairment.[34] Traces of tobacco can be found in prehistoric human remains. Various stimulants, including cocaine, have long been popular as work and study aids. Freud's use and study of cocaine are legendary. He wrote in his notes: "You perceive an increase of self-control, possess more vitality and capacity for work. This result is enjoyed without any of the unpleasant aftermaths which accompany exhilaration through alcoholic means."[35] Amphetamines, first synthesized in Germany in 1887, are popular among students in the form of Ritalin (methylphenidate) and Adderall (dextroamphetamine). In May 2006, the Partnership for a Drug-Free America reported that 2.25 million middle and high school children, about 10 percent of the total, were using stimulants such as Ritalin without a prescription.[36]

Modern researchers continue the search for substances to enhance cognition. In 1998, the FDA approved a drug called Provigil (modafinil) to treat narcolepsy, and in 2004, the agency broadened the approval to include treating sleepiness associated with obstructive sleep apnea / hypopnea syndrome and shift work sleep disorder. Long before this it had become clear that the drug made healthy people more alert; it was reported that company executives, for example, were taking the drug to offset jet lag.[37] Stories in the press and word-of-mouth led to significant sales for these so-called unapproved or off-label uses. In 2006, the manufacturer, Cephalon, announced that sales of the drug had reached 10 million prescriptions for more than $2 billion in cumulative revenue.[38] Much of this income is believed to come from unapproved uses.[39]

Ampakines are a new class of drugs believed to improve alertness and memory by boosting the activity of the neurotransmitter glutamate.[40] Jonathan Moreno, author of *Mind Wars: Brain Research and National Defense,* describes one study that showed that one drug in this class, CX_{717}, eliminated 15 to 25 percent of the performance deficit in sleep-deprived rhesus monkeys and another study in which 16 men who were given the drug after having been deprived of one night's sleep improved their scores on memory and attention tests.[41] A developer of ampakines, Professor Gary Lynch at UC Irvine, claims that animal experiments suggest that the drugs "enable the brain to rewire itself or make neural connections between different regions that normally people cannot make," and the United Kingdom Academy of Medical Sciences already has an expert group looking into the potential medical and social impacts.[42]

Many of the breakthroughs in the science of cognition enhancement are likely to come from research on Alzheimer disease. The federal government alone is spending more than $480 million a year on Alzheimer research, and the FDA already has approved a number of drugs to treat its symptoms, including donepezil (Aricept), rivastigmine tartrate (Exelon), galantamine HBr (Reminyl), and memantine (Namenda). Preliminary results from federally funded and industry-supported randomized trials showed that donepezil improves the performance of airline pilots in flight simulators.[43] These drugs may not simply maintain wakefulness or improve recall; some of them also may improve executive function, "the orchestration of basic cognitive processes during goal-oriented problem solving."[44] The same may be true of modafinil. One researcher who tested modafinil in 60 healthy volunteers two hours after giving them the drug saw "quite strong improvements in performance, particularly when things got difficult. That was interesting—as problems got harder, their performance seemed to improve."[45]

There even is a cognition-enhancing drug for dogs, Pfizer's Anipryl, approved for the treatment of "canine Cognitive Dysfunction Syndrome, an age-related neurologic syndrome characterized by various cognitive impairments such as disorientation, reduced social interaction, changes in sleep and activity patterns, and loss of housetraining."[46] No information is available about whether the drug is used (or prohibited) in dog shows.

Enhancing Mood, Creativity, and Spirituality

In its quest for happiness, mankind often relies on biomedical interventions to produce or intensify positive emotions. Classic mood-enhancing drugs include stimulants such as amphetamines and cocaine; opiates; marijuana; hallucinogens, such as mescaline and psilocybin; and alcohol, which produces varying effects depending on the dose and the individual's emotional state. Tranquilizers, such as the benzodiazepines, improve mood by reducing anxiety. The first benzodiazepine, chlordiazepoxide (Librium), was introduced in 1963. By the late 1970s, benzodiazepines had become the most widely prescribed drugs in the world, led by diazepam (Valium).[47]

A brain chemical called serotonin has a powerful effect on mood. Psychedelic drugs, such as psilocybin, mescaline, and LSD, mimic the effects of serotonin. Other drugs increase the release of serotonin. One of the most powerful of these is 3,4-methylenedioxymethamphetamine (MDMA), otherwise known as Ecstasy. First synthesized in Germany in 1912, the drug, which induces euphoria, became popular in the United States in the late 1980s at dance parties called raves.

Other drugs increase the amount of serotonin by reducing its reabsorption or "reuptake." These are the antidepressants known as selective serotonin reuptake inhibitors, or SSRIs, the best-known of which is Prozac. Philosopher Carl Elliott describes people who use SSRIs as saying that they feel "energized, more alert, better able to cope with the world, and better able to understand themselves and their problems."[48] A different type of antidepressant, bupropion (Wellbutrin), enhances mood by inhibiting the reuptake of the brain chemicals dopamine and norepinephrine. According to one 29-year-old lobbyist who takes bupropion every day, "It makes me feel great. Wellbutrin makes me feel clear-headed, much more able to focus. I don't think it means that I don't ever experience any sadness, but I think it makes me experience sadness in a very healthy way."[49] More recently, deep brain stimulation, whereby electrodes are implanted in the brain, has been shown not only to reduce depression but also, by increasing the flow of current, to cause some patients to become elated.[50]

Enhancements are used by some to stimulate the imagination and expand creativity. Writers long have relied on alcohol. Donald Goodwin, the author of *Alcohol and the Writer*, observes that, of the seven Americans who had won the Nobel Prize for Literature as of 1988 (Toni Morrison won in 1993), four—Sinclair Lewis, Eugene O'Neill, William Faulkner, and Ernest Hemingway—were "clearly alcoholic," and a fifth, John Steinbeck, was "probably alcoholic." According to Goodwin, this is "surely the highest rate of alcoholism in any precisely defined group known to exist."[51] A 1974 study of 316 college students found that more frequent marijuana users were more creative and adventuresome; the study was replicated in 2006, with the same results.[52] Astronomer Carl Sagan also credited marijuana with improving his creativity.[53]

Drugs long have been employed to facilitate the search for spiritual truths. Native Americans incorporate peyote and its hallucinogenic alkaloid, mescaline, in their religious practices. Since the 1960s, many people claimed to have had spiritual experiences while taking LSD.

Foods also contain substances that can enhance mood. Complex carbohydrates, folic acid (found in spinach and other leafy vegetables), and tryptophan (found in meats), can increase serotonin levels. Selenium, found in Brazil nuts, is believed by some to improve mood.[54] In 2002, a Scottish company began selling a "mood-enhancing" brand of ice cream called "Vibrant," which contained an essence of an orchid that grows in Alaska.[55]

Enhancing Combat Effectiveness

It should come as no surprise that the largest research program on biomedical enhancements is run by the U.S. military. Many of the studies are funded by the Defense Advanced Research Projects Agency (DARPA). DARPA's research program, which began in the early 1990s, is extramural, meaning that the research is done by scientists outside of the military on DARPA money. The Dana-Farber Cancer Institute in Boston, for example, is conducting DARPA-sponsored research on substances to make soldiers more energetic. Columbia University is studying how soldiers can make do with less sleep. Agricultural experts in Ames, Iowa, are developing bacteria that, once ingested, enable soldiers to obtain nutritional value from normally indigestible substances like cellulose.[56] According to bioethicist Jonathan Moreno, DARPA is spending $100 million on research to counteract sleep deprivation alone.[57]

One area of intense interest is metabolic enhancement. Moreno describes a DARPA project called "Metabolic Dominance," which is trying to develop a super-nutritional pill that, according to DARPA, would permit "continuous peak performance and cognitive function for 3 to 5 days, 24 hours per day, without the need for calories." In response to concerns that antienhancement forces would make Congress or President Bush stop the project, DARPA changed its name to "Peak Soldier Performance."[58] Tony Tether, DARPA's director, has tried to downplay how far the agency's research efforts are intended to go. "You know the old Army saying, 'Be all that you can be'?" he has explained. "Well, that's really what we're doing." According to Tether, his agency is simply trying to maintain the level of strength and endurance that soldiers achieve at the peak of their training, a level that, while "extraordinary," is not "any better than their body can be."[59]

The U.S. military is not alone in its interest in metabolic enhancement: a 2007 report by the Science and Technology Committee of the British House of Commons discloses that the UK Ministry of Defence awarded a three-year, £1.5 million grant to drug giant GlaxoSmithKline to produce an energy drink called "Lucozade Sports Body Fuel" for soldiers' 24-hour operational ration packs.[60]

Much of the focus of military research is on increasing alertness. Until recently, the enhancement of choice was amphetamines. They were used widely by American, German, and British forces in World War II and again by the U.S. forces in Korea.[61] Beginning in 1960, the Air Force sanctioned them on a limited basis for the Strategic Air Command and, in 1962, for the Tactical Air Command. The Vietnam War sparked large-scale amphetamine use, with Air Force and Navy pilots using them to extend their duty day and increase vigilance while flying. According to one Cobra gunship pilot, "uppers" were available "like candy," with no control over how much people used. During the invasion of Panama (Operation Just Cause), the drugs were administered in smaller doses under much more careful medical supervision, and in contrast to Vietnam, where pilots who used them frequently suffered from nervousness, loss of appetite, and inability to sleep, fewer side effects were reported during Operation Just Cause.[62]

The Air Force continued to dispense "speed" during Desert Shield and Desert Storm. A survey of 464 fighter pilots in the first Gulf War found that, during the six-week operation, 57 percent reported that they took Dexedrine at least once, with 58 percent saying they used it occasionally and 17 percent admitting that they used it routinely. Sixty-one percent of those who took the drug felt that it was essential to enable them to complete their missions.[63] In 1991, the Air Force Chief of Staff, General Merrill A. McPeak, banned the use of amphetamines because, in his words, "Jedi Knights don't need them."[64] The ban lasted until 1996, when Chief of Staff John Jumper reversed the policy when missions were being flown in Eastern Europe.[65] In 2002, the Air Force was dispensing 10 milligrams of amphetamines for every four hours of flying time for single-pilot fighter missions longer than eight hours and two-pilot bomber missions longer than twelve hours. Asked why military pilots were permitted to use amphetamines when they were prohibited by commercial airlines, Colonel Peter Demitry, chief of the Air Force Surgeon General's Science and Technology division, explained: "When a civilian gets tired, the appropriate strategy is to land, then sleep. In combat operations when you're strapped to an ejection seat, you don't have the luxury to pull over."[66]

Amphetamine use became controversial in 2002 when four Canadian soldiers were killed and eight wounded in a friendly fire incident in Afghanistan. They were hit by a 500-pound laser-guided bomb dropped from an Air Force F-16 being flown by pilots who, returning at eighteen thousand feet from a 10-hour mission, thought they were attracting small-arms fire.[67] When they learned of their mistake, the pilots claimed that they were jittery because they had taken Dexedrine for so many hours.[68] One of the pilots had been an instructor in the Illinois National Guard and had graduated from the Navy's Top Gun school. The fatalities were the first Canadians to die in combat since the Korean War.[69]

In an effort to find a safer alternative to amphetamines, the military is turning to modafinil, the alertness drug described above. According to Jonathan Moreno, U.S. troops first used modafinil during the 2003 invasion of Iraq. The British press reports that the U.K. Ministry of Defence purchased 24 thousand modafinil tablets in 2004.[70] Research has shown that the drug improves the performance of helicopter pilots in flight simulators.[71] Moreno reports on a modafinil study that the Air Force's Office of Scientific Research conducted in 16 volunteers who, over a four-day period, stayed awake for 28 hours, then slept from 11 a.m. until 7 p.m.; the modafinil group did significantly better on cognitive tests than subjects who took a placebo. Other research showed that modafinil enabled pilots to remain alert for 40 hours, and experiments at Walter

Reed Institute of Research have been carried out on soldiers who were sleep-deprived for as long as 85 hours.[72] (The moral and legal propriety of doing this research on military subjects will be discussed later.)

While the military is actively investigating new alertness drugs like modafinil, it continues to employ that old standby, caffeine. New U.S. Army "first stroke" rations contain caffeine-laced chewing gum, with each stick providing the equivalent of a cup of strong coffee.[73]

Military uses of enhancements are not always directly connected with combat effectiveness. A plastic surgeon in Sydney, Australia, claims the Australian navy paid him to perform breast augmentation on two female sailors for "psychological reasons."[74]

Finally, it is important to bear in mind that biomedical enhancements that result from military research can find their way into general use. For example, the military developed Lasik surgery, which athletes and other individuals use to correct their vision to better than 20/20.

Preventing Aging

Many of the cosmetic surgery techniques described earlier, such as facelifts, tummy tucks, and Botox injections, are aimed at restoring or maintaining youthful appearance. But a substantial research enterprise is attempting to develop the ability to combat the aging process itself.

There are three possible goals of this research. One is simply to prolong human life. For instance, researchers are seeking to confound a prediction by biogerontologist Leonard Hayflick that cells are programmed to divide no more than 50 times—the Hayflick limit, as it is called—which would impose a genetic limit on the lifespan of any organism.[75] But as many commentators have recognized, extending lifespan would hardly be desirable if it merely allowed individuals to suffer infirmity for a longer time. In a previous article, colleagues and I called this a state of "prolonged senescence"; Francis Fukuyama calls it the "national nursing home scenario."[76] The most famous account is perhaps Jonathan Swift's parody of the Struldbrugs in *Gulliver's Travels,* whom he described as "opinionative, peevish, covetous, morose, vain, talkative, but incapable of friendship, and dead to all natural affection." They can remember only things that happened during their youth and middle age and cannot read, because they can't recall the beginning of a sentence when they reach the end; at the age of 90, they lose their teeth, hair, and appetite.

A preferable objective to prolonged senescence is "compressed morbidity."[77] The idea is for people to lead long lives free of chronic disease and disability, and then die quickly as their organ systems shut down upon reaching the natural limits of the human lifespan. This is the main goal of geriatric medicine and of many gerontologists, who search for ways to combat the ravages of disease in older patients.

The most ambitious antiaging objective is "decelerated aging."[78] This can comprise both prolonged youthfulness or vigor and an extension of the lifespan. Its ultimate realization would be "arrested aging": eternal, or at least extremely long-lasting, youth. This was the dream of medieval alchemists, who sought not only to transmute base metals into gold but also to discover a "philosopher's stone" that would prevent aging. In the early twentieth century, men slept with virgins and ate hormone-rich monkey testicles (in powder form) to keep themselves young.[79] A promising approach began to appear in the mid-1970s with a growing understanding of telomeres, segments at the end of DNA strands in the cell nucleus that become smaller each time the cell divides. When they are small enough, telomeres prevent the cell from dividing any further, thereby ending the life of the cell; when enough cells die, the organism itself dies. In 1985, researchers discovered an enzyme called telomerase that kept the telomeres from getting smaller when cells divided. If injected into cells, could it enable them to continue to divide indefinitely? Was this the key to longevity? Unfortunately, there is a problem with this approach. We have a special name for cells that divide indefinitely; we call them cancer.

While no one appears to consume monkey testicles these days, Americans are estimated to spend more than $45 billion a year on antiaging products and services. One hormone that is popular for its alleged antiaging effects is human growth hormone. Originally, HGH was extracted from the pituitary glands of cadavers, and the NIH distributed the extremely limited amounts available free of charge to researchers and patients suffering from hormonal deficiencies. In early 1985, however, a process was developed to manufacture the hormone using recombinant DNA engineering. Although the supply is now almost inexhaustible, the companies making the substance (Genentech and Eli Lilly) charge high prices. Estimates are that twenty-five to thirty thousand Americans take injections of growth hormone for antiaging purposes, paying up to one thousand dollars a month.[80] This is especially striking because, as explained later in chapter 7, the sale of HGH to combat aging is a federal felony.

In 1993, two osteopaths, Ronald Klatz and Robert Goldman, founded the American Academy of Anti-Aging Medicine (A4M). This organization, which now boasts twenty thousand physician members, holds annual meetings and grants its own "certificates of board specialization." In 2004, Klatz and Goldman filed a $120 million suit for defamation against two academics, Jay Olshansky, a sociologist at the University of Illinois, and Thomas Perls, associate professor of medicine and geriatrics at Boston University, who criticized the members of the A4M as quacks. The suit was eventually settled. But some aging experts remain skeptical of the quest for the key to aging. Leonard Hayflick scoffs that "yesterday's prolongevists who searched for the fountain of youth, advocated sleeping with young virgins, encouraged grafting of monkey testicles, and ate yogurt, simply have been replaced with modern equivalents, who have equal probability for success."[81]

Serious research on aging is under way, however. In 2001, the National Institute on Aging at the NIH declared "Unlocking the Secrets of Aging, Health and Longevity" to be an important research goal in its official Strategic Plan, giving as its objective "to develop interventions to reduce or delay age-related degenerative processes in humans."[82] One of the experiments the NIH has funded is a form of extreme dieting known as "caloric restriction." Although the idea goes back to the 1930s, scientists have recently demonstrated that roundworms, fruit flies, and mice on diets with 30 percent fewer calories live an average of 40 percent longer. In 2001, the National Institute on Aging began funding human studies, and a few researchers are self-experimenting with long-term caloric-restriction diets. But consuming such a low-calorie diet is likely to be extremely difficult for most people, so the race is on to develop drugs that will produce the same effect without the effort. One substance of interest is resveratrol, which is refined from grape skins and is believed by some to be one of the reasons that the French of widespread anecdote can consume rich diets without suffering a proportionate increase in heart problems.[83]

Reproductive Enhancement

In the past, enhancement during reproduction was limited to mate selection through courtship rituals, matchmaking, and arranged marriages. This still takes place, of course. One example is that of basketball player Yao Ming, whose conception followed a marriage orchestrated by Chinese sports officials between two unusually tall basketball players, a 6′7″ father and a 6′1½″ mother.[84] For many mate-seekers, human matchmakers have been supplanted by computerized dating services, in which participants select one another according to desirable traits. One such service, eHarmony.com, provides information about 29 personal characteristics, including appearance, intellect, industriousness, ambition, family background, education, and character.[85]

Reproductive enhancement has become much more sophisticated with the development of assisted reproductive technologies. Originally aimed at treating infertility, these techniques also have enhancement applications. One avenue they have opened up is enhancement surrogacy—the use of eggs and sperm, or "gametes," with especially desirable heritable characteristics, obtained from someone other than the mother-to-be and her mate. This has given rise to a huge egg and sperm industry. At Fairfax Cryobank, in Fairfax, Virginia, the most requested sperm donor is described as handsome, with hazel eyes and dark hair, and is pursuing a Ph.D.[86] The Genetics and IVF Institute provides the following information about egg donors: adult photos, childhood photos, audio interviews, blood type, ethnic background of donor's mother and father, height, weight, whether pregnancies have been achieved, body build, eye color, hair color and texture, years of education and major areas of study, occupation, Scholastic Aptitude Test (SAT) scores and grade point averages, special interests, family medical history, essays by donors, and personality typing.[87] The California Cryobank company gives purchasers of donor sperm a 26-page donor profile.[88] A company called Fertility Alternatives pays a premium to "exceptional" egg donors. To qualify, the donor must have graduated from or currently be attending a major university, preferably one in the Ivy League; have a GPA of 3.0+; SAT scores of 1350+ or ACT scores of 30+; and have a documented high IQ.[89] These enterprises follow in the path of a sperm bank called the Repository for Germinal Choice, started in 1979 by millionaire Robert Graham and known as "the Genius Sperm Bank" because it sought out donations from Nobel laureates and other highly prized sources. Before it closed in 1999, 217 children were born with "genius sperm." The few who have revealed their identities do have exceptionally high IQs.[90]

An assisted reproductive technology with especially profound implications for reproductive enhancement is in vitro fertilization (IVF), the technique whereby eggs are fertilized with sperm in the laboratory, which enabled the birth in 1978 of Louise Brown, the first "test tube baby." IVF adds several capabilities that facilitate reproductive enhancement. First, it enables embryos to be created entirely outside of the woman's body with donor gametes. The Abraham Center of Life in San Antonio, Texas, for example, sells embryos "made to order" from gametes selected on the basis of the race, educational attainment, appearance, and personality of donors.[91] IVF also permits embryos to be tested for traits before they are implanted in the womb, through a technique known as "preimplantation genetic diagnosis" (PGD). What happens in IVF is that a number of eggs are fertilized in the lab, but only a few of them are implanted in the uterus and given a chance to develop. PGD is used to select the ones that will be implanted. Currently, PGD, with one exception, is used primarily to test embryos for genetic diseases and disorders. Unlike amniocentesis and ultrasound, which parents have used since the 1960s to test developing fetuses for genetic diseases and disorders, PGD avoids the need for an abortion. The same approach could be used to select and implant the embryos with the best nondisease traits.

The one exception is sex selection, in which preimplantation testing is used to identify the gender of embryos and only those that have the desired gender are implanted. Another technique is to fertilize eggs with sperm of the desired gender, identified, for example, by a technique called sperm sorting, which relies on the fact that sperm with male chromosomes weigh less than sperm with female chromosomes. A fertility clinic that offers sperm sorting claims that one experimental sperm-sorting technique called MicroSort can shift the male-female ratio of sperm to either 88 percent female or 73 percent male.[92] Another technique is to use PGD. This is much more expensive than sperm sorting, and involves discarding the embryos of the wrong sex, but it allows for the full range of PGD testing before implantation. Sex selection also can be accomplished without IVF by using ultrasound or prenatal tests such as amniocentesis or chorionic villus sampling to determine the gender of a fetus, followed, if necessary, by aborting a fetus of the wrong sex. Gender selection can be performed for medical reasons to reduce the chances that a child will be born with a genetic disease that is more likely to occur in children of one sex or the other. When it is sought for nonmedical purposes, however, gender selection is extremely controversial. Critics object that the practice disparages females, because for the most part it is aimed at producing male children, and complain that it could cause serious population imbalances if widely employed. But a

2006 survey of IVF clinics found that 42 percent of the clinics responding had performed sex selection for nonmedical purposes.[93]

Genetic Modification

Over the last 15 years, researchers have made a concerted effort to decode the human genome. In 2000, they pretty much completed the sequencing of human DNA. The focus now is on understanding how DNA accounts for the myriad structures, functions, and dysfunctions of the human body. This journey has been breathtaking in its disappointments as well as in its accomplishments. When he announced the success of the Human Genome Project in a White House ceremony in 2000, President Bill Clinton charted the next steps: "We must sort through this trove of genomic data to identify every human gene. We must discover the function of these genes and their protein products, and then we must rapidly convert that knowledge into treatments that can lengthen and enrich lives." To everyone in the East Room of the White House, the president made it seem like this would not take long. After all, one year earlier, Francis Collins, who had led the government research endeavor, had predicted that by 2010 we would be in the midst of the era of "genomic medicine," in which young patients would learn the diseases to which they were genetically predisposed and stave them off with a combination of lifestyle changes and genetically tailored drugs.

There always had been skeptics, who pointed out that a person's environment was also an important factor in producing disease and other physical and mental characteristics, and insisted that most important traits undoubtedly resulted from the operation not of one gene but of many, significantly complicating the process of understanding and influencing them. Still, the optimists forged ahead with their rosy forecasts.

Then came a series of stunning revelations. It had become commonplace to assume that there were approximately one hundred thousand genes in the human genetic code. This figure was based on the understanding that the genes code for the manufacture of proteins and the assumption that each gene coded for a specific protein. Because there were approximately a hundred thousand human proteins, that meant that there were a hundred thousand human genes. But the Human Genome Project revealed that there were only about twenty-six thousand stretches of human DNA that actually were genes; the same gene, it turned out, could code for multiple proteins. A second major discovery was that the DNA that lay between the genes, once called "junk DNA" because it was believed to have no purpose, in fact contained critical instructions that controlled the workings of the genes. A third breakthrough was the realization that the genes were not lined up on the DNA molecule as once thought, but instead overlapped, so that the same genetic material could function as part of more than one gene.

At the same time, experiments attempting to treat genetic disorders with gene therapy were turning out to be more difficult than expected. In 1998, an 18-year-old boy named Jesse Gelsinger died after being injected with a virus that was being tested as a means of inserting healthy genes into patients suffering from a genetic immune deficiency disorder. Shortly afterward, French scientists who had announced the first completely successful gene therapy for another type of immune disorder learned that a number of the infants in their experiment had developed leukemia. All of this made it clear that, while genetic science had made great strides, it was going to be much more complicated than some had imagined, and therefore it would take far longer to unravel and be put to good use.

Researchers nevertheless continue to develop genetic technologies, including ones that enhance human capabilities. A prime example is in sports. One of the earliest practical applications of genetic engineering was the development of recombinant DNA, in which DNA instructions are inserted into a genome of a different organism. This can reprogram organisms to manufacture unlimited quantities of a foreign substance, such as human hormones that previously were extremely scarce. One example is HGH, discussed earlier in the chapter on performance enhancement.

Another hormone made using recombinant DNA engineering is erythropoietin (EPO). As mentioned earlier in this chapter, this is a naturally occurring hormone that influences how many of a person's blood cells are red. It is desirable to increase the number of red blood cells, because the more of them you have, the more oxygen is carried to the tissues. Recombinant DNA technology clones the human EPO gene and implants it into hamster ovary cells, which then make the protein. A third hormone that has potential value to athletes and is synthesized using recombinant DNA is insulin-like growth factor-1 (IGF-1).

Genetic technology already has gone past this stage, however. Reengineered genes not only can produce synthetic versions of naturally occurring substances, they can also be inserted into organisms and programmed to turn on and off. A company called Oxford BioMedica has created a product called Repoxygen. This is an EPO gene under the control of a gene that, when inserted into muscle cells, acts as a switch to turn the gene on to produce EPO in the presence of low amounts of oxygen. The company developed the product for the treatment of anemia, but it holds obvious interest for athletes, because they can obtain the benefit of EPO only when they need it, and more important, they may be able to avoid detection by antidoping testing when the gene is turned off. This presumably was its attraction for a German track coach named Thomas Springstein, who spoke approvingly about it in the course of being tried in 2006 for giving performance-enhancing drugs to minors, including a 16-year-old female hurdler, for which he was given a 16-month suspended sentence.[94]

NIH funding is not available for research on genetic enhancement in human subjects.[95] But in May 2007, NIH scientists announced that they had identified a genetic mutation in racing dogs that helps explain why some dogs run faster than others. The mutation is in the gene that codes for a muscle protein called myostatin. The researchers found that whippets with one mutated copy of the gene were the fastest racers, while dogs with two mutated copies had oversized muscles that slowed them down. Although the research was in dogs, Elaine A. Ostrander, the leader of the research team, acknowledged that it "could have implications for competitive sports in dogs, horses and possibly even humans."[96] Medical researchers are seeking ways to turn off or counteract the production of myostatin to treat muscle-wasting diseases such as muscular dystrophy. They have developed an antibody that blocks myostatin in adult mice.[97] The same techniques could enable healthy individuals to grow bigger muscles.

The target of this research, the protein myostatin, has long been of interest in connection with muscle enhancement, because it retards the growth of skeletal muscle tissue. As early as 1807, reports appeared of cattle with unusually large muscles. The meat of these so-called double-muscle animals was still tender. Starting in the 1950s, Belgian cattle breeders began selecting for this trait, and the new "Belgian Blue" cattle breed took over the Belgian cattle industry. In 1997, researchers discovered the reason for the trait: a mutation in the myostatin gene that inactivates it.[98] In 2004, a baby boy came to public attention whose mother had been a professional sprinter and was missing one myostatin gene, so that her body produced a small amount of the protein.[99] The boy, who looks like a miniature weightlifter, is missing both genes.[100] When he was not yet 5 years old, he could hold a 6.6-pound dumbbell aloft with each arm stretched out; most children that age can only lift one pound.[101] Another child has been discovered in Michigan who has a similar condition called myostatin-related muscle hypertrophy. When he was only 2 days old, he could stand up and support himself if someone held his hands for balance. At 5 months, he was able to suspend himself between two hanging rings with his arms held out horizontally, an extremely difficult gymnastics skill called an "iron cross." At 19 months, he could hang upside down by his feet and perform inverted sit-ups. Along with tremendous strength, however, comes an abnormally rapid metabolism that produces almost no body fat. The child is constantly hungry and eats six full meals a day.[102]

Another field of genetic research being watched closely by athletes involves genes that code for fast- and slow-twitch muscles. Fast-twitch muscles are associated with sports that require short bursts of energy, such as sprinting and weightlifting. People with more developed slow-twitch muscles are better at endurance sports, such as long-distance running. The discovery of genetic variations associated with the two different types of muscles is already affecting the sports world. Researchers have identified one variant of the ACTN3 gene in humans that codes for a protein called α-actinin-3, which is associated with slow-twitch muscles. People who do not have this variant, called R577X, tend to have fast-twitch muscles. An Australian company is selling a genetic test that detects the variant for ninety-three dollars.[103] One person with a great deal of interest in ACTN3 is Jason P. Gulbin, who coauthored an article in 2003 in the *American Journal of Human Genetics* entitled "ACTN3 Genotype Is Associated with Human Elite Athletic Performance."[104] Gulbin, it turns out, is the coordinator of scouting activities for the Australian Institute of Sport, which helped develop the ACTN3 test. As he explains it, "Multitalented athletes only have a short time in which to decide which sporting areas will suit them best, so knowing their genetic make-up could help them make informed decisions about which discipline to focus in."[105] The ACTN3 test is likely to be followed by many other performance-associated genetic indicators. In 2006, one group of researchers published a human gene map for "performance and health-related fitness phenotypes," or traits. It contained more than a hundred entries.[106]

Another frontier of genetic research with important implications for athletes is pharmacogenetics—the study of the interaction of genes and drugs. Investigators are discovering genetic variations that decrease or facilitate drug activity and that increase or decrease adverse reactions. This helps explain why certain people respond better than others to specific drugs and will enable doctors in the future to reduce the trial and error that characterizes much of their current prescribing practice. The same knowledge can be applied to the use of performance-enhancing substances by athletes. Because of their genes, some athletes are likely to respond better to certain of these substances than to others. Not only might this increase the impact of the substance on performance, but athletes may also be able to avoid many if not most of the side effects.

Genetic enhancement research is targeting traits besides athletic ability. Scientists at McGill University in Montreal, for example, have discovered a gene that codes for a memory-blocking protein, eIF2α.[107] Mice with a mutation that blocks production of the protein performed better than normal mice at remembering how to swim to a hidden platform and did better on a "fear-conditioning" test that measures their recall of a stimulus that precedes a mild foot shock. One researcher observed that "if a person were reading a page of a textbook, it might take several times to memorize it. A human equivalent of these mice would get the information right away."[108] The NIH itself sponsored a study to determine if a drug for Parkinson disease called tolcapone improved memory in people with schizophrenia. The subjects included a number of normal individuals acting as controls who were grouped based on differences in a particular gene, catecholamine-*O*-methyltransferase (COMT). The investigators reported that the drug significantly improved executive function and verbal episodic memory in subjects with one variant of the gene, while it impaired these abilities in subjects with another variant.[109]

Genetic enhancement by actually inserting or deleting DNA remains a more distant prospect, because it faces the same hurdles described at the beginning of the chapter that beset gene therapy. Yet in 2004, a team of U.S. and South Korean researchers, led by Ronald Evans at the Salk Institute, announced the creation of a "marathon mouse" that can run twice as far as a normal mouse. The researchers were able to increase the activity of a "master regulator" called the PPARdelta gene, which decreased the production of fast-twitch muscles in favor of slow-twitch muscles. One key question was whether the genetic manipulation would disrupt the animals' reproductive capacity, but the mice remained fertile and the mutation was inherited by offspring.[110] Researchers at the University of Pennsylvania also claim to have genetically engineered a strain of "smart" mice by boosting their production of a protein called NR2B that controls the brain's ability to associate one event with another, and Boston University scientists report that the mice maintain their superior learning and memory function into old age.[111] In an interesting aside, after the Penn results were published, a report claimed that the mice had suffered a severe side effect that made them significantly more sensitive to pain than normal mice. But the original researchers pointed out that the way pain sensitivity is measured in the mice is to heat the floor of their cages and record at what temperature they respond by pressing a lever to turn off the electricity. To the critics, the fact that the smart mice turned the electricity off at lower temperatures than normal mice showed that the smart mice were especially sensitive to the heat. To the original researchers, it merely confirmed that the mice were smarter, because they learned more quickly to stop the discomfort.[112]

As we will see in the next section of the book, no type of biomedical enhancement generates more concern than human germline genetic enhancement, whereby changes in an individual's DNA would be passed on to their offspring. The earlier section on reproductive enhancement described some basic ways this already takes place. When athletes reproduce with one another, for example, they pass to their children whatever genes they possess that help give them their athletic prowess. IVF coupled with PGD for nondisease traits would be a somewhat more sophisticated technique, because it would allow parents to select embryos with specific sets of genetic characteristics from a series of fertilized eggs, and only those embryos would have the chance to grow up and reproduce. But true, active germline genetic engineering, by targeting and manipulating specific genes and shortcutting the normal patterns of inheritance, would be far more versatile. One way this could happen would be if genetic material were manipulated at an early enough stage of embryonic or fetal development that it showed up in the DNA of the resulting individual's gametes, or reproductive cells.

So far as is known, the direct manipulation of DNA to produce germline enhancement has not yet occurred in humans, although as illustrated by the preceding discussion of the marathon mouse, it has been accomplished in animals. Germline genetic manipulation for medical purposes occasionally does occur, however, although inadvertently. One experiment to treat hemophilia by inserting corrected genes was delayed after the virus used to transport the genes was detected in the seminal fluid of a 64-year-old subject, suggesting that the altered DNA also might show up in the sperm. Another example is oocyte transfer, which remedies a certain type of infertility that is caused by deficiencies in maternal cytoplasm—the material in the egg surrounding the nucleus. Oocyte transfer takes a donor egg and replaces its nucleus with a nucleus from one of the mother's eggs. The resulting hybrid egg has healthy cytoplasm from the donor egg and nuclear DNA from the mother. But it also has another type of DNA, called mitochondrial DNA, from the cytoplasm of the donor egg. The new egg has DNA from three people instead of the usual two, so it is a genetic modification. Moreover, the triple-source DNA will be found in all of the cells of the resulting person, including their reproductive cells, so it will be passed on to that person's progeny. Hence, it represents a germline change.

Biomedical enhancement is thus extremely varied. It ranges from Botox to blood doping, from strengthening the arms of weightlifters to calming the hands of surgeons. Its technologies are as simple as a cup of coffee and as complicated as reconfigured DNA. When we reach the fledgling forms of germline genetic engineering, we are gazing at the technological horizon. Far more sophisticated enhancements are certain to lie beyond.

But are these technologies good? Do they pose an unacceptable risk of harm to users or to third parties? Do they actually provide the benefits they claim, or are the benefits uncertain or illusory? Would enhancements make us all better off, or just the privileged few who already occupy the top socioeconomic tier of the population? Do they threaten our liberty or our democratic values? Could they threaten the integrity of the human species itself?

In considering these questions, it is helpful to split the use of biomedical enhancements into two broad categories. The first is their use by individuals solely for their own satisfaction or fulfillment. People might use enhancements for the sheer enjoyment of doing or looking better, to obtain a more positive feeling about the task at hand or about themselves. The other main reason that people might use biomedical enhancements is outwardly directed: being better at doing things might yield competitive advantages and societal rewards—the approval of others, a higher salary, Olympic medals.

The goals of self-satisfaction and social reward are sometimes difficult to disentangle. Self-satisfaction may generate self-confidence, which in turn might bring about greater social reward. At the same time, obtaining social rewards is likely to make someone feel self-satisfied. Indeed, the same technologies that might make someone feel self-satisfied also could bring them social advantages. Yet each of these objectives raises a different set of objections and concerns, and therefore it makes sense to begin by considering them separately.

Chapter 2

Self-Satisfaction

THE 2006 DOCUMENTARY FILM *Wordplay* is about people who like to do crossword puzzles. One of them is filmmaker Ken Burns, who explains: "I don't drink coffee, smoke cigarettes, or need a drink at the end of the day. What I need to do is the *New York Times* crossword puzzle, in ink, every day." For puzzle aficionados like Burns, it's all about figuring out the clues to a difficult puzzle not only quickly but also definitively. Hence, the ink.

Many people have no patience with puzzles. They never seem to be able to finish them. They don't have the time. They find them too much of a struggle. But if they could complete a puzzle with the same zest as Ken Burns, perhaps puzzles would give them enjoyment and satisfaction. If people looked in the mirror and saw prettier faces than a few weeks earlier, they might feel happier and more self-confident. Maybe a weekend jogger could take pleasure in being able to run twice as far.

A chorus of critics, however, claims that modifications that come about through the use of biomedical enhancements should not produce such feelings of self-satisfaction. Why do they believe this, and how convincing are their arguments?

Many of the reasons asserted by opponents of the use of biomedical enhancement to increase satisfaction are difficult to comprehend. The President's Council on Bioethics—the largely conservative advisory group headed at the time by Leon Kass—in a 2003 report complained, for example, that an enhanced performance is "utterly opaque to [one's] direct human experience" and "unintelligible to one's own self-understanding."[1] At another point, the Council stated that, in contrast to the decision to employ a better training program, the use of steroids to enhance athletic performance "is a calculating act of will to bypass one's own will and intelligibility altogether."[2] Bill McKibben similarly objects that genetic enhancement would rob a child "of the last possible chance of understanding her life."[3] These arguments sound profound, but they are, at best, obscure. Why can't the critics articulate them more clearly? One possibility is that they are referring to human dimensions that are so subtle that it is impossible to speak of them with greater clarity. As Carl Elliott explains, "Many of us feel uneasy . . . , without being quite able to say why."[4] The other possibility is these arguments are largely obfuscation.

Other criticisms, while more comprehensible, are readily dismissed. One is so weak that it is difficult to take it seriously: that enhancements are "unnatural." Clearly, the fact of a phenomenon occurring in nature does not make it good or desirable. Many scourges of humanity, from floods and famine to Alzheimer disease and cancer, are naturally occurring phenomena, yet we do not object to measures to combat them like sandbags, humanitarian food aid, Aricept, or chemotherapy. Similarly, that a phenomenon does not occur in nature does not make it bad, or else we would eschew everything from shoes to the wheel. Moreover, many biomedical enhancements such as caffeine, HGH, and EPO do occur in nature.

The President's Council states that a person who is enhanced is "less obviously *human* than his unaltered counterpart," but it is not clear why this is so.[5] True, some types of biomedical enhancement may change the way the individual appears to others, and in the case of extreme forms of enhancement such as the creation of chimeras, the result may be less human. But this is not true of all enhancements. Many of the changes they produce are modest or subtle, and as we saw earlier, an individual can be enhanced and still remain within the familiar norms of the species. The Council might be using the phrase "less human" simply as a pejorative to mean that the effects of enhancements are invariably evil, but it is hard to accept this as true. Indeed, how often have we heard somebody say that they are "not themselves"—that is, not human—until they have had their morning coffee?

Another unpersuasive contention is that an improvement made with the aid of an enhancement is not "real." The President's Council on Bioethics states, for example, that "the performance seems less real," that "we may lose sight of the difference between real and false excellence."[6] As discussed below, the Council clearly does not believe that enhanced performance is "real" in the sense that it deserves to be valued. But the Council cannot claim that the improvement in performance is merely imagined. There is no question that the muscle growth facilitated by steroids, for example, is real, in the sense that we can measure both its size and its effect on performance.

An objection that also emphasizes realness is that enhancement leaves a person less his real self, or as the President's Council says, "less obviously *himself*."[7] In his antitranshumanist tome *Enough,* Bill McKibben goes even further, claiming that "we stand on the edge of disappearing . . . as individuals."[8] McKibben is especially concerned about genetic engineering. If we use genetic enhancement to transcend the limitations of our genes, then in his opinion "we are snipping away at the very last weight holding us to the ground, and when it's gone we will float silently away into the vacuum of meaninglessness."[9] This is similar to the objection that certain enhancements, such as those that alter mood, produce a less "authentic" person. As Carl Elliott explains, "It would be worrying if Prozac altered my personality, even if it gave me a better personality, simply because it isn't *my* personality."[10] But this ignores the fact that we often *want* to change our personalities. The resulting personality may not be the same as before, but that doesn't make it any less mine. Nor is a personality change necessarily bad even when it is sudden and radical. Epiphanies, conversions, miracles, and turning over a new leaf—all of these are not usually causes for alarm but for celebration.

Another objection to enhancement is that it is not necessarily good to feel better. In their book *Talking Back to Prozac,* Peter and Ginger Ross Breggin worry, for example, that "increasingly life is becoming a contest between pills—exemplified by Prozac—and life itself. People are giving up on life in favor of pills. They are abandoning the struggle to embrace life for the ease of swallowing a pill."[11] Gerald McKenny extends this objection beyond mood alteration when he says that "to the extent that enhancements overcome, or lead us to deny, the vulnerability of the body, they also foreclose the kinds of self-formation that our awareness of vulnerability makes possible."[12] The belief that suffering and struggle build character, although not universal, certainly is widespread and no doubt helpful in overcoming adversity.[13] But in the same way that it does not warrant leaving people clinically depressed, it does not justify refusing to allow them to become happier or more satisfied.

The President's Council on Bioethics also criticizes changes brought about by enhancements as not "self-directed." "By turning to biological agents to transform ourselves in the image we choose and will," it states, "we in fact compromise our choosing and willing identity itself, because we are choosing to become less than normally the source or the shapers of our own identity."[14] Elsewhere the council notes that "on the plane of human experience and understanding, there is a difference between changes in our bodies that proceed through self-direction and those that do not, and between changes that result from our putting our bodies to work and those that result from having our bodies 'worked on' by others or altered directly. This is a real difference, one whose importance for the ethical analysis . . . may prove decisive."[15] But surely competent individuals who choose to use enhancements for self-satisfaction can do so in a self-directed manner. The Council concedes that the decision to employ enhancements is an act of will but calls it "a choice to alter oneself by submitting oneself to means that are unintelligible to one's own self-understanding and entirely beyond one's control."[16] But why are decisions to use enhancements out of our control? Why are they "unintelligible"? The council does not say.

Another of the council's themes is spiritualistic. Biomedical enhancement, they say, "neglect[s] our embodiment" and frustrates our longing for "something transcendent."[17] Bill McKibben grounds his plea of "Enough!"—that we must place limits on our pursuit of technological self-improvement—on our religious heritage. "In the Western tradition," he explains, "the idea of limits goes right back to the start, to a God who made heaven and earth, beast and man, and then decided that it was enough, and *stopped*."[18] Michael Sandel puts forward a more extensive development of this spiritualistic theme by objecting to enhancements on the ground that they negate "the gifted nature of human powers and achievements."[19] Sandel's primary agenda is to reinforce the hegemony of natural talent, which is addressed in the next chapter. But philosopher Eric Parens puts Sandel's deontological adulation of giftedness in proper perspective by placing it alongside a rival conception of our life's task: to "mend and transform ourselves." As Parens points out, "as one side emphasizes our obligation to remember that life is a gift and that we need to learn to let things be, the other emphasizes our obligation to transform that gift and to exhibit our creativity."[20] Each side, as he shows, finds inspiration in our ethical and religious traditions.

A final philosophical objection is that an achievement produced with the aid of enhancements is not earned and therefore should not be valued highly by the enhanced individual. The Council describes enhanced performances, for example, as less dignified or worthy of admiration.[21] Athletes who use steroids are "getting their achievements 'on the cheap,' performing deeds that *appear* to be, but that are not *in truth*, wholly their own."[22] The idea seems to be that, when we use enhancements, we are cheating ourselves. This is different than saying that biomedically enhanced performances should not be rewarded by society, but because the argument is the same, it will be addressed more fully in the following chapter. What is noteworthy here, though, is that the contention that enhancement-aided performance should not be valued by the individual is not the same as saying that the individual *does not* value the performance.

Consider rock climbing. Some climbers use artificial aids such as bolts and ladders to support their weight. Some ascents cannot be made in any other way due to the absence on the rock face of hand- and footholds. So-called free climbers use safety ropes to hold their weight in the event of an accident but eschew the use of artificial aids. Other climbers "free solo," meaning that they use special shoes and special gripping chalk but neither artificial aids nor safety ropes. Based on the arguments of the President's Council on Bioethics, the free soloists should feel the greatest satisfaction, and the artificial aid users little or none. Yet all climbers clearly derive satisfaction from the sport, and each group applauds and defends its own approach. Free and free solo climbers call artificial aids cheating and complain that they disfigure the climbing surface. Free solo climbers are denounced as crazy thrill-seekers.

Another intuition is that the critics are conflating a sense of self without enhancement with what the sense of self ought to be. In other words, because in their judgment the sense of an able self made possible by enhancements is new and different, they think it is less worthwhile. Parens calls this an argument from precedent.[23] True, if enhancements were entirely new, the only previous source of self-satisfaction would have been unenhanced traits. But that would only reflect what people had been used to. It would not mean that enhanced traits were to be less valued. Moreover, as Ronald Cole Turner points out, new sources of ability don't eliminate the quest for self-satisfaction but only relocate it: "The fact that I write at a computer makes writing easier by eliminating retyping and other frustrations, but writing itself is still an intense struggle, and it will remain so under any technological condition."[24] If you don't believe this, try climbing a mountain even with artificial aid. But all of this is largely beside the point. As demonstrated above, biomedical enhancement, in some form, is hardly new. The critics may prefer a world without it, but that world has never existed. This is not to say that certain types of biomedical enhancement do not raise troubling issues. But the critics are not selective: all enhancements earn their disapproval, a position that ultimately is indefensible.

But biomedical enhancements raise other concerns that are not as easily dismissed. What if they don't work? A person would not derive self-satisfaction from a biomedical enhancement that did not produce the desired effect. Moreover, they would suffer the adverse effects without any offsetting benefit. The risk that enhancements may not work is heightened by unscrupulous entrepreneurs who fabricate or misrepresent their effectiveness. One dietary supplement website, for example, hawks "memory supplements," "prostate healthy nutrients," "heart healthy nutritional supplements," and "herbs for menopause" and lists supplements that "boost the immune system," "interrupt the replication of many pathogens," are "anti-inflammatory," and can ameliorate "diabetic nerve damage."[25] None of these claims is supported by rigorous scientific evidence.

An even greater concern is that biomedical enhancements may cause injury. Some side effects may be relatively minor. Caffeine is a diuretic, and in large amounts or in especially sensitive people it can cause insomnia, irritability, nervousness, and headaches, but these effects are not usually serious and a person would need to drink 50 to 100 cups of coffee in a short time to suffer a fatal overdose.[26] When researchers attempted to place genetically engineered "factories" in primates to produce the hormone EPO, it caused a total shutdown of blood production, leading to lethal anemia.[27] Some side effects, while not physically damaging, are surprising. One experiment reported, for example, that people who ingested caffeine were more susceptible to persuasion.[28] Moreover, some people believe that the use of enhancement drugs is a precursor to experimenting with dangerous recreational drugs, a claim we will consider in more detail later.

In addition, individuals may feel under so much outside pressure to use enhancements that they make what seem like unwise decisions about the risks involved in a potential increase in self-satisfaction. People may find themselves dissatisfied with their appearance or performance unless it is as good as or better than those of others. The desire to look younger may override safety concerns. The enhancement industry no doubt will borrow a page from drug marketers and stimulate demand through advertising, including direct-to-consumer outreach.

As the demand for enhancement grows, so will its commercial attractiveness to the biomedical industry. Some commentators already complain that drug companies are beginning to neglect research on drugs for serious illnesses in favor of research on enhancements.[29] Greater numbers of health care professionals are specializing in enhancement medicine, where the patients are relatively easy to care for and pay out-of-pocket, so that practitioners can avoid the fee limits and other inconveniences of managed care. This could reduce the number of professionals available to care for the ill. Sociologist Arthur Frank argues that "technoluxe medicine distorts the allocation of medical services and distracts medicine from its original and still-predominant purpose."[30] Indeed, some physicians believe that providing access to enhancements should be outside the proper practice of medicine altogether. A two-time Olympic rower, who is pursuing a residency in rehabilitation medicine at Harvard, is quoted as stating, for example: "I have ethical problems with it as a doctor. I can't see where someone would provide a drug or medication to someone for a problem that doesn't exist."[31]

Another concern that I have focused on in previous writings is that the cost of enhancements might place them beyond the means of all but the relatively affluent. We tolerate innumerable sources of satisfaction that are affordable only by the few, such as fancy automobiles, exotic vacations, and first-class restaurants. But some may feel that the satisfaction obtainable with biomedical enhancements is so important that they constitute a necessity rather than a luxury.

In sum, the use of biomedical enhancement for self-satisfaction elicits some valid objections. But there are a number of possible responses. One is to let people make their own decisions about whether or not to use them. Another is for the critics to try to persuade people to desist from using them and to express their disapproval through social behavior, such as by refusing to associate with enhanced individuals. These approaches rely on essentially private decisions. A third option, however, is public action—invoking the power of government to curtail private behavior. As we will see, many opponents of enhancements favor some form of government intervention. The question is whether the objections to using enhancements for self-satisfaction are sufficiently compelling to justify the use of state power.

The starting point for any discussion of government control of behavior is the presumption in favor of personal liberty. Competent, well-informed individuals ordinarily have the right to conduct themselves as they see fit. Supreme Court Justice Harlan observed that "our Nation [is] built upon postulates of respect for the liberty of the individual."[32] This extends to a right of control over one's body. As Judge (later Justice) Benjamin Cardozo stated in 1914: "Every human being of adult years and sound mind has a right to determine what shall be done with his own body."[33] Liberty also includes the right to realize one's "character and potentialities as a human being."[34] This in turn encompasses the right to enhance one's capabilities, presumably including the use of biomedical technology.

The principle that competent individuals have the right to make voluntary decisions about whether or not to use enhancements for self-satisfaction is not without limit, of course. It is well accepted that societal intervention would be appropriate if an enhancement posed a significant risk of harm to third parties. If an enhancement drug made people dangerous drivers, for example, the government would be entitled to prevent people from driving while under the influence. If the potential harm to the gene pool from germline genetic enhancement were sufficiently dire, it would be legitimate for the state to try to prevent germline enhancement from taking place.

There is much less agreement on whether the government may intervene when the only persons harmed are the individual users themselves. Here again, there are some areas of general agreement. For example, most people undoubtedly approve of state action to protect individuals who are not competent to make choices for themselves, such as when they are too young or when their mental faculties are compromised. We will discuss this in more detail later in the book. But what about competent persons? Is government action appropriate to prevent them from what others regard as harming themselves?

Arguably, even competent persons cannot make good choices unless they have an adequate understanding of the potential consequences of their decisions. If adequate information about the risks and benefits of biomedical enhancements is lacking, then the government arguably has a legitimate role in ensuring that the necessary information is made available. But what if individuals do not have the information, either because of their own failure to obtain it or society's failure to produce it? Many would say that government action restricting individual choice may be appropriate. Joel Feinberg calls this "soft paternalism."[35] Soft paternalism is said to be consistent with the principle of personal liberty because it prevents people from making only the harmful choices that they presumably would not make if they were properly informed. For example, we place boundaries on the use of biomedical interventions when there is a lack of safety and efficacy data. It is unlawful, for example, to sell drugs or medical devices that have not been approved by the FDA on the basis of scientific studies purportedly demonstrating their safety and effectiveness. Moreover, many drugs and medical devices can be obtained lawfully only by prescription, on the premise that they are dangerous enough that the decision to use them should be left with a person with professional medical expertise.

Of course, excessive soft paternalism can destroy personal liberty. Therefore, we leave people free to accept some risks. Our regulatory system limits access to certain biomedical interventions, such as prescription drugs, on the grounds that they are too dangerous to be used without physician oversight. But some drugs are deemed safe enough that they can be purchased "over the counter" (that is, without a prescription). Some enhancements are in this category, caffeine being an obvious example.

Furthermore, when it comes to determining whether the potential benefits of biomedical enhancements outweigh the risks, some people question whether physicians have sufficient insight that they deserve to be given control over individual access. The President's Council on Bioethics, no friend of biomedical enhancement, even has expressed some doubt: "There are difficulties when medical practice moves beyond therapy. Where the goal is restoring health, the doctor's discretion is guided by an agreed-upon and recognizable target. But a physician prescribing for goals beyond therapy is in uncharted waters. Although fully armed with the means, he has no special expertise regarding the end—neither what it is nor whether it is desirable."[36] If physicians have no special ability to decide whether the benefits of using enhancements for self-satisfaction exceed the risks, a good argument can be made that their role should be limited to providing biomedical information, watching out for adverse effects that might not be obvious to the enhancement user, and, when asked, acting as an advisor. In that case, a strong case can be made that the ultimate decision of whether or not to use enhancements should be left up to the individual even when they do not have good information about the benefits and risks.

Given these reservations about the legitimate scope of soft paternalism, it may come as a surprise that some people believe that society has an obligation to protect people from harming themselves even when they are competent and fully informed. Joel Feinberg calls this viewpoint "hard paternalism." Unlike soft paternalism, which assumes that people will make the right decision if they have adequate knowledge and expertise, hard paternalism rests on the belief that "the subject has the wrong set of preferences and 'does not know what is good for him,'" so those who do know what is best should make the decision.[37]

Hard paternalism harks back to Aristotle, who believed that people should strive to live a good life and that individuals like him who know what such a life comprises should urge it on the unenlightened. Aristotle's view is a form of what is known in moral philosophy as "perfectionism." It turns out that the best way to make sense of the more obscure objections to enhancements made by Leon Kass and the Council on Bioethics quoted earlier, as well as to understand Michael Sandel's argument about giftedness, may be to regard them as arguments based on perfectionism: People who believe that enhancements can help them feel self-satisfied are misguided because the use of enhancements is inconsistent with the good life.

Now we come to a crucial distinction. Under the principle of personal liberty, Kass and Sandel have every right to offer their conception of the good life to others and to try to persuade them not to use enhancements. It is another thing entirely, however, for those who believe that enhancements are incompatible with a good life to make them illegal. Suppose that a competent adult wanted to use a relatively inexpensive, widely available, highly effective, and relatively safe enhancement that did not pose any physical risks to third parties and did not alter the germline, and suppose that the adult's desire was not in response to undue external pressure. Would the happenstance that some people regard this as inconsistent with "the good life" warrant making enhancement use against the law? Aristotle clearly thought that the state had a duty to try to make people live a good life. As he wrote in his *Politics*, "The legislator must labor to ensure that his citizens become good men.

He must therefore know what institutions will produce this result, and what is the end or aim to which a good life is directed."[38] But enforcing hard paternalism through the power of the state is diametrically opposed to the principle of personal liberty. As the Supreme Court has emphasized, "At the heart of liberty is the right to define one's own concept of existence, of meaning, of the universe, and of the mystery of human life. Beliefs about these matters could not define the attributes of personhood were they formed under compulsion of the State."[39]

Bioethicist Daniel Callahan learned this lesson about hard paternalism firsthand when he attempted to apply his approach to intergenerational justice to the allocation of health care resources. In his book *Setting Limits,* Callahan urged people to reject biomedical interventions that would make it possible for them to outlive their natural, active lifespans. In his opinion, desperately searching for longevity was no way to live. Callahan's arguments were sincere and, no doubt to some individuals, persuasive. But he didn't stop there. Although he didn't suggest making it illegal to give life-saving treatments to the extreme elderly, he proposed that the Medicare laws be changed so that the program would no longer pay for such treatments. Poorer people with a different viewpoint, who wanted to go on living but could not afford to purchase the treatments on their own, would no longer be allowed to live. Hardly anyone supported this suggestion. When he moved from exhortation to government mandate, Callahan's arguments failed.

In the light of the strength of the principle of personal liberty, opponents of enhancements for self-satisfaction have come up with a way to avoid confronting it directly: They revert to the obligation to avoid harming others. The "others" here is society itself. People who do not live a good life are acting immorally, they argue, and immorality harms society. Therefore, society has a right to protect itself by restricting the freedom of those who would act immorally by using enhancements.

The question of whether immoral behavior that does not directly harm others is a sufficient threat to society to justify making it illegal has long occupied legal scholars and political theorists. A classic clash occurred between two British legal theorists, Patrick (later Lord) Devlin and H. L. A. Hart. Their quarrel broke out over the 1957 Report of the Departmental Committee on Homosexual Offences and Prostitution, known as the Wolfenden report after Lord Wolfenden, who chaired the committee. The report recommended repealing the laws that made homosexuality between consenting adults a crime in Great Britain. In a lecture to the British Academy denouncing the report, later published as *The Enforcement of Morals,* Devlin argued that homosexuality was immoral and that its immorality injured society by weakening the bonds that held society together. "Society," he asserted, "means a community of ideas; without shared ideas on politics, morals, and ethics no society can exist. . . . If men and women try to create a society in which there is no fundamental agreement about good and evil they will fail; if, having based it on common agreement the agreement goes, the society will disintegrate." Devlin followed this with the language for which he is best known: "For society is not something that is kept together physically; it is held by the invisible bonds of common thought. . . . The bondage is part of the price of society; and mankind, which needs society, must pay its price."[40] Having lived through World War II, Devlin dramatized his position with the chilling observation that "a nation of debauchees would not in 1940 have responded satisfactorily to Winston Churchill's call to blood and toil and sweat and tears."[41] For Devlin, there was no zone of privacy beyond the reach of society, because it is "no more possible to define a sphere of private morality than it is to define one of private subversive activity." In short, "there can be no theoretical limits to legislation against immorality."[42]

H. L. A. Hart, Oxford professor of jurisprudence, openly disagreed with Devlin in remarks first broadcast over the radio, then in a series of lectures at Stanford, and eventually in his book, *Law, Liberty, and Morality.*[43] Hart was vehement in likening Devlin's "absurd" views to those of the Emperor Justinian, who believed that "homosexuality was the cause of earthquakes."[44] Morality is not static, Hart insisted. It often changes for the better, and in any event, a change in social norms does not destroy society.[45]

Devlin's principle that society has the right to legislate the morals of its members is reflected in some versions of a doctrine called "communitarianism." Two bioethicists who embrace communitarian principles are Canadian professor Charles Taylor and Princeton professor Robert George. Taylor argues that society defines who we are: "Our identity is always partly defined in conversation with others or through the common understanding which underlies the practices of our society." He adds that "since the free individual can only maintain his identity within a society/culture of a certain kind, he has to be concerned about the shape of this society/culture as a whole."[46] George, a member of the President's Council on Bioethics, believes that "sound politics and good law are concerned with helping people to lead morally upright and valuable lives." Accordingly, "a good political society may justly bring to bear the coercive power of public authority to provide people with some protection from the corrupting influence of vice."[47]

Whether it rests on ideas of perfectionism or communitarianism, hard paternalism encounters a major difficulty: how do we tell what set of moral principles is correct? Aristotle's answer was vague: the proper moral principles are those that enable one to live a good life. The communitarian answer is that they are the moral principles shared by the members of society. But this confuses what people believe with what they should believe.

The solution that some critics of enhancement have adopted is to turn from reason to emotion. We can identify immoral arguments and behaviors, they say, by our emotional reaction to them. Specifically, we find them repugnant. Leon Kass, for example, states that "in crucial cases . . . repugnance is the emotional expression of deep wisdom, beyond reason's power fully to articulate it."[48] He applies this approach to the ethics of human cloning: "We are repelled by the prospect of cloning human beings not because of the strangeness or novelty of the undertaking, but because we intuit and feel, immediately and without argument, the violation of things that we rightfully hold dear. Repugnance, here as elsewhere, revolts against the excesses of human willfulness, warning us not to transgress against what is unspeakably profound."[49] The argument from repugnance was enunciated by the Victorian jurist James Fitzjames Stephens, an opponent of John Stuart Mill who held that "the custom of looking upon certain courses of conduct with aversion [is] the essence of morality."[50] Devlin too recognized a connection between morality and sentiment, referring to the "intolerance, indignation, and disgust" with which people react to highly objectionable behavior.[51]

Yet whether it rests on a sense of shared morality or a feeling of repugnance, the view that the state should make behavior illegal even though it does not cause tangible harm to others is dangerous. The presumption of personal liberty would be erased if society were entitled to intervene whenever anyone felt vexed by the actions of others. As numerous commentators have pointed out, just about anything is likely to annoy somebody. A racist might be upset by having to live in an interracial society. Some Catholics might be aggrieved by the proximity of a drugstore selling Plan B emergency contraceptives. The aggrieved undoubtedly have the right to try to convince others to live in segregated communities or to fill their prescriptions at another drug store. But they do not have a right to forbid miscegenation or to make the sale of Plan B illegal. Clearly, we must think carefully before we decide to regulate individual behavior that does not cause tangible harm to others.

Competent adults have a presumptive right to employ biomedical enhancements for their own satisfaction. The state may curtail this right to prevent serious, tangible harm to others. There also is a legitimate role for government in protecting those who cannot make voluntary, informed decisions; in providing information on risks and benefits to help individuals make decisions; and perhaps in facilitating access for those who cannot afford them. Beyond that, it becomes hard to argue that limiting the freedom to use enhancements purely for one's own enjoyment is necessary for the public good.

But the internal reward of self-satisfaction is not the only reason that people might enhance themselves. They may do so to obtain greater external, or social, rewards. The same enhancements that increased self-satisfaction also could increase a person's chances of social success. An improvement in self-esteem made possible by cosmetic surgery could make a person more employable. A cognition-enhancing drug that enables people to zip through the crossword puzzle might enable them to score higher on a college entrance exam. The rarer such enhancements are, the greater the impact for any individual user who benefits from them. Users might obtain a decisive competitive advantage.

A new set of troubling issues arises when we shift from the use of enhancements for self-satisfaction to their ability to yield social rewards. The question is no longer whether to restrict individual freedom for purely paternalistic reasons. As the next chapter explains, the use of enhancements to obtain social benefits can have a much more evident adverse effect on others, because in most cases, there is only a limited amount of social goods to go around, so one person's social success almost certainly comes at the expense of another. The ways in which access to enhancements is distributed thus becomes critical. At the same time, the need to succeed, and the pressures from those who stand to benefit collaterally, could undermine an individual's ability to make rational choices about whether or not to use risky enhancement techniques, in which case they no longer may retain the presumption of individual autonomy. All of these considerations might call for a more vigorous exercise of public power to produce public good.

Chapter 3

Social Reward

WHEN BIOMEDICAL ENHANCEMENTS are used for self-satisfaction, users, if they can be said to be in competition, are competing against themselves. They are hoping to be faster, stronger, smarter, and more beautiful than they were before. But enhancements might enable them to be faster, stronger, smarter, or more beautiful than the next person too. The negative by-products of this one-upmanship are more than vanity and envy: society rewards people who are better than others. They get better jobs, houses, food, clothes, toys, health care, vacations, and educations. Enhancements that improve a person's capabilities could well be a key to higher living.

It therefore comes as no surprise that people use enhancements to give them a competitive advantage. The most obvious example is in sports, where elite and professional sports organizations wage a constant battle against athletes, coaches, and disreputable chemists in an effort to stop the use of performance-enhancing drugs. But the competitive advantages of enhancements extend well beyond sports. As jobs get scarcer and the premium for high performance continues to swell, the use of enhancements in the workplace is bound to expand. On-the-job use of alertness drugs like modafinil is growing. Musicians steady their hands with beta blockers before competitions. Businesspeople as well as actors are getting cosmetic surgery to boost their careers. The *New York Times* tells the story of a stockbroker who got a facelift to be able to compete with her younger colleagues.[1] In 2004, the American Academy of Facial Plastic and Reconstructive Surgery reported that 22 percent of men and 15 percent of women who sought plastic surgery did so for work-related reasons.[2] It is well known that less-attractive workers earn less. One study found that employees of average beauty earned 10 to 15 percent more than those of below-average beauty.[3] Experiments have identified a substantial "beauty premium" attributed to three factors: attractive workers are more confident, they have better communication and social skills, and they are judged by their employers, incorrectly, to be more capable.[4]

In what many perceive to be a cutthroat, winner-take-all society, biomedical enhancements may become essential to enable people just to survive economically, never mind to move forward. The old recipe for success, a combination of natural talent, hard work, and good luck, could become no longer sufficient. The objections to enhancements discussed in the previous chapter may seem to wither in the face of marketplace realities and employer demands for growing productivity. Businesses that now test employees to make sure they do not use drugs may soon test them to make sure they do.

The incentive to use enhancements is hardly weaker outside of the workplace. Beauty contestants use cosmetic surgery to augment their natural endowments. College students use stimulants when they write papers and take exams. Parents get doctors to prescribe amphetamines to help normal children do better in school. Sales of caffeinated energy drinks are soaring. An Australian study in 2001 found that children as young as 11 were drinking up to five cans of Red Bull and similar products before sports matches. "The coaches are encouraging them," bemoaned the study's author, "and parents are buying it for them."[5] A reporter for the *San Francisco Chronicle* claimed in 2004 that Little League coaches were giving Red Bull to preteen players.[6]

The demand for enhancements is being fueled by the enhancement industry. A prime target is baby boomers, who are eager to embrace products that claim to make them fitter in body and mind. Not only are boomers keenly aware of the onslaught of aging, but they also have a strong desire to outperform one another. The industry is only too happy to oblige. As one marketer of "fitter-brain" products explains, "boomers . . . have a marked propensity to push the envelope on personal development," adding "and not incidentally, to compete with one another by any personal-development measure available."[7] At the moment, boomers probably value enhancements largely as an aid in maintaining a vim-and-vigor lifestyle, but as lifespan increases and the population refuses or cannot afford to retire, the competition for jobs will make enhancements that lengthen the workspan crucial for boomers' economic survival.

Clearly, then, enhancements are poised to become a larger part of daily life, not only to give people greater satisfaction but also to bring them greater social rewards. Like all changes in the way we live, the new order of things may take some getting used to. It may feel strange at first to wake up not only by drinking a cup of strong coffee but also by swallowing a handful of "peppers," "brainers," and "moodies," the dosage conforming to one's schedule at the office, school, or factory.

But just because the use of enhancements becomes an indispensable part of the day does not tell us whether their use should be controlled by society rather than by the users themselves. Clearly something is not bad simply because it is new. Therefore, we must examine the use of biomedical enhancements for competitive advantage with the same critical eye with which we considered the ethical objections to the use of enhancements for self-satisfaction. What, if anything, is wrong with it?

Let's take sports as the starting point.

A simplistic answer to what's wrong with the use of biomedical enhancements for social reward is that it may be cheating. The use of certain biomedical enhancements violates the agreed-upon rules of such sports organizations as the Olympics, the National Collegiate Athletic Association, the National Basketball Association, Major League Baseball, the National Football League, and the Paralympics, as well as the International Chess and the World Bridge federations. This makes the use of biomedical enhancements no different than the practice of corking bats in baseball (replacing some of the wood with cork to make the bat lighter and therefore easier to swing) or coming in first in a marathon race by slipping onto the course near the end, like Rosie Ruiz, who in 1980 was the first woman to cross the finish line in the Boston Marathon but later was determined to have entered the race only a mile from the finish line. Enhancements even violate the rules for animals. An article in the *Pittsburgh Post-Gazette* entitled "There's Hell Toupee for Bad Cows" reports that three livestock exhibitors at the 2003 Ohio State Fair were disqualified for moving tufts of their Holsteins' hair to their backs to make their backs appear straighter.[8] Urine and hair samples are collected from prize cattle and tested for banned drugs, and in 2007, the owner of the grand champion steer at the Geauga County fair in Ohio forfeited the award after the animal tested positive for steroids.[9]

As we will see, these rules are not without their detractors. Some question whether or not they are necessary or appropriate. There is some controversy about how infractions should be detected (for example, should drug testing take place outside of competitions) or whether alleged wrongdoers should be afforded proper procedural protections. More important, as we will see, the rules are highly arbitrary: Sports permits athletes to use many types of enhancements, both biomedical and otherwise, and as we will see, there may be little difference from an ethical standpoint between the ones it allows and the ones it prohibits.

But the real reason that this explanation, that enhancements in sports is wrong because it breaks the rules, is too simplistic is that it begs the question. Why are biomedical enhancements against the rules?

Unsafe Reward

One of the standard objections to the use of enhancements in sports is that they are unsafe. When the Olympics in 1967 first started trying to stop doping, it listed "protecting the athletes' health" as one of the three rationales. (The others were "respect for medical and sports ethics" and "ensuring an equal chance for everyone during competition."[10]) Biomedical enhancements continue to raise safety concerns. Consider steroids. The National Institute on Drug Abuse (NIDA) lists the following major side effects resulting from the abuse of anabolic steroids: "liver tumors and cancer, jaundice (yellowish pigmentation of skin, tissues, and body fluids), fluid retention, high blood pressure, increases in LDL (bad cholesterol), and decreases in HDL (good cholesterol). Other side effects include kidney tumors, severe acne, and trembling." NIDA adds that "steroid abuse," which includes all enhancement uses, produces a number of gender-specific side effects, including shrinking of the testicles, reduced sperm count, infertility, baldness, development of breasts, and increased risk for prostate cancer in men; and in women, enlargement of the clitoris and male characteristics such as growth of facial hair and deepened voice. Other steroid risks mentioned by NIDA are HIV/AIDS and hepatitis from needle-sharing, aggression, psychiatric side effects such as mood swings, depression, paranoid jealousy, extreme irritability, delusions, impaired judgment, and insomnia and irritability so extreme that it frequently leads to the use of heroin to counteract it.[11]

The perception that steroids are extremely hazardous to one's health was reinforced in the 2005 congressional hearings on steroids. Senator Jim Bunning (R-Ky.), a former baseball player, testified that "it's important that the American public understand just how harmful steroids can be to someone's health."[12] Parents described how steroids made their sons commit suicide, an outcome that was "right out of the medical textbooks on steroids."[13] Olympic gold medalist Carl Lewis testified that one West German female athlete died after going "completely crazy, taking injections, injections, injections, one after another."[14] In 2007, when professional wrestler Chris Benoit killed his wife and 7-year-old child and then hanged himself from his weight machine, the presence of large amounts of testosterone in his urine and prescription steroids in his home led to claims that he had acted in a fit of "'roid rage."[15]

The truth is less clear, however. Many of the adverse health effects attributed to steroids by NIDA and other sources lack supporting evidence. Some, for example, pertain to an oral use of a class of compounds known as the 17-α-alkylated steroids. These compounds indeed can cause elevations in liver enzymes and an increased risk of liver cancer. But these effects exist because these compounds are orally ingested, which means that they are broken down in the liver. The same is not true of injected steroid compounds, such as the anabolic steroids used by athletes.[16] Anabolic steroids are metabolized too quickly in the liver to be effective, so they must be given by injection, which bypasses the liver and therefore does not cause liver problems.

Steroids, of course, are powerful hormones. The ones that build muscles are versions of the male hormone, testosterone. They not only have anabolic (that is, muscle-building) characteristics, but they also are androgenic (producing masculine physical characteristics). Over the years, efforts have been made to isolate the anabolic from the androgenic effects, but without success.[17] Anabolic steroids in women produce acne, voice deepening, hair loss, breast reduction, and enlargement of the clitoris.[18] In males, anabolic steroids suppress the natural production of hormones. This can cause testicular atrophy, decreased sperm production, sperm irregularities, and gynecomastia (male breast development).[19] The effects in males usually are reversible once steroid use is discontinued; in females, the changes may be harder to reverse.[20]

The evidence on whether steroids can cause more serious side effects is equivocal. One study showed that high levels of testosterone caused cell death.[21] An experiment in mice found that adult males given anabolic steroids for six months at doses comparable to those taken by bodybuilders had a 4.3 percent increase in mortality and that a year after exposure, 52 percent of them had died compared with only 12 percent of the controls.[22] Evidence from human use is especially scarce. One study found that powerlifters had a mortality rate of 12.9 percent over 12 years compared with 3.1 percent of the general population, but the study did not determine whether the subjects in fact had used steroids, did not measure the amount they used, if any, and did not control for other substances and behaviors.[23] There have been only three studies in which high doses of anabolic steroids (300–600 mg per week of testosterone enanthate) were injected into human subjects. One six-week study found that while steroids significantly increased muscle size and strength, they produced no adverse effects.[24] A second study lasting 21 weeks also found no serious adverse effects in 54 healthy males ages 18 to 35.[25] But a third study in 60 men ages 60 to 75 that lasted 20 weeks reported that eight subjects suffered side effects, enough to warrant discontinuing the study. Four of the subjects, one receiving 600 mg and three receiving 300 mg, had elevated hematocrit (red blood cell) levels. Two subjects in the 600 mg group developed edema (swelling) in the legs or water retention. Prostate cancer was discovered in two other subjects, leading the investigators to speculate that testosterone may stimulate growth in previously undetectable cancers.[26] Clearly steroids are not a good idea for men over 60. Nor are they appropriate for children and adolescents, whose bones have not yet fully formed, since steroids can cause bone growth plates to close prematurely.[27]

In terms of psychiatric effects, the evidence also is murky. Some studies report effects on mood and aggression, others do not.[28] Although abnormal amounts of testosterone showed up in wrestler Chris Benoit's system after his suicide, the chief medical examiner of Georgia refused to attribute Benoit's behavior to "'roid rage," and an autopsy later showed that he had chronic traumatic encephalopathy, a degenerative condition produced by repeated concussions that is usually seen in boxers, and that causes depression and erratic behavior.[29]

It also is noteworthy that, as steroid opponents complain, an enormous number of people are reported to be using steroids. One account puts the number of U.S. athletes using steroids at up to three million, which may include as many as one million adolescents.[30] Athletes are subject to frequent and thorough medical examinations. Given how rampant anabolic steroid use is believed to be and how long many athletes have been using them, one would expect to see far more frequent reports of serious health problems among athletes if steroids were as hazardous as NIDA and others make them out to be.

The gaps in the available data have led some scientists to conclude that the health hazards of steroids, at least in the age group of the athletes who are most likely to use them, have been overstated, that serious health effects are rare, and that the most common side effects are reversible and benign.[31] Other researchers go further, stating that the only adverse effects firmly supported by experimental data are potentially unfavorable effects in blood lipid profiles and an increased risk for mood changes and aggression.[32]

One thing that appears fairly clear is that there are few, if any, confirmed deaths from steroid use. Carl Lewis's story about the West German female athlete who died from steroid injections is called into question by his follow-up remark that the area where the athlete had been injecting steroids "was hard as a rock. They couldn't even put a needle in it."[33] How does someone die from injecting steroids if they can't insert a needle? The truth behind a father's claim in the 2005 baseball hearings that steroids made his son commit suicide is a little more complicated than the father made it sound. The boy, who was 17 when he died, had been diagnosed with low self-esteem and depression, for which he was taking the antidepressant Lexapro. He was especially ashamed of being skinny, because his family was deeply into sports, so he started using steroids to become big enough to compete successfully. He killed himself after his parents caught him using drugs and stealing.

Even assuming that steroids and other performance-enhancing substances are dangerous, it is curious that they are singled out for such opprobrium when society allows adults, not to mention youths, to suffer so many injuries from sports in general. Professional, college, and high school football players suffer three hundred thousand concussions a year, and 60 percent of college soccer players sustain at least one concussion annually.[34] Researchers report that children who play hockey, football, lacrosse, and baseball risk sudden death from hard blows to the chest even if they wear protective equipment. An examination of 184 cases of fatal ventricular fibrillation (abnormal heart rhythm) in child athletes between 1995 and 2005 found that 47 percent took place during practice or competition in organized sports, with 39 percent occurring despite protective gear. The average age of the decedents was 15. Fatal chest blows were delivered by baseball pitches of no more than 30 miles per hour.[35] The Centers for Disease Control and Prevention estimates that from June 2000 to June 2001, 4.3 million people visited hospital emergency rooms for nonfatal sports-related injuries.[36] There is no evidence that the risks from enhancements exceed or are out of proportion to these other dangers.

Of course, this is not to say that people should use steroids. The difficulty of obtaining lawful supplies of these substances forces athletes to use underground preparations of uncertain identity, strength, and purity, at uncontrolled dosages, without proper medical supervision. In view of this, what is surprising is not that there are a few reports of serious or even fatal effects but that athletes do not appear to be dropping like flies. Even with steroids of known strength and purity, there clearly are safety issues, especially in children and older men. Other enhancement substances also raise health concerns. Human growth hormone also has not been subjected to careful, long-term testing in people with normal natural levels of the hormone, but short-term studies suggest that it may cause insulin resistance, glucose intolerance, decreased natural production of HGH, carpal tunnel syndrome, water retention, and perhaps cardiovascular effects.[37] Excessive amounts of EPO can cause the blood to thicken dangerously, especially during exercise.[38] EPO is suspected in the deaths of five Dutch cyclists in 1987 and of 18 other cyclists between 1997 and 2000.[39]

It also must be borne in mind that latent adverse effects may turn up later, even many years after use. The adverse effects of giving the synthetic estrogen diethylstilbestrol (DES) to pregnant women were not discovered until their daughters developed cervical cancer upon reaching puberty. Moreover, it is a truism of pharmacology that no drug is completely safe. No matter how benign the substance seems to be, it is always possible for it to cause harm. A 17-year-old track star in 2007 died from using too much Bengay.[40] People die from drinking too much water. So the ultimate question is not whether steroids are "safe" but whether, given the known and unknown hazards, the risks are outweighed by the benefits. But as we saw in the previous chapter, unless we embrace the liberty-quenching approach of hard paternalism, the answer to this question may be that, at least in the case of competent adults, the determination is best left up to the individual.

But what about children? Performance-enhancing substances can be especially dangerous for them. In adolescents, as noted, steroids can cause irreversible, early closure of growth plates.[41] As NIDA points out in one of its rare evidence-based claims, steroids halt growth "prematurely through premature skeletal maturation and accelerated puberty changes. This means that adolescents risk remaining short for the remainder of their lives if they take anabolic steroids before the typical adolescent growth spurt."[42] Children also are presumed to lack the capacity to make informed, rational choices. Clearly, therefore, restrictions on enhancement use by minors would be appropriate. Yet even so, it should be pointed out that we allow children to play tackle football, hockey, and skateboarding—all activities with relatively high risks of injury. Moreover, some performance-enhancing drugs may be reasonably safe even for children. And there is value in enabling a child to play sports better, even at some risk. Ask any adult who is not good at sports the torments provoked as children. Finally, children who can play better may actually reduce their risk of injury.

The question of whether it is appropriate to give biomedical enhancements to children is addressed in a later chapter as part of a larger discussion of enhancement use by groups of individuals who may lack the capacity to make voluntary choices. These groups, as it happens, sometimes include athletes. But a separate question is whether the special safety considerations that apply in the case of children should prevent the use of enhancements by adults. Those who want to ban doping in sports point to the influence that athletes have on children. Rep. John Sweeney (R-N.Y.) testified in 2004, for example, that "as athletes have become more creative, turning to substances such as andro and its muscle building cousins, our children have become more susceptible to the allure of performance enhancing substances. While the integrity of sports is significant, the use of steroids in sports would not be of such profound concern if it did not impact children so drastically."[43] One worry is that children will take adult athletes as role models and copy their use of performance enhancements in sports while still children. The chair of the House Committee investigating steroid use in baseball emphasized this when he said that "our primary focus remains on the message being sent to children. Children who play baseball. Children who idolize and emulate professional baseball players."[44]

There also is the fear that the use of enhancements will lead children to partake of illicit recreational drugs. Senator Joseph Biden (D-Del.) maintained in 1989 hearings on steroid use in football that "steroids could become another 'gate-way drug,'" a phrase that's now being used to refer to the use of one drug that leads to the use of other, more objectionable drugs like marijuana and cocaine.[45]

But there are no data showing that the use of performance enhancers leads to illicit drug use. Conceivably, children who perceived that there were benefits from one type of prohibited substance would be inclined to try their luck at other types. But the problem may be caused more by the illicit status of the performance-enhancing drugs rather than by any tendency to improve performance. Both children and adults use all sorts of legitimate medications without, it seems, concluding that if one type of drug is good, all drugs must be good.

Moreover, adults engage in many behaviors that are deemed bad or deleterious for children, such as drinking, smoking, and sex. Even role models are entitled to personal freedoms. Adult athletes need to make it clear that the rules are different for adults and children and should refrain from actively promoting enhancements to audiences that may include a substantial number of youngsters, such as on television. But concern about an indirect effect on children does not necessarily justify constraining the liberty of an adult. As philosopher Robert L. Simon argues, "Why restrict the freedom of top athletes rather than increase the responsibility for supervision of youngsters assigned to coaches, teachers and parents? After all, we don't restrict the freedom of adults in numerous other areas where they may set bad examples for the young."[46] As a ski patroller, I deal with lots of injured kids who "just wanted to see if they could do that flip like the guy on TV." This does not mean that we should eliminate freestyle skiing from the Olympics.

Futility

Another standard objection to allowing the use of performance enhancements in sports is that it would ultimately be futile. If one athlete uses an enhancement to get ahead, the argument goes, then everyone will have to use it to keep abreast, and the first athlete will not gain any advantage. And if the enhancement poses a health risk, then the athlete who begins using it—as well as everyone who follows suit—will be subjected to the risk for nothing.

Bill McKibben makes this point in connection with parents enhancing their children. In his opinion, enhancements "are the most anti-choice technologies anyone's ever thought of." Imagine what happens, he asks, after "the first few hundred parents on New York's Upper East

Side decide that they will indeed spend some of their spare cash on upgrading their offspring. Almost immediately, at precisely the moment the first cover story on the subject appears in *New York* magazine, every other well-off couple of childbearing age in Manhattan will be forced to decide whether, like it or not, they're going to have to follow suit. If not, their kids may *lose*—may not get into the right preschool, may not get into Brearley, may not get into Harvard. What choice will these parents have?" McKibben then turns to sports. "Very few kids," he asserts, "grow up thinking: 'I'm going to do steroids so I can hit home runs.' But at some point young athletes reach a level at which a couple of other kids are sticking needles in their butts to build their biceps, and as a result they're hammering it over the fence, and as a result they're moving up to the majors. You have a *choice*, sure," McKibben observes. "But really it was only the first few guys who had a *free* choice."[47]

Yet as Robert Simon and others have pointed out, this is not just true of biomedical enhancements.[48] The same can be said for any method for improving performance. If one athlete trains an extra hour a day, the other athletes have to as well, or they will fall behind. Barring the possibility that the additional training will benefit some athletes more than others, no one will obtain an advantage; given the number of injuries caused by training, particularly overtraining, there may well be an increase in the risk of harm. This appearance of futility accompanies any advance in performance technology. If one athlete or coach devises a new method of psychological preparation or a piece of equipment, then everyone will adopt it, and no one will gain any advantage. Some of these new technologies may reduce the risk of injury, such as better football helmets. But others, such as faster bobsleds or racing skis, increase the risk.

A good illustration is the development of the modern tennis racquet. In 1967, the first all-metal tennis racquet was introduced, and Jimmy Connors used one, the T-2000 made by Wilson, to win at Wimbledon in 1974. Howard Head, who had previously developed the metal ski, turned his attention to tennis in the early 1970s after his retirement from the ski industry. Recognizing that tennis had no limits on racquet size, he patented a new racquet that not only was made of metal but also boasted a 50 percent increase in head size to enlarge the "sweet spot." Head purchased the Prince Sports Manufacturing Company to produce and market his new design.[49] The racquet achieved notoriety when a 16-year-old named Pam Shriver used it in 1978 to defeat the reigning Wimbledon champion, Martina Navratilova, in the semifinals of the U.S. Open. (She later lost to Chris Evert in the finals.) After that, oversized racquets began being constructed of composites, including graphite and Kevlar. Now virtually every professional tennis player uses an oversized racquet. It enables them to play better than the old wooden racquet. When the International Tennis Federation adopted the first rules for the dimensions of racquets in 1981, the specifications accommodated the new racquet design.[50]

Oversized composite tennis racquets are an example of equipment that enhances sports performance. This book focuses on enhancements that employ biomedical technology. Later we will consider whether there is any difference between the two that would justify treating them differently under the rules of sports. But one thing is clear: neither of them is futile. They both enable athletes to improve their performance.

Unearned Reward

In 2005, baseball commissioner Bud Selig wrote to Donald Fehr, head of the players' union, that "steroid users cheat the game."[51] Not just the rules, but the game itself. What is it about enhancements that, even if they were legal, would make victories achieved with their help unworthy? A standard answer is that the victories would be unearned. As Attorney General John Ashcroft stated in announcing federal indictments following revelations about steroid use in baseball, "the tragedy of so-called performance-enhancing drugs is that they foster the lie that excellence can be bought rather than earned."[52] Why are victories with the aid of enhancements unearned? Because, it is said, they enable athletes to play better without hard work.

Yet victories in sports are always won not by dint of hard work alone. An important factor is luck: the luck not to slip on a wet or icy patch, be distracted by a fan, or suffer an injury during training. For example, Olympic skiers, it is reported, "regard Olympic races like any other, subject to the whims of luck, seeding, and weather conditions."[53] Athletes even employ good luck charms. The first Japanese woman to win an Olympic gold medal in track-and-field had a small Shinto charm clipped to her running shorts.[54] To boost the Canadian hockey team's chances of beating the United States and winning its first Olympic gold medal in 50 years, Wayne Gretzky, the executive director of the Canadian team, had the Canadian company that prepared the ice bury a $1 Canadian coin at the center of the rink. "We got two gold medals out of it," said Gretzky, announcing that he planned to donate the "Loonie" to the Canadian Olympic Hall of Fame.[55] Except in the minds of those who believe that God rewards good works and punishes evildoing, good luck is not earned and bad luck is not deserved. They happen. To the extent that they contribute to success in sports, they do not entitle athletes to take credit for their success. In that sense, athletes who are lucky are no different from athletes who use performance enhancements.

Good fortune extends much farther than the vagaries of fate during training or on the day of competition. Successful athletes benefit from the luck of having been born into wealthy or supportive families. It is common, especially during Olympic telecasts, to hear the lengths to which families go in helping their children pursue sports: pre-dawn practices, expensive equipment, special schools and camps, private trainers, the enormous investments in time. Sarah Hughes, who won an Olympic gold medal in figure skating in 2002, had a skating rink in her backyard. Resource-strapped coaches in foreign countries envy their American counterparts because American athletes have wealthy parents who finance their training.[56] The *New York Times* described the advantages enjoyed by one 16-year-old prospect: "The parents of Beau Fraser have spent $30,000 to help him become a better athlete. From the time Beau was 10, his parents, Gayle and Brian Fraser of Aptos, Calif., have paid for professional coaches, private trainers, athletic testing, baseball camps, tournaments and travel with elite teams—not to mention travel costs for the entire family to watch him play. The extra help may or may not transform Beau into a professional baseball player, but, at 16, he is a starting catcher on his high school team."[57]

Beyond the luck of good nurture is the good luck of nature. Sandel is right that skillful athletes have a gift. This was initially demonstrated through twin studies, which create registries to track the lives of pairs of identical infants separated at or near birth and raised by different families. Because the children are virtually identical genetically but differ in the environment in which they are brought up, the researchers can discern the degree to which differences in their behavior can be attributed to genes or environment. Twin studies indicate that performance-related fitness characteristics (such as static strength and running speed) and health-related characteristics (such as flexibility and maximum oxygen uptake) are moderately to highly heritable.[58] This means that much of the variation in athletic talent in the population is attributable to differences in people's genetic endowment. With the added knowledge from the Human Genome Project, researchers are slowly identifying the specific genetic combinations that account for this variation. Athletic individuals most likely have inherited genes for exceptional height, strength, coordination, fearlessness, and slow- or fast-twitch muscles. Unathletic individuals most likely have not.

Take Lance Armstrong. How can a 34-year-old man win the grueling Tour de France bicycle race, especially after surviving testicular cancer that had metastasized to his brain? No doubt much of his success is attributable to his relentless training regimen. This alone can account for the fact that his heart is 30 percent larger than average, and that his "VO2 max," the maximum amount of oxygen that his lungs can absorb, is also among the highest ever measured in elite cycling. But he also possesses an unusual genetic characteristic. When a normal person exercises hard, lactic acid builds up in the muscles, causing pain and fatigue. Armstrong produces about half as much lactic acid as the average person. According to the director of the Human Performance Lab at the University of Texas, Armstrong's lactic acid levels are the lowest he has ever seen.[59] As a result, Armstrong doesn't get as tired, and he recovers from fatigue faster, than competitors. Researchers at Case Western Reserve University recently reported that they had duplicated Armstrong's lactic acid levels in mice by genetically engineering them to overexpress an enzyme called PEPCK-C.[60] More than likely, Armstrong has a similar genetic anomaly.

Also, technology has always played an enormous role in sports. Sports equipment has steadily evolved, as illustrated by the earlier description of the development of the modern tennis racquet. Invariably, equipment changes are made in order to improve performance. Pole vaulters originally used poles made of bamboo. When the game switched to fiberglass and carbon fiber poles in the early 1960s, the world record overnight jumped by three feet. The change in aerodynamics produced by dimpling golf balls lengthened the distance of a typical drive from about 160 to 220 yards. Tennis uses not only high-tech racquets but also "space age" stringing with synthetics instead of gut to give players more power and heavier spin on the ball. Gustavo Kuerten, an unseeded player ranked 66, won the first of three French Open titles in 1997 using a brand of synthetic string called Luxilon.[61] Since 1971, metal bats have replaced wooden bats in Little League baseball.[62] In slow-pitch baseball, a new bat with twin, multi-braced aluminum walls enables players to smash longer hits.[63] (Allegations that the harder hits that result cause too many injuries led one legislator to introduce a bill in New Jersey to outlaw the use of metal, titanium, and composite bats in league baseball and softball games by players 17 and younger.[64]) Downhill ski racers can shave time by wearing special aerodynamic racing suits. Spyder Active Sports in Boulder, Colorado, makes one out of fabric that has silver threads woven into the backing; the threads are knit into a special pattern that evens out the fabric, reducing wind resistance. To get the desired result, the company tested prototype swatches in a facility at the University of Buffalo ordinarily used to analyze the aerodynamic properties of ballistic missiles.[65] Changes in equipment also affect performance in sports that permit the use of performance-enhancing drugs. A controversy in nontested powerlifting involved uniforms made out of stiff denim that helps raise the arms when lifting weight.

One of the most important types of performance-enhancing equipment is technology to improve eyesight. Slugger Mark McGwire has been pilloried for using a dietary supplement called androstenedione that produces steroidlike effects after being metabolized—but not for his specially made contact lenses that give him 20/10 vision.[66] One prominent sports medicine physician states that, with the exception of pitchers, virtually all baseball players have better than 20/20 vision, either naturally or with the help of contact lenses and eye surgery, and that this is critical to being able to hit fastball pitches at speeds that can exceed 100 miles per hour.[67] Tiger Woods, who has worn corrective lenses since he was a child, got his 20/15 vision from Lasik surgery, with the result, according to one sports writer, that "when he putts, the hole looks bigger than it used to. When he stands over a shot, the face of the club looks bigger."[68] Yet as Charles Krauthammer notes, "I have yet to see a banner at the Masters saying: 'Nicklaus did it by squinting.'"[69]

A newcomer among vision enhancements is MaxSight soft contact lenses by Bausch and Lomb, which have colored rings that reduce glare and make vision sharper. The lenses, introduced in August 2005, come in two tints, grey-green and amber. According to the manufacturer, these are "tuned to different sporting needs. Grey-green is for sports played in bright sunlight, where visual comfort is a concern, and amber is for sports like tennis that require tracking a fast-moving ball."[70] But the rings are also designed to give players a threatening look. One of the smallest players on the Penn State football team, Jordan Norwood, says, "I need something to look a little intimidating, so I throw those in." A sportswriter comments: "Norwood can be downright scary on game days, displaying the look of someone who just stepped out of central casting of a horror movie."[71] By June 2006, the lenses were being worn by golfer Michelle Wie, baseball players Ken Griffey Jr. and A.J. Pierzynski, the U.S. men's soccer team, and the Texas Longhorns.[72]

Athletes also rely on sports psychology to improve performance. The team psychologist for the Houston Texans football team uses "stress inoculation" and other "mental toughness" techniques, such as pumping noise into a special indoor practice field at 130 decibels—the volume of a jet engine—to inure the players to the somewhat less noisy conditions in the actual stadium.[73]

Sports psychology is but one adjuvant among a number of high-tech training methods. In a 2007 report, the Science and Technology Committee of the British House of Commons listed biomechanics ("improving understanding of mechanics of movement"), immunology, nutrition and hydration, and physiology as legal "human enhancement technologies."[74] The U.S. Olympic Committee operates a sports science facility in Lake Placid, New York, which it uses to train team members in biathlon, bobsled, figure skating, ice hockey, luge, skiing, speed skating, boxing, canoe and kayak, judo, rowing, synchronized swimming, taekwondo, team handball, water polo, and wrestling. According to the USOC, "Equipment in the sport science laboratory includes sport-specific ergometers for canoe/kayak, biathlon, cross-country and speed skating. There is an extra large treadmill with the capacity to study running, roller skiing and in-line skating. Athletes' physiological capabilities can be measured with a computerized system, which scientifically evaluates their maximal oxygen uptake. The Sport Sciences Division also utilizes cinematography to analyze the biomechanical aspects of sport performance."[75] The U.S. Tennis Association is planning to centralize its player development program at a new complex at the Evert Tennis Academy in Boca Raton, Florida, which will feature 23 courts, dorms, and a staff of 30, including a "mental conditioning coach." The cost per player will be $42,000 a year.[76]

But the U.S. sports program pales before Australia's. The Australian government runs a National Talent Search Program to identify the 180,000 14- to 18-year-olds who are in the top 10 percent of the population in terms of athletic ability so that they can begin training for the Olympics and other elite competitions.[77] This program is run by the same government agency that helped conduct the search for the

ACTN3 genetic variant, described earlier, which distinguishes between a propensity for slow- or fast-twitch muscles.[78]

Long-distance runners and other endurance athletes have long used carbohydrate loading to increase the amounts of glycogen, an energy-producing sugar, that are stored in their muscle tissue. Now the diets of elite competitors are regulated by experts according to state-of-the-art nutritional science. Then there are dietary supplements, with sales to athletes estimated at $4 billion a year. The top seller is creatine, an amino-acid compound stored in muscle tissue that aids in producing phosphocreatine (PCr), an important fuel for short, intense exercise. Many dietary supplements are of doubtful effectiveness, but not creatine. An Army study found that males taking creatine could bench-press 14 percent more repetitions than a placebo group, and female soccer players who took creatine in a 2002 Australian study ran faster sprints.[79]

All of these innovations share two features: they improve athletic performance, and the improvement is not "earned." This leads one sports philosopher to observe that "it seems artificial indeed to draw the line at drugs when so much of today's training techniques, equipment, food, medical care, even the origin of the sports themselves, are the product of our technological culture."[80] Yet critics of biomedical enhancement are adamant that they are distinct from other performance-improving technologies. Some point to the fact that enhancements are taken internally, while training and equipment occur externally, as if this were ethically significant. One baseball commentator confidently asserts that cheating through the use of spitballs and hollowed-out bats is not as objectionable as using performance-enhancing drugs because the former "are on-the-field, organic manipulations of the actual rudiments of the game," whereas the latter "originate off the field, taking the outside world where it doesn't belong."[81] A common theme is that unlike enhancement, areas like training, equipment, and diet involve "human agency." Conceding that enhancements may involve some agency on the part of the athlete, the President's Council on Bioethics distinguishes between "intelligible agency" or "getting better because of what we do," which characterizes acceptable technologies, and "unintelligible agency," or "getting better because of what is done to us," which it says characterizes biomedical enhancements.[82] Michael Sandel agrees, stating that "as the role of enhancement increases, our admiration for the achievement fades—or, rather, our admiration for the achievement shifts from the player to his pharmacist. This suggests that our moral response to enhancement is a response to the diminished agency of the person whose achievement is enhanced."[83]

But why are sports psychology, high-tech diets, and computerized training aids any more things done *by* us and less things that are done *to* us than steroids or erythropoietin? True, eating food is an act of agency, but so is injecting a drug or swallowing a pill. It is not as if these things are done without the athlete's agreement and participation. In fact, they seem to involve a greater degree of agency than being attached to a training machine to measure ergonomic output or being bombarded by the noise of a jet engine. The arbitrariness of this distinction is exemplified by the policy of the American Association of Pediatrics. The use and promotion of performance-enhancing substances, it claims, "tends to devalue the principles of a balanced diet, good coaching and sound physical training."[84] Why are diet, coaching, and training valued principles—but not other ways of enhancing performance? It can't be because of meaningful differences in agency.

Ironically, the ultimate rebuttal to the objection that the social reward obtained from biomedical enhancement is unethical because it does not involve effort is provided by the critics' chief pariah, steroids. Listening to them, you would think that steroids grow bigger muscles without effort, even when the athlete sleeps. What steroids in fact do is allow athletes to work harder without injuring themselves, which has the effect of increasing the size of their muscles. Steroids do this by increasing the number and size of muscle fibers so that they are stronger and thereby able to tolerate more exertion and by blocking the effects of cortisol, which produces fatigue and breaks down muscle fibers during exercise.[85] In short, steroids do the opposite of enabling athletes to avoid hard work. Steroids achieve their effect only because athletes work.

Unfair Reward

A separate criticism lodged against biomedical enhancement is that the reward they provide, whether earned or not, is unfair. One of the Olympic Medical Commission's three original rationales for banning performance-enhancing drugs in sports, it will be recalled, was "maintaining equal opportunities for all at the time of competition."[86] If athletes do not have an equal opportunity to win, the point seems to be, the competition is unfair. A concern about fairness is echoed by other critics of enhancement. The American Association of Pediatrics states "the intentional use of performance enhancement is unfair, and therefore morally and ethically indefensible."[87] Peter Roby, director of the Center for the Study of Sport in Society at Northeastern University, asserts that "this whole issue calls into question the integrity of sports. The last thing they want people to think is that they can't trust the results. That the performances they're seeing on the field are not truthful and fair."[88]

But what is unfair about enhancements? In an obvious sense, it would be unfair if some athletes didn't abide by the rules and used prohibited substances. (Note that if everyone broke the rules, there would be no potential for unfairness in this sense.) But that assumes that performance enhancements are against the rules. If enhancements were not against the rules, what would be unfair about them?

Performance enhancements might well be unfair if they benefit some users more than others. But this may not be the case. Human growth hormone does not increase a person's height; it merely allows them to achieve it sooner. This is not generally considered unfair, presumably because by not lasting too far into the period in their lives when the social rewards are the greatest, it does not net them too much social reward. The situation is much the same for other enhancements. So far, there does not seem to be a lot of concern that some enhancements work differently in different people, boosting some more than others.

Things will not stay this way for long, however. Pharmacogenetics is revealing more and more information about individual reactions to drugs, including performance-enhancing drugs. Recall the NIH-sponsored study that found that a Parkinson disease drug, tolcapone, significantly improved executive function and verbal episodic memory in subjects with one variant of a particular gene, while impairing the same abilities in subjects who had a different variant. If the drug eventually were used to enhance cognition, some people would get a greater degree of enhancement from it than others, based on their genetic makeup. Unless there were other enhancements that the people with the less advantageous genes could get to offset the effect, this seems unfair. As pharmacogenetics advances, it therefore will become necessary to make a more concerted effort to determine how much of this unfairness should be tolerated, assuming something can be done about it.

In the meantime, perhaps athletes would be acting unfairly if they figured out a way to improve their performance but kept it secret from other athletes. I say "perhaps" because, since stimulating the discovery of new and better ways of improving performance is a positive good, athletes usually are permitted to use them even when no one else can. Thus, the metal tennis racquet burst on the scene in 1974 when Jimmy Connors used the Wilson T-2000 to win at Wimbledon. The oversized racquet achieved notoriety, as mentioned earlier, when 16-year-old Pam Shriver used it in 1978 to defeat the current Wimbledon champion, Martina Navratilova, who did not have one. The same thing happened in the late 1960s when Kenny Moore ran for a thousand miles wearing the first shock-absorbent running shoes.[89] (The result, celebrated in a small part in the film *Personal Best,* was the Nike company.) There are exceptions: Barrie Houlihan cites the Olympic prohibition on the use of fiberglass poles in the 1972 games because the poles were not widely enough available.[90] But in most instances, the first athlete to the punch with new enhancement technology gets to use it before anyone else. This would be unfair only if athletes were able to maintain a monopoly on a new technology for too long, if the time between its first use by an athlete and its availability to all were too great.

But what is fair about sports to begin with? An important factor in winning Olympic and World Cup alpine skiing events, for example, is having the best racing skis. These skis are not available to the general public. Nor are they available to all competitors. They are custom-made, and they are produced especially for that level of skiing. After testing them on speed tracks to find out which pairs are the fastest, the manufacturers dole them out to racers based on team favoritism and the racers' international rankings, with the fastest pair going to the highest-ranked skier on the most favored team, the next fastest pair to the next ranked skier on that team, and so on. For years, the premier racing ski manufacturer, the Atomic ski company, gave first pick to the Austrian ski team. Coincidentally, perhaps, the Austrians dominated the sport. In the early 2000s, U.S. racers began to obtain improved access to the top pairs of skis after the U.S. Ski and Snowboard Association made a concerted effort to woo Atomic executives. As a result, U.S. racer Daron Rahlves received second pick behind Austrian Stephan Eberharter, and went on to place first in the prestigious Austrian Hahnenkamm downhill race, the first American to do so in 44 years, while Eberharter finished fourth.[91]

The unfairness of the system for distributing racing skis is just one aspect of the broader unfairness in sports. Professor Roger Gardner at the University of Delaware observes that the entire process of pitting countries in different parts of the world and at different stages of economic development against one another in international competition is skewed: "Athletes from some countries gain an advantage in certain sports due to more favorable climates or sporting traditions. It is often commented in just such a context that countries such as Austria and Switzerland have an unfair advantage over America when it comes to winter sports. Or consider that American athletes, in a similar manner, would seem to have an unfair competitive advantage over third world athletes because of better facilities and sophisticated training techniques."[92] An anonymous Olympic coach echoes Gardner's views, stating simply: "Sports is not fair. It's not that way. Athletes have different talents, different genetic codes. They use different equipment. They use coaches with different backgrounds and different resources. They live in countries with different standards. Some places cannot afford food. Some places cannot afford shoes. Some places the coach doesn't know [anything]."[93] Gardner wonders what's fair about it "when, say, Steffi Graf [then] the world's number one ranked tennis player, is matched against the 128th ranked player; or when a basketball team that averages 6′10″ in height plays one that averages 6′2″? Such conditions of inequality and any ensuing advantages gained, although intuitively unfair, would appear to fall into a class of unfair but accepted (or at least tolerated) advantages in sport."[94] Or consider this from sportswriter Will Carroll: "I hear people say we need a level playing field. We don't have a level playing field. There are guys that are so much more talented than others. Or how about having virtual natural selection with a Bonds or a [Ken] Griffey Jr., whose parents were athletes? Bret Boone was third generation. They're virtually designed to be athletes."[95]

Opponents of biomedical enhancements believe not only that it would be unfair to reward athletes who used them even if they were allowed by the rules but also that it *is fair* to reward athletes for their natural talent. As Sandel states in a comment about genetic enhancement that he no doubt would apply to biomedical enhancements in general, "The real problem . . . is that they corrupt athletic competition as a human activity that honors the cultivation and display of natural talents."[96] Sandel celebrates natural talent because it is the result of the genetic lottery, and because this means that it is distributed randomly, like luck, anyone can be blessed with it, so it is fair to allow it to benefit the fortunate few.

This view rests on a principle that is ingrained in American ethics and jurisprudence, that it is fair to allocate scarce resources randomly. The classic illustration is a famous 1842 case in which a sailor was tried for manslaughter for throwing passengers overboard from an overcrowded lifeboat. The ship, the *William Brown,* struck an iceberg on its way from Liverpool to Philadelphia and sank. Forty-one people, including the first mate, eight seamen, and 22 passengers who were emigrants from Scotland and Ireland, got into a 22-foot longboat. The boat immediately began leaking. It was still afloat 24 hours later, but then the weather took a turn for the worse, and at the first mate's instigation, 14 male passengers were tossed overboard. (Two women jumped in voluntarily, apparently to join their brother who had been cast from the boat.) The next morning, the survivors in the boat were rescued by another ship. Public opinion was outraged that none of the crew had been sacrificed, and upon reaching the United States, Holmes, a sailor who had taken charge of throwing the passengers out, was indicted, convicted, and sentenced to six months in jail and a $20 fine.[97] His conviction was upheld by an appellate court.

The court's opinion became a landmark in American law. The judge declared that, when someone must be sacrificed to save others, "the selection is by lot. This mode is resorted to as the fairest mode, and, in some sort, as an appeal to God, for selection of the victim. . . . For ourselves, we can conceive of no mode so consonant both to humanity and to justice; and the occasion, we think, must be peculiar which will dispense with its exercise."[98] Courts also have upheld random systems for selecting which families should obtain access to limited public housing, and which stores should receive liquor licenses.[99]

If it is fair to decide who will survive in a lifeboat by a roll of the dice, it surely seems fair for the genetic craps game to decide who will benefit from natural talent. Just as people are entitled to their winnings from random state lotteries, so they ought to be allowed to keep the winnings from their genetic lotteries.

One problem with this argument is that the distribution of favorable genes is random only to a limited degree. As we shall see, prize children can be bred in much the same way as prize cattle, and new reproductive technologies like sperm and egg donation and preimplantation genetic diagnosis are increasingly giving parents the ability to select offspring with favorable characteristics. Talent, in short, is becoming less and less "natural." As genetic science advances, it may well give rise to genetic manipulations that actively design a child's genetic endowment. At that point, natural talent will all but have disappeared.

But even now, it cannot be said that allowing athletes to benefit from the distribution of natural talent is fairer than permitting them to make use of biomedical enhancements. If an enhancement is not against the rules, is relatively safe, and is readily available, then, as we have observed above, the expectation is that everyone will use it, just as all tennis players adopted oversized racquets. As a result, the enhancement will enable everyone to perform better. The benefit will be universal, rather than selective. Undeniably, it is fairer to allow all athletes to improve than to reserve high performance for the few.

Harvard law professor Einer Elhauge makes a further telling point. If everyone employs biomedical enhancements, and, as in the case of a new piece of equipment, they produce in everyone a comparable improvement in performance, then nothing has happened to decrease the rewards that flow from natural gifts. If steroids enabled weightlifters to hoist an extra 20 pounds, for example, than naturally strong competitors who were able to lift 300 pounds without steroids would be able to lift 320 pounds with. They would not be overtaken by less naturally talented steroid-users who previously could lift only 280 pounds, because even with the 20-pound advantage from the drug, they will be able to lift only 300 pounds. The only caveat is that there might be more or less fixed physical ceilings that enhancements could not transcend. Imagine a growth hormone that made basketball players taller—there is probably some height above which they would not be able to remain upright. This is alleged to be a concern with steroids, which might increase muscle mass to such an extent that it overtaxes the strength of an athlete's tendons, ligaments, and bones.

Record Keeping

In *The Thinking Man's Guide to Baseball,* the influential sportswriter Leonard Koppett wrote that "statistics are the lifeblood of baseball," adding that "it is entirely possible that more American boys have mastered long division by dealing with batting averages than in any other way."[100] Hang around any barbershop and you're bound to hear about batting averages, runs batted in, earned run averages, saves, and in more rarified salons, passed balls, the most runs in a season by a shortstop, the longest hitting streak by a catcher, and how many times teams have hit four consecutive home runs. Other sports, while perhaps not as compulsive about statistics, are also enamored of assist-to-turnover ratios (basketball), takeaways (football), hat tricks (ice hockey), and shots on goal (soccer).

Not surprisingly, then, any change that interferes with statistical comparisons upsets the aficionado. How can we tell if a player today truly beats Babe Ruth's home record, when Ruth never used steroids? In the 2004 Senate hearings on baseball, Senator John McCain (R-Ariz.) complained not only that the lack of stringent drug testing policies imperils players but also that it "calls into question the records set by those suspected of using performance-enhancing drugs."[101] Sportswriter Nick Cafardo of the *Boston Globe* is even more adamant, stating that "the use of illegal drugs is a major issue that should not go unpunished or unrecognized when it comes to statistical achievement, which is the major basis for a player's performance."[102]

When some athletes use banned substances and others do not, it is indeed difficult to compare their performances. But if enhancements were permitted by the rules, then the situation would be little different from any other change in a sport that affects the way it is played. In 1973, the American League adopted the designated hitter rule, which allows teams to employ substitute batters for pitchers. This makes it impossible to compare performances in the American League and the National League, because the National League did not change the rule. Yet fans have learned to live with the change, albeit not without grumbling.[103] Other sports have had to accommodate substantial modifications in performance as the result of new equipment. World pole-vault records of the bamboo era cannot match the heights attained by Olympians wielding fiberglass poles. Statistical tables for the sport therefore are divided according to the dates that the poles were made of different materials.[104] Having to place Barry Bonds's homers in a different category from Babe Ruth's may upset some enthusiasts, but it does not seem to be an insurmountable obstacle to permitting players to use biomedical enhancements.

This is not to downplay the importance of fan enthusiasm. As of 2007, estimates of the value of a baseball team franchise vary from $244 million for the Florida Marlins to $1.2 billion for the New York Yankees.[105] After Barry Bonds topped Hank Aaron's home run record, everyone who makes money on baseball anxiously watched opinion polls to gauge the potential effect of the steroid scandal on their future incomes. Are ticket sales up or down? What are the Nielsen ratings for games on TV? The Tour de France is struggling to retain sponsors after a wave of doping scandals and the cancellation of other cycling events in the wake of the charges against Floyd Landis.[106] A plan to place *Spiderman 2* logos on baseball bases was scrapped after it encountered opposition from fans.[107]

Fan disgust even can cause an entire sport to whither and die, or, in some cases, to be stillborn. Consider the XFL football league. On February 3, 2000, NBC and the World Wrestling Federation announced their concept for a new kind of football league, with fewer rules, trash-talking announcers, scantily clad cheerleaders, and an opening scramble for the ball instead of a coin toss.[108] The following year, the game debuted, complete with gimmicky camera techniques, behind-the-scenes looks at the cheerleader locker rooms, and player jerseys with nicknames like "He Hate Me."[109] The game immediately began to draw criticism. Commentators decried its gimmicks, theatrics, and misogynistic attitude. Fans thought it looked too much like pro wrestling.[110] Opening games drew large audiences, but even though the sport switched to real commentators and toned down its language, attendance at games and television ratings quickly plummeted. After the season-ending games drew some of the smallest audiences ever for prime time television, the XFL folded.[111] Following the cancellation, ESPN commentator Jay Mariotti offered his gratitude "to the masses for smacking down this farcical disgrace to civilized culture."[112] Another sportswriter called the league's folding "the year's most hopeful sign that we have a future as a society," and a headline in the *Seattle Times* proclaimed, "XFL benched, taste wins."[113]

So sports is wise to pay attention to how its fan base reacts to enhancements. But this is a matter of economics, not ethics. And as doping historian John Hoberman points out, scandal isn't always bad for business. After a Tour de France cycling team sponsored by Swiss watchmaker Festina was tossed out of the 1998 event because of widespread doping, the company reported that the negative publicity had increased sales.[114] Historian Catherine Carstairs notes, "doping scandals put sports on the front page of newspapers and at the top of the news, corralling a larger audience. The scandals provide viewers with an additional frisson of excitement—that of catching the dopers and deciding who is guilty."[115] As Hoberman caustically observes: "Call it the Howard Stern principle, but the sad fact is that public grossness and the sheer entertainment value it provides have been associated at times with increased revenues flowing back to the sewer from which the grossness emerged. Indeed, two weeks into the [Tour de France] scandal not one corporate sponsor had dumped its Tour team despite the carnage in the newspapers, a collective corporate decision that will not be lost on other potential investors in the sports carnival."[116]

Let's take stock of where we are in terms of the objections to enhancements in sports. If biomedical enhancements improve athletic performance; if at least some are safe enough that competent adult athletes should be permitted to decide for themselves whether or not to use them; if the rewards that they make possible are not significantly less earned than rewards in sports generally; if their use is not unfair because, like better equipment, they simply lift all boats; and if they do not necessarily confound record keeping or drive away fans, what objection remains to permitting their use? Opponents have one final philosophical objection to assert. They argue that enhancements violate "the spirit of sport."

The Spirit of Sport

Initially, as noted earlier, sports was hostile toward biomedical enhancements primarily on the grounds that they were risks to health. But eventually it became clear that opponents of doping also objected to enhancements that were relatively safe. Romanian gymnast Andrea Raducan was stripped of her gold medal at the 2000 Olympics because she took two tablets of Sudafed, a compound so safe that it is sold without a prescription.[117] For many years, the Olympics banned caffeine in concentrations in excess of 12 micrograms per milliliter of urine.[118] A 150-pound person would need to ingest about 600 mg of caffeine to exceed the 12-microgram level. This is the equivalent of one 16-ounce cup of Starbucks coffee and a couple of cans of Mountain Dew. In 2003, the World Anti-Doping Agency (WADA), the organization created in 1999 to oversee the war against doping in sports, abandoned all pretense that its antidoping stance rested fundamentally on a concern for athletes' health. It replaced the three rationales originally put forward by the Olympic Medical Commission with three different criteria for determining when a substance should be banned, and said that satisfying any two of them would be sufficient: (1) "It is performance-enhancing." (2) "It represents a risk to the health of the athlete." (3) "It is against the spirit of sport."[119] In short, enhancements as safe as Sudafed or caffeine can be banned if they are "against the spirit of sport."

What is the "spirit of sport"? Robert Simon provides an answer that is reminiscent of the objections discussed earlier against the use of enhancements for self-satisfaction. "We want athletic competition to be a test of persons," Simon explains. "If outcomes are significantly affected not by such features [as the "intelligent choices and valued characteristics of the other"] but instead by the capacity of the body to benefit physiologically from drugs, athletes are no longer reacting to each other as persons but rather become more like competing bodies." In short, "the use of performance-enhancing drugs in sports restricts the area in which we can be respected as persons."[120] Competition, whether with one's self or with other athletes, certainly is fundamental to sports, but it is not clear that athletes react less like persons and more like "competing bodies" when they use enhancements rather than relying on other ways to perform better. And saying that playing a sport with the aid of enhancements is not to be respected because it is not a "valued characteristic" is simply tautological. Another commentator who does not think that enhancements are compatible with the spirit of sport, Michael Lavin, also does not get very far in trying to explain why, and ends up resting on a belief that there is a consensus against enhancements that is based on "an unconsciously grasped ideal of competitive sport."[121]

In one of the earliest scholarly attacks on performance enhancement, Tom Murray, now a member of WADA and president of the Hastings Center, the premier bioethics think tank, claimed that "drugs and other performance aids should be banned because they do not reflect the forms of human excellence that sports are intended to honor."[122] For Murray, an activity qualifies as a sport only if it rewards determination, effort, natural talent, and luck. An activity in which competitors employ enhancements is by definition therefore not a sport. Instead, maintains Murray, it is a "spectacle."[123] English law professor Simon Gardiner seems to agree when he asserts that "it is questionable whether the drug taking athlete has competed in the first place."[124]

One tactic used by Murray and others to prove that an activity that allows enhancements is not a sport is to ask, "Would it still be a marathon if someone competed on roller skates?" followed by "Would you still consider it baseball if players took drugs that enabled them to hit the ball a mile?" Murray's argument seems to be that competing in a marathon on skates is not a marathon, and by analogy that playing baseball with the aid of enhancements is not baseball. That may well be true, if we define baseball as a game played without biomedical enhancements. But just because we might call baseball on steroids something else, say "strongball," doesn't mean that it isn't a sport. The *American Heritage Dictionary* defines a sport as "a physical activity that is governed by a set of rules or customs and often engaged in competitively." Strongball unquestionably would qualify. There are plenty of informal athletics, like intramural or street sports, that do not bother to test participants for drugs. But just try convincing the players in a pickup basketball or volleyball game that what they are engaged in is only a "spectacle."

In part, Murray's attitude toward enhancements stems from his disconsolation over what he perceives as the debasement of a cherished experience. Evidently there was a halcyon period, during which many older Americans came of age, when the use of drugs in sports was unremarked, if not absent. No doubt Murray has fond memories of watching his idols accomplish breathtaking feats of athleticism with passion and grit—when, so to speak, "men were men."

Murray is not alone in his nostalgia. During the Senate hearings on steroids in baseball, former pitcher and current senator Jim Bunning stated: "Mr. Chairman, maybe I'm old fashioned. I remember when players didn't get better as they got older. We all got worse. When I played with Hank Aaron and Willie Mays and Ted Williams, they didn't put on forty pounds of bulk in their careers, and they didn't hit more homers in their late thirties than they did in their late twenties."[125]

But as documented above, the use of performance-enhancing substances in sports has a long tradition. In fact, as we shall see, only in the last fifty years or so has the notion that drug use is incompatible with sports become fashionable. It is not as if sports before modern biomedical enhancements was free of moral concerns. John McGraw, who dominated baseball at the turn of the twentieth century, "would grab the belt of a base-runner tagging up at third base on a fly ball and delay the runner's departure from the bag long enough to get him thrown out. Whitey Ford cut baseballs with a razor blade to give pitches an unusual break. Ty Cobb sharpened his spikes and slid in high to bases to deliberately injure fielders."[126] Cobb also was "a hard-drinking, hard-fighting racist who is reputed to have killed a man. Babe Ruth was a womanizing alcoholic who once charged into the stands to assault one of his critics. Ditto for Mickey Mantle, whose liver gave out when he was 53. The all-time hit king, Pete Rose, was a compulsive gambler who was jailed for tax evasion."[127]

Another sense in which performance enhancements may strike their opponents as incompatible with the "spirit of sport" is that they may seem to overemphasize competitiveness, the importance of winning over sportsmanship. This view of sport can be traced back at least as far as the Victorian era, when the upper classes emphasized "amateurism" and viewed sports as a refined, gentlemanly pursuit, characterized by sportsmanship and fair play, rather than ruthless competition. For Victorians, this attitude was more than just a manifestation of good breeding. "Amateurism" was a means by which the upper class sealed itself off from athletic competition from the lower classes. According to British sports historian Mike Huggins, "amateurism, accompanied by snobbishness, hypocrisy and double standards, became emblematic of class. . . . The key distinction was between 'gentlemen' and the rest, limiting and stabilising the democratic thrust of Victorian society." The Victorian middle class emulated the upper class, Huggins explains. "As the sports boom accelerated middle-class members, playing 'for sport alone,' experienced rowdy and partisan crowds, prepared to pay to watch and fanatical in their support, exhibiting very different working-class norms." Money became important: "Cash prizes for challenges were a standard expectation in working-class communities, and money in working-class hands was threateningly disruptive, a potential source of moral corruption. Professionals had to satisfy spectators, employers or patrons by winning, so the result was more important than aesthetic pleasure or entertainment." The gentleman's feigned distaste for lucre and his unease at the growing power of his social inferiors led him to portray the new competition as dishonorable: "Working-class players supposedly had no respectable reputation to lose. . . . Amateurs pointed to professionals' win-at-all-costs mentality, their more aggressive and violent approach and their sharp practice, deceit and cheating."[128]

The founder of the modern Olympic movement, Baron de Coubertin, was a product of the Victorian era, and when he revived the games, he insisted that only "amateurs" be permitted to compete. As Barrie Houlihan states in his book *Dying to Win,* "The promoters of the modern Olympics sought in the history of the early Olympics a rationale which would legitimise their preferred method of athletics which was designed to maintain the social position and interests of a privileged leisure class."[129] Coubertin's vision formed the foundation for the rules of amateurism that controlled Olympic eligibility for most of the twentieth century. Under these rules, for example, track-and-field star Jim Thorpe forfeited his Olympic gold medals from the 1912 Stockholm games when it was learned that he had earned $25 a week playing semiprofessional baseball two summers earlier.[130] But like the Victorian upper-class notions of sports propriety from which it emerged, the Olympic emphasis on amateurism faded as interest in the games expanded, and the International Olympic Committee dropped the amateur requirement for eligibility in 1981, leaving it to individual sports federations to regulate athletes' earnings. Nevertheless, the idea that sports should be gentlemanly rather than cutthroat, devoted to enjoying the contest rather than vanquishing the opponents, persists. The *Oxford English Dictionary* continues to reflect this notion in its definition of sport as "an activity involving physical exertion and skill in which an individual or team competes against another or others *for entertainment*" (emphasis added). Even Barry Bonds thinks that sports primarily should be about pleasure. "What is cheating?" he asked at a news conference in 2005. "We need to forget about the past and let us play the game. We're entertainers. Let us entertain."[131]

This brings us back to the question: Is biomedical enhancement incompatible with the spirit of sport? Murray's vision of sport has much to recommend it. Shorn of its class-based origins, the Victorian ideal of sport is admirable. Perhaps it would be better if athletes were not so bent on winning at all costs. But would it be so bad if athletes upheld the Olympic motto of "faster, higher, stronger" not only by training on new exercise machinery, being born into a wealthy family, eating carefully programmed meals, and using a new type of racquet, but also by taking relatively safe performance-enhancing drugs? And would it be better for rewards from sports to be reserved for those with natural talent, as Murray would prefer? Because if so, as the next chapter explains, class is not really out of the picture.

Chapter 4

The Hegemony of Meritocracy

The concerns raised by the use of biomedical enhancement for social reward have to be understood in their social and historical context. So far the discussion of these concerns has been confined to sports. But the rewards made possible by biomedical enhancements would extend far beyond sports: to better houses, health care, vacations, toys, education, careers, and mates. Enhancement even could be a key to political power.

It is against this expanded role for enhancement that its transformative potential must be assessed. Critics of enhancement do not limit their objections to sports, although it suits them to play on the nostalgia that sports evokes. Society as a whole would be imperiled, in their view, if people were permitted to benefit from enhanced performance. Instead, they say, societal benefit should be distributed according to the same rules that enhancement opponents insist on for sports: as a reward for effort, natural talent, and good luck.

In previous sections, I have questioned whether this formula was appropriate for sports. We observed that neither natural talent nor good luck is deserved. We saw that the point of enhancements is not necessarily to enable athletes to excel without hard work and that allowing all athletes to use enhancements could be fair and not necessarily contrary to the spirit of sport. Ethically, there does not seem to be any compelling reason to prevent reasonably competent adults from using relatively safe enhancements.

But once we step outside of sports, the critics' formula does not merely have ethical implications. It has social impact. It seeks to preserve a particular social hierarchy, in much the same way as did the glorification of the amateur gentleman athlete. The critics' distaste for biomedical enhancement is an attempt to maintain a certain power structure.

This power structure rests first on the principle of work. The idea that hard work is good came from our Puritan forefathers and their Calvinist forebears. As numerous scholars have pointed out, including Sharon Beder in *Selling the Work Ethic: From Puritan Pulpit to Corporate PR,* the ancient Greeks did not think much of work.[1] Socrates, Plato, and Aristotle all felt that work interfered with more virtuous pursuits like philosophy and government. This view persisted until the Reformation, when, in part as a rebellion against the profligacy of the Catholic Church, religious thinkers began to associate work with virtue. The Puritans elevated work to the status of a fundamental religious tenet in a particularly clever fashion. Only the elect, they believed, went to heaven. Hard work would not make you one of the elect, because whether or not you were one of the elect was preordained. But working hard was a sign that you had been chosen. Work therefore became a means of demonstrating to yourself, and to those around you, that you had been pre-selected for eternal bliss. The harder you worked, the easier it was to believe that you were destined for heaven. Work therefore reinforced your faith, which in turn strengthened your belief in the value of work. In effect, the Puritans invented true "faith-based initiative."

When the Puritans made it to America, they brought their work ethic with them. The United States came into being with a notable repudiation of lineage as the arbiter of social standing. From its cradle, the infant nation trumpeted its founding principle to the world, that all men are equally entitled to the happiness derived from a good life. How was one to achieve the good life other than by being born to it? The ostensible American answer was: through work. Thus arose the American Dream. Horatio Alger, a Unitarian clergyman forced to leave the pulpit following allegations of pedophilia, wrote books with titles such as *Strive and Succeed, Risen from the Ranks,* and *Bound to Rise,* in which the hero invariably pulled himself up the social ladder through honest effort. As Professor Beder writes, "America's reputation as a land of opportunity rested on its claim that the destruction of hereditary obstacles to advancement had created conditions in which social mobility depended on individual initiative alone." The dream was made real time and again by the rags-to-riches odysseys of men like the butcher's son, John Jacob Astor; Andrew Carnegie, son of a weaver; Cornelius Vanderbilt, who quit school when he was 11 to work on ferry boats; Henry Ford, born on a farm; and John D. Rockefeller, whose father was a traveling salesman. Observes Beder: "The self-made man, archetypical embodiment of the American Dream, owed his advancement to habits of industry, sobriety, moderation, self-discipline, and avoidance of debt."[2]

But hard work clearly is not enough. Many people work hard without getting very far ahead. In addition, one needs good fortune, the lucky break that brings the obscure clerk to the boss's attention. But that too does not suffice; the lucky break does the clerk no good if he is incompetent. To succeed, then, one also needs talent.

This, then, is the traditional American formula for social success, the ticket to the American Dream: natural talent, luck, and hard work.

It is debatable which of these three elements is most determinative of success. What is not debatable is that only one, hard work, is a quality that the individual can actually take credit for, and even the capacity for hard work itself may stem from genetic or environmental factors beyond the individual's control. The other two, good luck and natural talent, are not earned at all, and therefore not deserved in any meaningful sense. To the extent that they produce societal rewards, the rewards are no more based on merit than the social status aristocrats attained due to their accidents of birth.

But, oh, how good it is to rule the roost. So those who benefit under the traditional formula are keen to fortify their social status so that their position in society is safe from those who do not measure up. Being highly talented, their methods are ingenious. First, they emphasize the role of effort and downplay the two undeserved elements, reformulating the recipe for realizing the American Dream so that it seems as if it can be attained by hard work alone. By and large, they succeed. A recent survey by the Center for Survey Research and Analysis (CSRA) at the University of Connecticut found that 75 percent of randomly selected respondents thought that it was possible to start out poor in this country, work hard, and become rich.[3] As the director of the Center for Survey Research and Analysis concluded, "The American people still believe in the American Dream, that success is achievable through hard work." And a year earlier, an Associated Press / Ipsos poll had found that a majority of Americans agreed that "almost anyone can get rich if he puts his mind to it."[4]

The second step America's success stories take to solidify their position is to transform natural talent into something to which they are entitled. Again they are ingenious: they do this in a way that appeals both to the spiritually minded and the rationally minded alike. For the spiritually minded, they make natural talent sacred. As we saw earlier, Michael Sandel characterizes natural talents as "gifts," and it is clear who he thinks is the Benefactor. Senator Joseph Lieberman (D-Conn.; today Independent) embodied this attitude when he announced his candidacy for president of the United States in the town where he had attended public high school: "It was here that my parents, Henry and Marcia, themselves children of immigrants, worked their way into the American middle class and gave my sister and me the opportunities they never had. And it was here that I first understood the power of the promise America makes to all its people, that no matter who you are or where you start, if you work hard and play by the rules, you can go as far in this country as your God-given talents will take you."

Sandel even brazenly attempts to link natural talent to altruism. The talented must appreciate that "if our genetic endowments are gifts, rather than achievements for which we can claim credit, it is a mistake and a conceit to assume that we are entitled to the full measure of the bounty they reap in a market economy. We therefore have an obligation to share this bounty with those who, through no fault of their own, lack comparable gifts."[5] By implication, if we do not revere natural talent and allow those who possess it to reap the rewards, they will become more selfish and those who lack talent will be worse off because they will get less charity. This overlooks, of course, that the winners in the United States—the wealthy—give a much lower percentage of their income to charity than the losers—the working poor.[6] More important, there is no reason to believe that those who succeed with the help of enhancements—something else that no individual can take personal credit for—would be any less inclined toward philanthropy than anyone else.

Sanctifying natural talent takes care of the righteous. To appeal to the rationalists, society's winners simply point to their superior abilities. What sets our new republic apart, they explain, is that the old aristocracies rewarded people for who they were, while ours rewards people for what they produce. The winners in society do not benefit because they are naturally talented but because they are good at what they do.

The really brilliant part is the concept that was appropriated to describe the resulting social system: "meritocracy." As in, "we deserve this." As Stephen McNamee and Robert Miller Jr. explain in their book *The Meritocracy Myth,* meritocracy is an ideology, and "ideologies are ultimately based on persuasion as a form of social power." McNamee and Miller observe that "it is not enough for some to simply have more than others. For a system of inequality to be stable, those who have more must convince those who have less that the distribution of who gets what is fair, just, proper, or the natural order of things. . . . In feudal societies, for instance, the aristocracy used 'birthright' and the idea of 'the divine right of kings' to justify power and privilege over commoners and peasants. . . . In industrial societies such as the United States, inequality is justified by an ideology of meritocracy."[7]

Ironically, the person who coined the term *meritocracy,* British sociologist and politician Michael Young in his 1958 book, *The Rise of the Meritocracy,* did not intend it to be complimentary.[8] The book is a satire; although written in 1958, it purports to be a retrospective written in 2033, and in it, Young, who had been the author of the British Labour Party's social agenda in the 1945 election that turned Churchill's Conservative Party out of office and paved the way for the British welfare state, uses *meritocracy* to describe a society in which the naturally talented leaders of the working class are coopted into the elite, leaving the lower classes with little ability to produce radical social change. Yet in the hands of the meritocrats, the term came to stand for the positive core value of American society. As Stephen McNamee and Robert Miller Jr. explain: "America is seen as the land of opportunity where people get out of the system what they put into it. Ostensibly, the most talented, hardest working, and most virtuous get ahead. The lazy, shiftless, and indolent fall behind. You may not be held responsible for where you start out in life, but you are responsible for where you end up. If you are truly meritorious, you will overcome any obstacle and succeed."[9]

Of course, meritocracy is not the worst way of distributing societal rewards. In contrast to an aristocracy, at least the winners in a meritocracy are good at what they do. But America is not really much of a meritocracy. There is far less upward mobility than is often supposed, and society allocates its rewards primarily on the basis of factors other than ability. The American Dream, for the overwhelming number of its population, is the American Myth.

As Stephen McNamee and Robert Miller Jr. point out, if America truly were a meritocracy, societal rewards would be distributed to individuals based on whether or not they had the "right stuff": "being talented, having the right attitude, working hard, and having high moral character."[10] Intelligence clearly is a key component of talent. Measured in terms of IQ, the distribution of intelligence in the population conforms to a normal distribution, or bell curve. Therefore, one would expect the distribution of income and wealth to be bell-shaped as well. But it is not. As McNamee and Miller point out, "Income and especially wealth are highly skewed, with small percentages of the population getting most of what there is to get."[11] Why is this? According to McNamee and Miller, societal rewards overwhelmingly go to those who come from privileged backgrounds, regardless of their natural talent or hard work: "The most important determinant of where people end up in the economic pecking order of society is where they started in the first place. . . . Instead of a race to get ahead that begins anew with each generation, the 'race,' if it could be called that, is more aptly described as a relay race in which children inherit different starting points from parents."[12]

It is well known that people with college degrees earn more. Yet the role of favoritism in access to higher education, giving preference to children of alumni, is notorious. The *Wall Street Journal* reports that "many of the top schools, including Harvard, Princeton, Stanford and the University of Pennsylvania, admit so-called 'legacies' at a rate two to four times that of their overall applicant pool."[13] Berkeley sociologist Jerome Karabel describes how this admissions policy affected one particular applicant. "In the fall of 1963," he writes, "George W. Bush was a senior at Phillips Academy in Andover, Mass., facing the same dilemma confronting his 232 classmates: where to apply to college. He had never made the honor roll, and his verbal score on the SAT was a mediocre 566. Although popular among his classmates, he was neither an exceptional athlete nor did he possess any particularly outstanding extracurricular talents. Looking over his record, Andover's dean of students suggested that the young Mr. Bush consider applying to schools other than Yale, the alma mater of his father and grandfather." But facing increasing applications, Yale decided to give a preference not only to legacies but also to those legacies whose families had contributed the most to the university and wielded the most influence in society. "As the son of a prominent Texas oilman then running for the United States Senate—and the grandson of a United States senator from Connecticut who had recently served as a member of the Yale Corporation," Karabel continues, "George W. Bush was no ordinary applicant. In April 1964, he was accepted to Yale—unlike 49 percent of all alumni sons who applied that year."[14]

Karabel describes how Yale sought to change its legacy policy two years later, only to be confronted with irate alums. One of them, the late columnist William F. Buckley, complained that Yale no longer was "the 'kind of place where your family goes for generations' and had been transformed into an institution where 'the son of an alumnus, who goes to a private preparatory school, now has less chance of getting in than some boy from P.S. 109 somewhere.'"[15] The attempt at change was scrapped by 1974, "just as a major fund-raising effort was beginning." Nor was Yale's flirtation with scrapping its legacy policy lost on Harvard and Princeton. According to Karabel, they recently admitted legacies three times as often as other applicants.[16]

Colleges thwarted meritocracy not only by favoring the offspring of alumni but also by discriminating against Jews. Around World War I, Malcolm Gladwell writes in *The New Yorker*, "the country's elite colleges faced what became known as 'the Jewish problem.' They were being inundated with the children of Eastern European Jewish immigrants. These students came from the lower middle class and they disrupted the genteel WASP sensibility that had been so much a part of the Ivy League tradition."[17] As one Harvard professor complained, "They were socially untrained and their bodily habits are not good." The source of the Jewish problem was that Jewish kids scored extremely high on achievement tests. For example, Columbia University used the New York State Regents Examinations as a key factor in its admissions decisions, "and the plain truth," Gladwell notes, "was that Jews did extraordinarily well on the Regents Exams." Not wanting to impose actual quotas on Jewish students, as other Ivy League colleges were considering, Columbia came up with the idea of making applicants take an aptitude test: "According to Herbert Hawkes, the dean of Columbia College during this period, because the typical Jewish student was simply a 'grind,' who excelled on the Regents Exams because he worked so hard, a test of innate intelligence would put him back in his place."

The premier college aptitude test, of course, is the S.A.T. In his book chronicling the history of the S.A.T., *The Big Test,* journalist Nicholas Lemann describes how it emerged from IQ testing, and how when he was president of Harvard in the 1930s, James Conant seized on the test as a tool that could overthrow the privileged WASP class by enabling talented kids to get into top colleges despite not having gone to good high schools.[18] How ironic that Columbia viewed aptitude testing in precisely the opposite way: as the means of *perpetuating* the privileged class. As Gladwell points out, "The great selling point of the S.A.T. has always been that it promises to reveal whether the high-school senior with a 3.0 G.P.A. is someone who could have done much better if he had been properly educated or someone who is already at the limit of his abilities. We want to know that information because, like Hawkes, we prefer naturals to grinds: we think that people who achieve based on vast reserves of innate ability are somehow more promising and more worthy than those who simply work hard."

The hero of Gladwell's story, incidentally, is Stanley Kaplan, because his successful coaching technique confounded Hawkes's presumption that aptitude tests measured innate ability. "In proving that the S.A.T. was coachable," states Gladwell, "Stanley Kaplan did something else, which was of even greater importance. He undermined the use of aptitude tests as a means of social engineering."

If, as the foregoing illustrates, the United States in many ways is not much of a meritocracy, it is vital to the meritocrats to make sure that as few people as possible realize it. An article in the *Washington Post* points out, for example, that *Forbes* magazine describes Fidelity Investments Chairman and CEO Edward C. Johnson III (net worth: $4.9 billion) as "self-made" even though "Johnson III took over Fidelity from his father, Fidelity founder Edward C. Johnson II." Forbes also insists on calling Viacom CEO Sumner Redstone (net worth: $9.7 billion) and financier Charles Bartlett Johnson (net worth: $2 billion) "self-made" even though the former got his start by taking charge of his father's drive-in theater business and the latter along with his brother inherited their father's mutual fund company.[19]

Yet the reign of meritocracy persists in the face of these realities. According to the 2006 Associated Press / Ipsos poll mentioned earlier, a majority of Americans believe that "people who make lots of money deserve it." As McNamee and Miller conclude, "In a non-meritocratic society, the socially advantaged wield meritocracy as an ideological instrument of subjugation."

This makes it readily apparent why so much scorn is heaped on biomedical enhancement. By enabling those who are deficient in natural talent to be better at what they do, enhancement means more competition for the gifted. Therefore it is critical for the gifted to attack this improvement in performance as unfair, inauthentic, destructive to "personhood," and above all, as cheating and unmerited. As Yale graduate George Bush declared in his 2004 State of the Union Message, steroids are "shortcuts to accomplishment."[20]

Given this appreciation of the impact of enhancement on meritocracy, efforts to prohibit the use of biomedical enhancements, such as doping bans in elite sports, lose much of their remaining ethical force. Instead of appearing to preserve the role of effort, opposition to enhancement can be seen as an attempt by the gifted and lucky to preserve their unearned hegemony. In this guise, biomedical enhancement is not a form of cheating but a means of creating greater equality of opportunity. When former senator George Mitchell released his 2007 report on steroid use in baseball, for example, one major league umpire acknowledged that most umpires were aware that many players were using performance enhancers, but "it didn't raise a red flag for them because they saw it as a way for the players to stay on the field": "I have some empathy for them, I admit," said the umpire. "The game at this level is so competitive. A lot of these guys, I'm sure they did what they did to recuperate from injuries, or to fight age."[21]

Indeed, one possible function of enhancements in sports could be to help level the playing field. Rather than prohibiting all competitors from using enhancements, the rules could permit athletes to use enhancements in inverse proportion to their natural talent and good luck. For example, the International Cycling Union (known by its French initials as UCI), concerned about reports that cyclists were using EPO to increase their number of red blood cells, adopted a policy that athletes whose percentage of red blood cells in their blood (or hematocrit level) exceeded 50 percent would be assumed to be using EPO and be suspended from competing. Because the average hematocrit level in males is in the neighborhood of 45 percent, in theory this would allow cyclists with a low natural hematocrit level to use EPO to increase it to 50 percent. (The Olympics now has a test that can detect synthetic EPO directly, obviating the need for the hematocrit threshold approach.)

A similar issue is raised by disabled athletes who want to compete in nondisabled events. Should they be allowed to use equipment that compensates for their disability, and if so, what limits should there be on the effectiveness of this equipment? The U.S. Supreme Court dealt with this issue in the Casey Martin case. Martin is a professional golfer who has Klippel-Trenaunay-Weber syndrome, a degenerative circulatory disorder that makes it impossible for him to walk an 18-hole golf course. To be able to play in the PGA Tour, he sought permission to use an electric golf cart, which is prohibited by the rules. After the PGA Tour refused his request on the grounds that a cart would "fundamentally alter" the competition, Martin sued under the Americans with Disability Act (ADA). In a 7-to-2 decision, the U.S. Supreme Court ruled for Martin on the basis that use of the cart would not fundamentally alter the event.[22]

The most interesting aspect of the case was Justice Antonin Scalia's dissenting opinion. He chided the justices in the majority for basing their decision in part on their finding that use of a golf cart would not give Martin an advantage over his competitors, because even with the cart, his physical impairment would leave him at least as fatigued as golfers who walked the course. In Scalia's judgment, this qualification plunges the courts into the quagmire of determining on a case-by-case basis whether an enhancement would do more than place a person on a par with competitors: "One can envision the parents of a Little League player with attention deficit disorder trying to convince a judge that their son's disability makes it at least 25 percent more difficult to hit a pitched ball. (If they are successful, the only thing that could prevent a court order giving the kid four strikes would be a judicial determination that, in baseball, three strikes are metaphysically necessary, which is quite absurd.)"

Track-and-field is being forced to confront this type of controversy in the case of a South African sprinter, Oscar Pistorius, who was born with lower legs but no feet. After injuring himself playing rugby on artificial feet, he took up running using a special prosthetic made with high-tech carbon-fiber leaf springs called "cheetah limb" by its manufacturer. In 2004, he broke the 22-second barrier in the 200-meter dash in the Athens Paralympics. This prompted him to apply to compete for South Africa in the regular 2008 Beijing Olympics—not the Paralympics. But the International Amateur Athletic Federation turned him down on the basis that his prostheses gave him an unfair advantage over "normal" runners. Specifically, tests showed that the springy prosthetics produced less vertical motion, allowing users to achieve the same speeds as normal competitors with the use of 25 percent less energy.[23]

Oscar Pistorius's apparatus thus appears to give him an advantage over naturally talented competitors, enabling him to outclass them despite his disability. But if naturally talented runners were permitted to use enhancements as well, wouldn't they outpace *him*? This brings us back to Einer Elhauge's observation that if enhancements were permitted, naturally talented people could use them as well, thereby maintaining their performance edge over those with less talent. If this is the case, what do the talented have to fear from enhancements?

One answer is that, outside of sports, maximum limits on excellence may be more prevalent. In beauty pageants, there is probably a limit on how beautiful cosmetic surgery can make contestants. Another possibility is that competitions outside of sports may be less discriminating in that they are willing to reward a basic level of competence. To win an Olympic event, an athlete needs to be the best. But though people need a considerable amount of talent to become successful lawyers, they don't have to be the best in their class in law school. Enhancements may increase a person's skill enough to pursue a successful career alongside attorneys with greater natural gifts.

Another eventuality that may trouble the talented is that, in competitions that have no absolute limit on accomplishment, such as the pursuit of wealth, or in which absolute limits have not yet been reached, any attempt to maintain their natural advantage with the aid of enhancements will only drive less talented individuals to pursue more powerful and potentially more dangerous means. The result would be an enhancement arms race in which everyone tried to be a step ahead of everyone else. But to a large extent, this is always true of societal competition. The only difference is that the contestants would have an additional set of technologies at their disposal.

Michael Sandel makes an important point, however, when he observes that even if performance enhancements can be said to be no different from many other methods that people use to compete, that does not mean that enhancements are desirable. In regard to genetic enhancement, he concedes that "improving children through genetic engineering is similar in spirit to the heavily managed, high-pressure child-rearing that is now common," but "this similarity does not vindicate genetic enhancement. On the contrary, it highlights a problem with the trend toward hyperparenting."[24] The last thing we need, it might be argued, is another respect in which everyone tries to keep up with the Joneses. We therefore need to consider whether the use of enhancements is so different from other competitive behaviors that it deserves to be singled out for opprobrium, and whether the power of the state legitimately should be invoked to ban the use of enhancements when the objections to them appear to be largely arbitrary.

But those who possess natural talent may not have to concern themselves with the prospect of an enhancement arms race at all. The less talented may never be able to use enhancements to pull themselves alongside. They may not be able to afford them.

Chapter 5

Access to Enhancements and the Challenge to Equality

IN OUR 1998 BOOK *Access to the Genome: The Challenge to Equality,* my coauthor, Jeffrey Botkin, and I observed that the high price of new genetic technologies, including genetic enhancements, would place them beyond the means of many people, leading to a dangerous performance gap between the genetic haves and have-nots. We even invented a term to describe the new aristocracy, the well-off families who had installed genetic enhancements into their germlines so that the improvements would be carried over to future generations. We called them a *genobility*.

As I warned in my 2003 book, *Wondergenes,* a widening gap between the enhanced and unenhanced segments of society could destroy our democratic political system. This might not happen right away or all at once, because there might be enough elasticity in the fabric of society to accommodate a degree of increased stratification. Just enough people in the underclasses may have the good luck to rise—or get snapped up by the upper class, as the originator of the term *meritocracy* predicted—that the promise of upward mobility cushions the reality. Just as we seem content to be ruled by elected officials who are significantly better off then the people they represent, so the unenhanced may allow themselves to be ruled by the enhanced, at least for a time.

But eventually the system would collapse. The enhanced would be tempted to aggregate more and more goods and power, just as the wealthy now compound the interest on their investments. There is no more reason to expect the enhanced to behave any more judiciously than the ancien regime in Europe, whose excesses provoked revolutionary democracy. Faced with growing unrest, the enhanced elite would resort to demagoguery, manipulation, and finally tyranny. Along the way, they undoubtedly would employ biomedical methods to calm the multitudes, as Aldous Huxley depicted in *Brave New World.* While *Wondergenes* focused on one particular type of enhancement, genetic enhancement, biomedical enhancement in general would have the same effect. The end result would be rebellion and chaos—or totalitarianism.

Nothing has changed since 2003 to provide encouragement that this dystopia can be avoided. Many popular enhancements are sufficiently expensive that they are not affordable to large segments of the population. The cost of cosmetic surgery techniques places them beyond the means of many. Surgeons' fees alone, not including anesthesia, facility fees, medications, and tests, average more than $3,500 for breast augmentation, $4,000 for a nose job, and $6,500 for facelifts.[1] Botox costs about $400 a treatment, and each treatment only lasts a few months. Caffeine is still relatively cheap, although designer coffees can run more than $5 a cup at chains like Starbucks. The lowest U.S. price for the alertness drug Provigil (200 mg/day) is almost $9 per day, or more than $250 a month.[2] Human growth hormone injections run more than $10,000 a year.

Enhancements on the horizon are likely to be equally expensive, at least initially. In September 2007, Craig Venter, the scientist/entrepreneur who competed with the NIH in the 1990s to sequence the entire human genome, announced that he had sequenced his own genome at a cost of about $70 million.[3] Researchers look forward to a "$1000 genome"—the ability to sequence a person's entire genetic endowment for $1,000.[4] This will enable researchers to identify regions of DNA that code for nondisease traits, a necessary step toward developing genetic enhancement technologies. But a $1,000 test is still out of the question for the poor. Genetic enhancements performed at stages of human development when they would be most likely to be effective would entail in vitro fertilization. According to the American Society for Reproductive Medicine, on average it takes two to three IVF cycles to become pregnant, and a single cycle costs an average of $12,440.[5] The cost of the genetic engineering component would be on top of this.

One reason for the high cost of these biomedical innovations is that the law blocks competition, which could drive down prices. The law does this in two ways. First, it grants the inventors patents, and lends the power of the courts to enforce them. Patent protection enables drug manufacturers to charge high prices for new products. As described earlier, human growth hormone originally was harvested by the NIH from cadavers and distributed free of charge to patients. Once drug companies figured out how to manufacture it synthetically using recombinant DNA technology, they patented it and sold it for thousands of dollars a dose. True, the hormone was once as scarce as hen's teeth and now is available in virtually unlimited quantities, but the enlarged supply does no good for those who cannot afford it.

Researchers even have filed patents on stretches of human DNA. This has allowed them to charge royalties for using the DNA sequences in research or genetic testing. One company, Myriad Genetics, has patented a gene associated with a risk for breast cancer. In 2004, the European Patent Office revoked the patent after objections from European clinicians and researchers, including complaints that the company had forced French physicians to send test samples to its lab rather than performing the tests themselves, which they could do more accurately and at a third the charge to patients.[6] Similar complaints have been voiced in the United States, where the Myriad patent continues to be enforced. Another alleged abuse is filing patents on pieces of DNA without knowing their function. In 2007, the House of Representatives passed a bill that would make it easier to challenge patent claims, but the legislation has triggered fierce opposition from biotech companies, drug manufacturers, and universities, all of whom bank on the future value of their patented discoveries.[7]

The idea that someone can own the rights to a piece of human DNA strikes many as outrageous. The U.S. patent system was supposed to prevent this by refusing to grant patents on "products of nature," but genetic researchers have circumvented the exclusion by claiming that what they actually are patenting are refined and isolated portions of DNA, rather than just the natural molecular material. Gene patents are all the more objectionable given that many of them were paid for with public funds. The research that led to Myriad's patent on the breast cancer gene, for example, used publicly available sequencing data that had been produced with government funding as well as a direct $5 million government grant.[8]

Patent protection isn't the only way the law limits competition in biotechnology. The FDA licensing system gives exclusive marketing rights to the companies that are first to obtain an FDA license to market a new product, and these companies maintain high prices for their products until the period of exclusivity ends and they begin to face competition from generic versions. Most enhancements regulated by the FDA are off-label uses of products that the agency has approved for therapeutic purposes, such as human growth hormone, erythropoietin, and steroids. Only a few licenses have been granted for actual enhancement uses, including for Botox, breast implants, and certain contact lenses. But this is likely to change, because FDA rules prohibit companies from promoting their products for off-label uses. If a company wants to advertise a drug as an enhancement, it has to obtain a license for the enhancement use of the drug. The cost of obtaining a license is huge because of the expense of conducting the necessary clinical trials, but as more enhancement products are developed and the demand for them increases, companies may decide that the price is worth it to enable them to market enhancements directly to consumers.

Although the prices of enhancement technologies may start out high, they may come down with time, just as prices have declined for electronic equipment such as televisions and computers. The price of cosmetic surgery might become less expensive, for example, as more and more procedures that formerly took place at high cost in hospital operating rooms followed by overnight stays come to be performed on an outpatient basis in surgeons' offices. Moreover, enhancements are paid for out-of-pocket rather than by public or private health insurance. (This is one reason why the renewed concern about the growing number of Americans who lack health insurance, as well as the growing chance that some type of universal insurance program will be created in the near future, will not necessarily increase access to enhancements.) This means that people have an incentive to shop around to obtain the lowest price, stimulating price competition among providers. The price of Lasik eye surgery, for instance, decreased by almost 30 percent over the first ten years.[9] As one plastic surgeon stated, consumers approach cosmetic surgery as a retail decision, "as if they were buying a cruise, a vacation, a car."[10]

Yet prices may not decline if the demand is strong enough. The cost of cosmetic surgery has not decreased, for example. Instead it has kept pace with inflation, with the exception of facelifts, the price of which has outstripped inflation, presumably due to its growth in popularity.[11] Moreover, prices may not decline fast enough to avoid the social dislocations that could result from widely unequal access.

Enhancement enthusiasts dismiss these concerns. Ramez Naam, author of *More Than Human,* argues that "legal enhancement technologies could benefit the poor almost as much as the rich [because of] the law of diminishing returns."[12] Applied to enhancements, the law of diminishing returns says that, while the first dollars spent on enhancements will produce substantial advantages, subsequent expenditures will yield fewer and fewer benefits. According to Naam, even though only the wealthy may be able to afford the most expensive enhancements, the advantages they will receive will not be that much greater than the benefits that less affluent people can obtain from less expensive enhancements. But Naam is assuming that enhancement benefit will be available at a sufficiently low cost that the well-off will not gain a significant social advantage. Yet the relationship between price and degree of benefit could be such that the wealthy would obtain an insurmountable advantage over the less wealthy.

The second argument Naam makes is that once patents expire, prices will drop "in proportion to the number of people who want" the enhancement in question. In short, "the greater the demand, the lower the price" such that "the most sought-after enhancements will be the cheapest." But the reality is far more complicated. Naam uses the example of penicillin, the price of which came down dramatically in price after its initial discovery. It is true that the high demand encouraged drug manufacturers to increase the supply of penicillin and that there was a tremendous reduction in price: from $3,955 a pound in 1945 to $282 a pound by 1950.[13] But the real reason for the reduction in the price was not the demand but the competitiveness of the industry, because the antibiotic was never patented (being a product of nature), and the costs for new manufacturers to enter the market were low.[14] If a market is not highly competitive, or the supply is limited, increases in demand will cause increases, not decreases, in price. Think of the increasing cost of a barrel of crude oil.

A more moderate proponent of genetic enhancement, Gregory Stock, concedes that the issue of access is problematic. Focusing on what he calls "germinal choice," or enhancement interventions in the reproductive process, he observes that "how germinal choice technology affects our future will hinge on who has access to it as well as on what it offers. If the technology is available to large numbers of people, it is unlikely to give rise to a narrow elite." His solution is universal access: "Provision of free universal access to major aspects of GCT would align better with our ideals of equal opportunity for children and might be surprisingly affordable. If the price of a full GCT procedure could be kept down to, say, $6000 a baby, this would be roughly equal to the average yearly expenditure on a student in public school in the United States."[15] However, Stock seems oblivious to the challenge of convincing the nation to spend as much on enhancement as it spends on public education. Public education is funded by property taxes. How many households would be willing to double the amount of property taxes they pay in order to provide parents with access to IVF and the ability to genetically engineer their offspring?

Proponents of enhancement also argue that the disparities that would result if enhancements are available only to the well-off would be no different from the disparities that already exist, which we seem able to accommodate without extremely negative social effects. For example, we allow parents who can afford it to send their children to elite private schools even though persons who attend private schools earn significantly higher wages than those who attend public schools.[16] We defend private schooling not only by invoking the principle of freedom of religion on behalf of parents who send their children to parochial schools but also by appealing to the constitutional right parents have to rear their children as they desire. Thus, the Supreme Court repeatedly has struck down state laws seeking to compel parents to send their children to public schools. In a landmark case involving an Oregon statute, for example, the Court emphasized that "the fundamental theory of liberty upon which all governments in this Union repose excludes any general power of the State to standardize its children by forcing them to accept instruction from public teachers only."[17] Private schooling also remains acceptable because we convince ourselves that the quality of a public education, for the most part, is adequate, perhaps even equivalent for the gifted student. We tout the exceptional public schools, such as the 1,300 that *Newsweek* magazine lists according to a formula that divides the total number of advanced placement tests taken each year at the school by the number of graduates.[18] And we rely on trivia from the

U.S. Department of Education, like the report in 2006 explaining that while private school students achieved higher levels of reading in eighth grade, public school students did better in math in grade four.[19]

Furthermore, the American social system so far seems to be able to survive despite enormous differences in wealth. Corporate executives earn hundreds of times more than their workers, compared to just an 11-to-1 ratio in Japan and a 22-to-1 ratio in Britain. In 2001, the top 1 percent of households held more than 33 percent of all privately held wealth, while the bottom 80 percent of households owned only 16 percent. The three hundred thousand Americans with the highest incomes earned 440 times more than those in the bottom half of the country, and their income almost equaled that of the bottom 150 million.[20] In 2006, just over half of household income was concentrated in the top 20 percent of Americans.[21] As Elizabeth Warren and Amelia Warren Tyagi observe in their 2003 book, *The Two-Income Trap: Why Middle-Class Mothers And Fathers Are Going Broke*, "The average two-income family earns far more today than did the single-breadwinner family of a generation ago. And yet, once they have paid the mortgage, the car payments, the taxes, the health insurance, and the day-care bills, today's dual-income families have less discretionary income—and less money to put away for a rainy day—than the single-income family of a *generation ago*."[22] In 2000, George Bush quipped to a wealthy audience: "What an impressive crowd: the haves, and the have-mores. Some people call you the elite; I call you my base."[23] But in February 2007, he acknowledged that "income inequality is real," adding that "the earnings gap is now twice as wide as it was in 1980, and it continues to grow."[24] A professor at the University of California puts it succinctly: "Just 10% of the people own the United States of America."[25]

Highly effective yet high-priced biomedical enhancements could exacerbate these disparities beyond the breaking point. Individuals who already possessed the most wealth and enjoyed the greatest social advantages would accrue even more for themselves. As I wrote in *Wondergenes*,

> The enhanced will be the most attractive, strongest, most graceful, most intelligent, most charismatic, and most inventive, and they will run the most successful businesses. All of these advantages will be rolled into the same persons. They will enjoy decisive advantages over everyone else in all realms of life—sports and beauty contests, game and talent shows, en-

> tertainment and the arts, admission to the best educational institutions, entry into the professions, political office and government appointment, getting rich or richer, and grabbing the most desirable mates. They will attain a monopoly over the best things in life, and their position at the pinnacle of society will be unassailable.[26]

Not only would the price of biomedical enhancements continue to place them beyond the reach of many, but also fewer and fewer people would be able to break into the ranks of those who could afford them.

At some point, the belief in equality of opportunity—the fundamental underpinning of the current system of inequality—would weaken beyond the breaking point. One commentator observes that "people have put up with all this because it happened so quickly and for the same reason that the great mass of losers in casinos put up with odds that favor the house: The spectacle of a few ecstatic big winners encourages the losers to believe that, hey, they might get lucky and win, too."[27] Once enough people accepted that they and their children had little or no chance of climbing toward the top of the social ladder, they might well withdraw their investment in the continued operation of the system, which then would collapse.

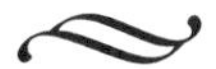

Chapter 6

Lack of Choice

NO BIOMEDICAL INTERVENTION is risk-free, and, as we saw in chapter 2, enhancements are no exception. The twin ethical principles of beneficence ("do good") and nonmaleficence ("do no harm") prohibit health care professionals from providing products or services that do more harm than good. Originally, the professionals themselves weighed the risks and benefits of interventions and selected the ones that they thought would be best for their patients. It gradually became clear, however, that while the professionals might be able to discern which interventions could not possibly provide any net benefits, a number of alternatives might be viewed as acceptable, and the optimal choice might vary from patient to patient depending on the patient's preferences and aversion to risk. The practice therefore developed of obtaining the patient's informed consent, that is, of presenting patients with the information that was known about the viable alternatives and allowing the patients to select the course of treatment they preferred. Informed consent accords with the third fundamental principle of modern medical ethics: promoting patient autonomy. It also promotes efficiency by avoiding waste. A good example is when a patient decides to forgo treatment. If a physician ignored the patient's wishes and treated the patient because that was what the doctor thought was best, resources that could be devoted to another patient would be wasted on someone who did not want them.

Informed consent has its defenders and detractors. It has been criticized on a number of grounds, including that patients can rarely understand the information they receive, that some patients might be better off if decisions were completely up to their caregivers, and that health care professionals might misuse the doctrine to avoid liability for unreasonable actions by arguing that, by giving informed consent, the patient had accepted the risks. But while there might be many ways in which the doctrine of informed consent might be improved, there are few calls to discard it altogether. It has become firmly entrenched in biomedical ethics, and there is no reason why it should not apply to biomedical enhancements as well as to health-oriented decisionmaking.

Persons cannot give informed consent if they lack the ability to make rational, voluntary choices, however. This can happen in two situations: when the person lacks the requisite mental capacity, and when the choice is too constrained to be considered truly voluntary. Judges struggle with the issue of mental capacity when deciding whether patients who have conditions such as retardation or dementia are competent to make treatment decisions. The courts' rulings reveal a striking willingness to bend over backward to deem patients competent. In effect, the law prefers to err on the side of autonomy rather than nonmaleficence. It is willing to restrict individuals' decisionmaking authority in order to protect them from making harmful choices that we presume they would not make if they were competent. But the law tries to avoid lapsing into hard paternalism, which would restrict individual choice even for competent persons on the ground that they do not know what is best for them.

It might be thought that the use of biomedical enhancements would not involve questions of mental competency because people who are not mentally competent would not be given what are properly considered enhancements—not because there would be no point in doing so, but because interventions that improved their functioning would count as therapy rather than enhancement. But as I noted at the beginning of the book, an intervention might not only correct a person's incapacity but also leave the person better than normal, in which case it would qualify as an enhancement as well as a therapy. Moreover, recall the category of "compensatory enhancement." A person with diminished mental capacity might be given an enhancement to improve a normal trait, such as appearance or athletic ability, in an effort to compensate for or offset the mental disability. (Mentally incompetent persons also might be used as research subjects in enhancement experiments, a topic that is addressed later.) In these instances, a problem would arise if, due to their mental impairment, the people given access to enhancements could not make an informed, rational choice of whether or not to use them.

Children

The law takes the view that a person under the age of majority (18 years old for the most part) cannot make binding contracts or any other kind of legally recognized decision, including giving informed consent to medical care. There are exceptions, such as when older adolescents are deemed to be "emancipated minors" because they are married or have had children and no longer live under their parents' control or when the law allows them to make specific decisions, such as whether to be treated for a sexually transmitted disease without notifying their parents. But usually the parents or legal guardian call the shots. Given that enhancements might be harmful, it stands to reason that children ordinarily should not be given enhancements without the permission of their parents or legal guardian. But when, if ever, is it inappropriate for parents to expose children to risks to their health or well-being with the aim of enhancing the child's performance, appearance, or capabilities? How serious do these risks have to be for society to be entitled to interfere with the parents' decisions?

Some say it would never be appropriate for parents to give biomedical enhancements to their children. In 2005, the American Academy of Pediatrics issued a policy statement condemning the use of performance-enhancing substances in children and adolescents and calling on schools and coaches to take strong stances against the practice.[1] The academy not only cited potential health risks but also claimed that enhancement use was "unfair, and therefore morally and ethically indefensible." Critics such as Jürgen Habermas charge that enhancements "instrumentalize" children, turning them into mere objects to be manipulated as parents desire.[2] Supreme Court Justice John Paul Stevens warned, for example, that "even a fit parent is capable of treating a child like a mere possession."[3] Enhancing children also is criticized as "commodification," or wrongly equating an individual with his or her capabilities. Michael Sandel states that when parents enhance their children, "the problem is not that parents usurp the autonomy of the child they design. The problem lies in the hubris of the designing parents, in their drive to master the mystery of birth."[4] Why is the attempt to master the mystery of disease not also hubris? Because, says Sandel, "medical intervention to cure or prevent illness or restore the injured to health does not desecrate nature but honors it." In Sandel's view, "Healing sickness or injury does not override a child's natural capacities but permits them to flourish."[5]

Critics also object when parents enhance their children in order to fulfill the parents' own fantasies or ambitions. This seems to fit the mindset of Neil Hoekstra, the adoptive father of the abnormally muscled Michigan child described in chapter 1 who was born with a deficiency in myostatin, a protein that retards muscle growth. During an interview in which he was described as "already dreaming big things for his adopted son," Hoekstra, a die-hard University of Michigan football fan, said: "I want him to be a football player. He could be the next Michael Hart," a reference to a star Michigan running back.[6]

Finally, critics of enhancing children complain that enhancements would deprive the child of an "open future." Joel Feinberg, the leading proponent of this view, asserts that "it is a duty of parents to keep as many as possible of a child's central life-options open until the child becomes an autonomous adult himself, and can decide on his own how to exercise them."[7] Bill McKibben describes the parent who genetically enhances a child "as god-king, laying down the channel through which the child's life must flow."[8] This criticism is extended to enhancements that take place during the reproductive process, such as the manipulation of a child's DNA and preimplantation genetic testing. Tom Murray urges us not to allow parents to use genetic testing to select the gender of embryos fertilized using IVF, because it would mean "giving in to a parental whim where that whim is not particularly significant, and when there's not a compelling reason for having more choice and control in children."[9]

Concerns about preserving an open future lead to widespread opposition to performing any sort of genetic testing on children, unless its purpose is to facilitate treatment, alert the parents to disorders that will strike the children early in life, or, in the case of older adolescents who are sexually active, provide them with information that may bear on reproductive decisionmaking.[10] Andy Miah and Emma Rich, for example, caution against testing children for genetically based athletic talent. "At most," they argue, "genetic tests should be used as a way of shaping advice about training rather than influencing the kind of sport a child decides to undertake."[11] One study found that children who were told that they had genetic profiles that were "neutral" in terms of athletic ability had higher self-esteem than children with "good" genetic profiles, the implication being that the children with good profiles did not feel that they could claim as much personal credit for their athletic prowess.[12]

While promoting a child's self-esteem certainly is worthwhile, a number of these objections to enhancing children are unconvincing. The American Academy of Pediatrics doesn't explain why it calls enhancements "unfair," but as we saw in chapter 3, there is nothing inherently unfair about them. Nor do the critics of enhancement testing to identify a child's talents explain why this would be any different, from an ethical standpoint, than the myriad other ways in which children are probed and pigeonholed. After conceding that genetic tests are different in that they permit talents to be identified before a person is born, Julian Savulescu and Bennett Foddy point out that "we already look to identify a person's particular talents when they are very young. Children with nimble fingers and perfect pitch are encouraged to play the violin, and children who grow tall at a young age are encouraged to play basketball."[13] An entire industry in fact is devoted to developing and marketing tests to assess athletic potential. One company, Sparq Training in Portland, Oregon, sells the Sparq Rating Test, which is given to 250,000 children a year.[14] The company claims that its test is "the first-ever system designed to measure sport-specific athleticism. Created to capture the key aspects of athleticism, these tests are combined and weighted in a unique proprietary formula."[15] Another company, Sports Potential, sells a test called "Smart" for $135 which measures the physical and cognitive skills of children 8 to 12 years old to determine their potential in 38 different sports.[16] As Savulescu and Foddy observe, "a parent who wants to oppress their child, to live through them to make their life miserable in some way can already do this with great efficiency without using genetic technology."[17]

Rather than trying to instrumentalize or commodify their children, parents who give them enhancements simply may feel that they are expanding their children's chances for success. Savulescu and Foddy point out that parents could use the results of genetic tests for athletic ability "to encourage a lazy or skeptical child to get involved in sports."[18] Sparq Training says that its test provides athletes with an invaluable tool for "staying motivated."[19] In *Wondergenes,* I described a couple who fed their toddler okra so that she would appear more sophisticated than other preschool applicants when the admissions interviewer asked her to name her favorite foods. Bizarre, perhaps, but undoubtedly intended to start the child down the path of a high-class education. Other parents go to the mat with teachers and school administrators to secure for their children more attention, better treatment, or higher grades. In a recent twist, some parents reportedly pretend that their children have a learning disability to gain them more time on tests. As a learning specialist at one New York City private school explained, "We have high-powered, savvy parents, and if they come in with a $3,000 evaluation, dead set on getting extra time, it's very difficult to turn them down." This has led the College Board to tighten its requirements for establishing that a student is entitled to extra time when taking the SAT.[20]

That enhancements may expand rather than contract a child's options is at odds with the notion that they deprive children of an open future. Take ACTN3 genetic testing for sports ability. If the test identified only one or two sports that a child could play well and a child was steered toward those sports only, it indeed could narrow the child's future options. But the ACTN3 test merely purports to indicate whether a child's genome tends to produce muscle types conducive to endurance sports rather than sports that rely on shorter bursts of effort. Such a test would identify a whole range of athletic activities at which the child might excel. This makes it harder to consider the test to be a limitation rather than a liberation from futility and disappointment.

At a minimum, then, we ought to distinguish enhancements that extend a child's options from those that reduce them. Human growth hormone might restrict children's futures, because if it actually could make them grow extremely lanky and tall, that would suit them well for basketball, tennis, and volleyball and less so for football, wrestling, horseracing, or spelunking. A drug that enhanced cognition, however, would seem to be just like education, opening up a wide array of future possibilities. Insofar as Michael Sandel acknowledges that medical care "does not override a child's natural capacities but permits them to flourish," the same might be said of enhancements giving children additional abilities without simultaneously circumscribing others. For example, one woman surveyed by a group of experts from the British Academy of Medical Sciences about her attitude toward cognition-enhancing drugs stated, "If, in the future, there are cognition tablets for exams and

I wasn't happy for my children to take them, would I be disadvantaging them against those children that actually take them?"[21] Indeed, this suggests that, in the same way that parents are required to give their children proper medical care or face public censure, they may come to be expected to give them biomedical enhancements to avoid being considered "unfit."

Moreover, some people believe that the role of parents is not so much to leave their children's futures as open as possible as to shape their futures. Political scientist Shelley Burtt says that "the question is not how little impact a parent can make on a child's view of the world (how neutral parenting can be) but how fully parents can discharge their obligations to guide children to a productive, satisfying adulthood."[22] Even if enhancements did channel a child's development in certain directions, then, this would be appropriate if it propelled children toward a good life.

Even if we accept the premise that parents should not enhance their children if it means increasing some options at the expense of others, it is not clear that society legitimately can intrude into this realm of parental decisionmaking. Parents routinely enroll their children in music, art, religious, and sports lessons, even though these activities take time away from other pursuits, including schoolwork, and represent a choice to develop certain talents at the expense of others. In some cases, the amount of time, energy, and resources devoted to these activities is so great that it precludes children from experiencing what might be considered a "normal" childhood. Children with acting or musical careers or who are being groomed for elite sports, for example, have little room for other extracurricular activities or sometimes even for childhood friendships. Joan Ryan, the *San Francisco Examiner* columnist and author who studied young athletes for her book *Little Girls in Pretty Boxes: The Making and Breaking of Elite Gymnasts and Figure Skaters,* found that these pressure-cooked girls could be emotionally stunted: "Many of these girls had problems expressing emotion, and some had real problems with men. They'd go with domineering, even abusive men, because that's what they'd become used to. And they were very immature socially because their lives were so sheltered. I talked to one girl in her mid-20s who wanted only to date high school boys because she was petrified of guys her own age."[23] And yet while we may be concerned about these kids, and perhaps disapprove of what their parents are allowing them to go through, we don't put our collective foot down to stop it.

The principle that parents in the United States enjoy broad authority to raise their children as they see fit is entrenched in the law and embodied in a long line of Supreme Court cases. "The interest of parents in the care, custody, and control of their children," the Court has declared, is "perhaps the oldest of the fundamental liberty interests recognized by this Court."[24] In 1923, the Court struck down a state law that would have prohibited teaching languages other than English in public schools, an effort by Nebraska to discourage the teaching of German in response to World War I. In the Court's judgment, this would interfere with the right of parents to "bring up children."[25] Two years later, in declaring unconstitutional an Oregon statute that would have required all children to attend public schools, the Court reaffirmed that parents are entitled "to direct the upbringing and education of children under their control."[26] Although in 1944, the Court upheld a state law barring child labor, it once again recognized the fundamental nature of the parental right of control: "It is cardinal with us that the custody, care and nurture of the child reside first in the parents, whose primary function and freedom include preparation for obligations the state can neither supply nor hinder."[27]

Pediatric bioethicist Douglas Diekema offers several reasons for upholding this parental prerogative. Parents can sort out intra-family conflicts over how to raise children. A generous degree of parental discretion is required in order for the family unit to flourish.[28] Most important, a child's parents usually are in the best position to "understand the unique needs of their children, desire what's best for their children, and make decisions that are beneficial to their children." The Supreme Court has picked up on this last theme, stating in 1979 that the law historically has recognized "that natural bonds of affection lead parents to act in the best interests of their children."[29]

Furthermore, the constitutional right of parents to rear their children extends even to exposing the children to known health risks. As the Supreme Court has pointed out, "Simply because the decision of a parent . . . involves risks does not automatically transfer the power to make that decision from the parents to some agency or officer of the state."[30] Judges have upheld parents who refused to consent to corrective surgery for a heart defect; withheld consent to chemotherapy; denied permission for psychotropic drugs to be administered to their children even when the parents no longer had custody; blocked a spinal tap for meningitis on a 5-week-old infant; and donated a child's kidney to a sibling.[31] For four years, the public in Northern Ohio followed the saga of leukemia patient Noah Maxim as his parents successfully fought the state to stop chemotherapy three months into the course of a three-year treatment regimen, even though the treatments were supposedly able to give the boy an 80 percent chance of long-term survival. Believing that the side effects from the chemotherapy were too harsh, the parents instead sought treatment from a doctor specializing in "holistic medicine," who put the boy on a special diet. When the chemotherapy treatments were started, the boy's cancer had been in remission, but four months after they were discontinued, his cancer returned. The parents then put him back on chemotherapy, but by then his chances of survival had dropped, and he died less than four years later.[32]

The right of parents to expose their children to health risks also extends beyond making health care decisions. Parents routinely permit their children to play hazardous sports. At the elite level, the danger can be acute. For example, a 2003 CNN program entitled "Achieving the Perfect 10," reported on nine preteen girls at a Pennsylvania gym who were vying to be selected in a national search to be groomed for the Olympics.[33] These kids practiced six days a week for 50 weeks a year. All were home-schooled. The parents of one 7-year-old kept her going through training by giving her rewards, including hamsters, a cat, and new bedroom furniture. When it came time to compete for the national selection, the 7-year-old completed her routine despite having torn ligaments and an ankle broken in two places. Later in the year she broke her other ankle, which may have cost her a shot at the Olympics. Another child landed on her head during a practice, resulting in what she referred to as "a little bit of a concussion." She competed in the selection contest despite tendonitis, fever, and inflammation of the growth plate in her heel. When asked what her coaches had told her to do about her heel, she replied: "Suck it up." As her coach observed, "The ability to deal with pain separates the champions from the rest." This was reinforced by the gym physician, who explained that "we can't do what we do to the average athlete or a high school athlete, and put them at rest, and let them heal. If we do that, she'll lose her season." Two of the children selected for Olympic grooming after the tryout ended up missing the U.S. championship competition; one broke her hand during practice, and the other broke her leg.

The parents of these gymnasts clearly exposed young children to significant health risks. But parental authority is not unlimited. At the same time that it emphasizes the need to protect parental prerogatives, the Supreme Court recognizes that "a state is not without constitutional control over parental discretion in dealing with children when their physical or mental health is jeopardized."[34] Even when parents claim constitutional protection for their decisions based on the free exercise of religion, the Court is willing to limit their power "if it appears that parental decisions will jeopardize the health or safety of the child, or have a potential for significant social burdens."[35] As the Court put it in a 1944 child labor case, "parents may be free to become martyrs themselves. But it does not follow they are free, in identical circumstances, to make martyrs of their children before they have reached the age of full and legal discretion when they can make that choice for themselves."[36] Courts have intervened when parents failed to obtain treatment for a 5-week-old infant with two broken arms; when a mother exposed a child to second hand cigarette smoke during visitations; and when a Norwegian-born mother tried treating her seriously burned daughter at home with wheat germ oil, Golden Seal, comfrey, myrrh, and cold water rather than taking her to a hospital.[37] A vegan couple was sentenced to life in prison after their 6-week-old baby died of malnutrition after being fed a diet of soy milk and apple juice.[38]

Where the exact boundary lies between martyrdom and permissible risk, however, is not clear. The Supreme Court says that the state should not intervene "so long as a parent adequately cares for his or her children (i.e., is fit)."[39] The California court that ordered the Norwegian-born parent of the burned child to provide proper treatment and take a first aid course noted that the family had an "alternate lifestyle" but that this was not the government's concern "unless that lifestyle places a child at risk for abuse or neglect."[40] Diekema states that "under U.S. law . . . , parents or guardians are generally empowered to make [health care] decisions on their [children's] behalf, and the law has respected those decisions except where they place the child's health, well-being, or life in jeopardy."[41] Diekema similarly approves of state intervention only when the parents fail to provide adequate protection from "justiciable maltreatment," which he defines as treatment that amounts to "abuse and neglect."

"Abuse and neglect" is indeed the prevailing legal standard that defines culpable parental behavior. State abuse-and-neglect laws vary somewhat, but the Ohio statute is representative. It lists a number of specific prohibitions: parents are forbidden to "abuse the child"; "torture or cruelly abuse the child"; "administer corporal punishment or other physical disciplinary measure, or physically restrain the child in a cruel manner or for a prolonged period, which punishment, discipline, or restraint is excessive under the circumstances and creates a substantial risk of serious physical harm to the child"; "repeatedly administer unwarranted disciplinary measures to the child, when there is a substantial risk that such conduct, if continued, will seriously impair or retard the child's mental health or development"; "entice, coerce, permit, encourage, compel, hire, employ, use, or allow the child to act, model, or in any other way participate in, or be photographed for, the production, presentation, dissemination, or advertisement of any material or performance that the offender knows or reasonably should know is obscene, is sexually oriented matter, or is nudity-oriented matter"; allow the child to be on or within 100 feet of premises where illegal drugs are being cultivated or manufactured; or operate an automobile under the influence of drugs or alcohol when a child is in the car.[42] But none of these prohibited acts specifically covers giving a child a biomedical enhancement. The Ohio statute also contains a general provision that forbids parents from creating "a substantial risk to the health or safety of the child, by violating a duty of care, protection, or support." If biomedical enhancements created "a substantial risk" to the child's health or safety, then administering them to one's children would constitute abuse and neglect. But the statute does not define when a risk is "substantial."

Some commentators take an expansive view of governmental intervention, saying that it is called for whenever it is necessary to assure that parents act in their children's "best interests."[43] Others take a more narrow view. Deville and Kopelman argue that there has to be "clear and convincing evidence" that parents' actions or decisions represent "likely and serious harm" to the child.[44] Joel Feinberg would bar parents from substantially interfering with a child's entitlement to physical health and vigor, integrity and normal functioning of one's body, absence of absorbing pain and suffering or grotesque disfigurement, minimal intellectual acuity, and emotional stability.[45] The American Academy of Pediatrics Committee on Bioethics comments that the state should require treatment over parental objections "only when treatment is likely to prevent substantial harm or suffering or death."[46] The California appellate court in the case involving the Norwegian mother agreed with her "that since the parent-child relationship is so important, the state should exercise great care before intervening and the state should not intrude into the relationship merely because it believes a certain kind of care or treatment is preferable." The court added that "it is only when a child's health is actually and seriously threatened that the state should intervene."[47]

In short, from a legal standpoint it seems relatively clear that parents can enhance some of their children's traits at the expense of others, and that they can decide which traits to enhance, even if this appears to serve the parents' own goals rather than the children's. (A separate question is how far parents can go in forcing children to use enhancements against the children's wishes.) It also is plain that parents can provide enhancements to their children that pose some degree of risk to the children's health. Under current laws, state intervention seems to be appropriate only when the children's use of enhancements would amount to parental "abuse"—that is, when they would face a significant risk of substantial harm to health.

It might be supposed that the standpoint of the law is not the correct perspective from which to assess parental conduct and that it should instead be judged by moral standards, even if those standards are not operationalized by the law. But remember that we are talking about when the state (that is, the law) should intervene in the parent-child relationship. The legal perspective is the correct perspective, although we may feel the need to revise the law if we thought that it was morally deficient.

Parents are not the only sources of authority in a child's life, however. Schools might exert pressure to make children use enhancements. Schools are known to pressure parents to give drugs to children—especially boys—to make them more docile in class. A story in the *Washington Post* recounted how the principal of an elite private school told the parents of a fidgety 5-year-old to have him evaluated by a psychologist recommended by the school or else be expelled.[48] Not surprisingly, the psychologist diagnosed the boy as having attention-deficit hyperactive disorder (ADHD) and told the parents he might need Ritalin. The parents were suspicious because the boy had perfect eidetic memory of everything that had ever been read to him and could sit still for hours doing science and art projects. So they obtained a second opinion. The second psychologist told them the boy was too young for a definitive diagnosis of ADHD. Two years later he was found to be dyslexic; he couldn't sit still in school because he couldn't understand written words. A report in the *Wall Street Journal* explains that "teachers, counselors, administrators and even parents have incentives to label—or mislabel—boys who, in prior times, would just be considered overly active, eccentric, dreamy or in need of adult attention. These incentives include a $420 federal bounty for each student labeled 'disabled,' a bonus some think is at least partly responsible for the recent disabilities bulge."[49]

If schools succumb to the lure of $420 to make parents medicate their children for what in truth is often normal behavior, imagine how compelling it would be to medicate pupils to enable them to do better on standardized tests, especially if the test results might trigger financial rewards and penalties for teachers and administrators and ultimately affected the fate of the school itself. Under the federal No Child Left Behind program, for example, a school that accepts program funds but fails to make the necessary progress on standardized tests is subject to progressively harsher punishment. As University of Virginia law professor James Ryan explains,

> After two consecutive years of failure, schools must develop a plan for improvement and are supposed to receive "technical" assistance. Students in those schools are also allowed to choose another public school, including a charter school, within the same district. After three years, students who have not already departed for greener pastures must be provided with tutoring services from an outside provider, public or private. Those schools that fail to make AYP [adequate yearly progress] for four consecutive years must take one of several measures, including replacing school staff or instituting a new curriculum, and those that fail for five years in a row must essentially surrender control to the state government, which can reopen the school as a charter school, turn over management to a private company, or take over the school itself.[50]

A school facing a for-profit or government takeover obviously has a powerful incentive to get its students' test scores up by means that are not necessarily acceptable, including making them take biomedical enhancements.

Workers

Another venue in which people may lack choice about whether or not to use risky enhancements is the workplace. Enhanced performance could benefit an employer in two ways: it could cut down on workplace accidents and injuries, and it could increase the firm's productivity and competitiveness. Consequently, employers may try to insist that employees use them as a condition of getting hired, remaining employed, or being promoted. Even if an employer objected to enhancement use for ethical reasons, it would feel overwhelming pressure from commercial rivals to go with the flow. Indeed, James Canton of the Institute for Global Futures thinks that the use of biomedical enhancements in the workplace is the key to America remaining globally competitive in the future.[51]

Can employers legally require employees to use enhancements? The answer is unclear. Section 5(a)(1) of the Occupational Safety and Health Act, known as "the General Duty Clause," requires employers to "furnish to each of his employees employment and a place of employment which are free from recognized hazards that are causing or are likely to cause death or serious physical harm to his employees." If an enhancement were that dangerous, an employer could not force its employees to use it. But what about less dangerous interventions? Employers have a substantial amount of leeway in imposing requirements on employees that are related to their health. This even extends to off-work behavior. An employee-benefits company in Michigan called Weyco (now part of Meritain Health) prohibited employees from smoking on their own time, and in 2005 fired several workers who refused to submit to random nicotine testing. Employees who test positive are suspended for a month without pay. If they fail a second test, they lose their job. The company even has extended its reach to spouses of employees, subjecting them to monthly nicotine screening. If a spouse tests positive, the employee is fined $80 a month until the spouse takes a smoking cessation course and tests negative.[52] In 1989, according to an organization that monitors workers' rights, an Indiana corporation that bans the use of alcohol by its employees fired one after he admitted that he had had a few drinks in a bar several years earlier.[53] These practices appear to be legal, but some states have reacted by enacting laws prohibiting employment discrimination against smokers and, in some cases, on the basis of any legal off-duty activity.

Employers also can establish wellness programs for employees, including asking them questions about disabilities and giving them medical examinations, so long as employee participation is voluntary. According to the Equal Opportunity Employment Commission, which enforces laws prohibiting workplace discrimination, this means that the employer can neither require participation nor penalize employees for nonparticipation in the program.[54] But an employer can require an employee to participate in wellness programs, including making the employee submit to periodic physical examinations, if the employer can show that the requirements are "job-related and consistent with business necessity." Could enhancements be so essential to job performance that they meet this standard? This too is unclear, because there is no definitive definition of the standard. The desire to prevent injury and improve productivity generally may be sufficient to indicate that enhancement use is consistent with business necessity, but it will be harder for an employer to show that enhancement use is related to the performance of an employee's specific job. An employer could conceivably establish a job requirement that its employees perform at a level that is unattainable without the use of enhancements. This might be permissible so long as the enhancements that the employee had to use were not so dangerous that the employer violated the General Duty Clause of the Occupational Safety and Health Act, mentioned above.

Finally, employers are allowed to control employees' lives to some degree even for reasons unrelated to their health. For example, employers can impose so-called appearance and grooming standards, such as dress codes and rules regarding wearing tattoos and facial hair. The EEOC permits these restrictions so long as they are "adopted for nondiscriminatory reasons, consistently applied to persons of all racial and ethnic groups, and, if the standard has a disparate impact, it must be job-related and consistent with business necessity."[55] In short, so long as an enhancement is relatively safe, there may be nothing in present employment laws that would prevent employers from requiring employees to use it to improve their on-the-job performance. For example, it is conceivable that some employers might be able to mandate the use of caffeine.

The Military

Chapter 1 told the story of the use of alertness drugs by the military, including the unfortunate Air Force pilots who, after taking amphetamines, accidentally dropped a smart bomb on a group of Canadian soldiers in Afghanistan. The military insists that amphetamine use by its members is entirely voluntary and points to an informed consent form that they have to sign. After disclosing that the FDA has not approved Dexedrine to alleviate fatigue, the form states that the drug nevertheless has been found to be effective in treating the symptoms of chronic fatigue and recites the possible side effects and drug interactions. The form then attests that the signer's decision to take Dexedrine is voluntary, adding: "I understand that I am not being required to take the medication. Neither can I be punished if I decide not to take Dexedrine."[56]

So far it would appear that pilots are free to decline the drug without fear of being disciplined. But the form doesn't stop there: "However," it goes on, "should I choose not to take it under circumstances where its use appears indicated, I understand safety considerations may compel my commander, upon the advice of the flight surgeon, to determine whether or not I should be considered unfit to fly a given mission." In other words, use amphetamines on long flights or you'll be grounded. Think about this from the pilot's perspective. You are a military pilot, one who is unlikely to get very many chances to fly combat missions in a world without major conventional conflicts, whose chances for promotion and glory are contingent on flying such missions in the rare event they become available, whose *main goal in life* is to fly those missions, but you can sacrifice all this to avoid popping a pep pill. The pilot's freedom to refuse to use amphetamines under these circumstances is, to say the least, questionable.

In other cases, it isn't so much a question of giving up the one thing you've trained for all your life as disobeying the command of a superior officer. During the Gulf War, it was feared that one of the biological weapons that the Iraqis might use would be the aerosolized version of the anthrax bacterium. The germ spores would have to be "milled" into a tiny size (1 to 3 microns) and coated with an electrostatic powder to prevent them from clumping together and falling to the ground. The result would be an infectious agent that was dispersed in the air, readily inhaled deep into the alveolar sacs of the lungs, and highly lethal. Inhalation anthrax causes overwhelming pulmonary edema and septicemia; the victim dies from a combination of massive blood poisoning and drowning in his own fluids, usually within seven days after exposure.[57] In 1979 the Soviets accidentally released a bunch of aerosolized anthrax spores at a biological warfare facility in Sverdlovsk. Of the 79 people who became ill, 68 died.

To prevent such a bioweapon from decimating our troops, the military initiated a mandatory vaccination program. Many veterans of the conflict claim that as a result, they suffer from a condition known as Gulf War Syndrome. In 1996, a presidential advisory commission concluded that it was unlikely that any health problems that the veterans experienced could be attributed to the anthrax vaccine. Accordingly, in 1998, Secretary of Defense William Cohen ordered all soldiers on active duty to be vaccinated, using a product produced by a new manufacturer, BioPort. When some troops resisted, they were court-martialed.[58]

As described in chapter 1, the Defense Department is heavily invested in the development of biomedical enhancements to improve the performance of its personnel. The fruits of these research programs can be expected to be distributed to the troops in the field as they become available. These soldiers are no more likely to be able to refuse to use them than their predecessors have been able to resist amphetamines and the anthrax vaccine.

Athletes

Athletes may face overwhelming pressure to use biomedical enhancements from sponsoring organizations, teams, coaches, trainers, and fellow athletes. The likelihood that they will be unable to resist this pressure is especially great if they are young and impressionable.

The most notorious example is the East German doping program during the 1970s and 1980s. Begun by Manfred Ewald, the leader of the East German sports federation, it was run by the East German secret police, the Stasi, on behalf of the government.[59] To disguise its true nature, it was called "State Planning Theme 14.25" and referred to biomedical enhancements as "supporting means."[60] It is estimated that as many as ten thousand athletes were given enhancements.[61] Many of them were children. Some of the athletes apparently knew what was happening, especially when their voices deepened or they grew excessive body hair. The athletes in the know kept taking the drugs and competing for "glory, cars, apartments, travel, secure futures."[62]

Most of the East German athletes, however, insist that they were not aware of the doping program. They claim that they were told that the blue pills they were given, "the innocent color of robins' eggs," were vitamins. In fact they were steroids, principally dehydrochlormethyltestosterone, sold under the trade name Oral Turinabol, which was developed and manufactured by a state-owned East German drug manufacturer.[63] "Taking pills was normal, though I had no idea what I was taking," recalls Rita Reinisch, a German Democratic Republic swimmer who won three gold medals at the 1980 Moscow Olympics. "My coach told me, 'That's good for you, it will help your body recover quicker after training,' and I trusted him blindly."[64] Two-time Olympic gold medal figure skater Katarina Witt admits that "you heard rumors as an athlete, but you never asked," adding that "there is an East German mentality where you say, that's just the way it is and you can't do anything about it."[65]

Steroids weren't the only enhancements being used by the East Germans. In 1979, as the Olympics developed better testing methods to detect steroids, the East Germans constructed a hidden underground bunker that simulated high-altitude training by depressurizing to the equivalent of the atmosphere found at thirteen thousand feet above sea level. The two-story chamber contained treadmills, exercise bikes, weight-lifting devices, and rowing practice pools.[66]

The East German strategy worked. In the 1968 Summer Olympics, before their doping program began, East Germany won 25 medals and the United States won 102. In 1976, after the program had been put into effect, East Germany won 90 medals, including 40 gold medals, and despite only having a population of 17 million people, beat out the United States for the first time on both counts. At the 1988 Olympics in Seoul, East German athletes won 102 medals; the United States won only 94.[67] By 1987, most of the top 21 competitor countries had accepted in principle a proposal by Canada's minister to establish an international antidrug charter. One of the main holdouts was East Germany.[68]

The East German experience raises an important philosophical issue: At what point does external pressure become impermissible coercion? Clearly giving steroids to minors and pretending that they are harmless vitamins is abhorrent. So would be threats of violence against an athlete or the athlete's family, which were allegedly made by the East German secret police against recalcitrant competitors and those who might reveal the secret government program.[69] But what about older athletes who knew what they were taking and who consented to do so for "glory, cars, apartments, travel, secure futures"? In their classic *History and Theory of Informed Consent*, Ruth Faden and Tom Beauchamp define *coercion* as occurring when "one party intentionally and successfully influences another by presenting a credible threat of unwanted and avoidable harm so severe that the person is unable to resist acting to avoid it."[70] In their opinion, coercion must be kept distinct from an irresistible offer; while an offer may be manipulative, only the prospect of a decisively *negative* future event can be considered a threat. Hence, according to Faden and Beauchamp, that East German athletes were offered tangible and intangible benefits does not make it coercion. They were still able to make a voluntary decision about whether or not to use steroids.

High-Pressure Situations

The pressure to use enhancements may not come only from other individuals or organizations, such as parents, schools, employers, military superiors, or sports teams. It also may be an internal response to the external environment. Students driven to seek better grades do not need to be prodded by parents or schools. Employers don't have to pressure employees who view enhancements as a means of securing better jobs. A company that sells training materials to teach people how to be effective negotiators, for example, says, "It's like steroids for your career." Soldiers hoping to get promoted or merely to stay alive on the battlefield may decide that the potential benefits of enhancements outweigh even dire health hazards despite not being explicitly ordered to use them. As for athletes, a survey of world-class contenders supposedly found that a sizable majority would take a drug that allowed them to win for five years and then killed them.[71] The story may be apocryphal, but there is no question that many athletes use steroids and other performance-enhancing substances without being urged to do so by coaches or trainers. Given the drive to win, this is no more surprising than the frequency with which injured athletes insist on returning to playing before they are healed. As Penn State professor Charles Yesalis explained to Congress in testimony in 2005, "Philosophically, many in our society appear to have taken a 'bottom-line' attitude and consider winning the only truly worthwhile goal of competition. If we accept this philosophy, then it becomes easy to justify, or be led to the belief, that one should win at any cost. At that point doping becomes a very rational behavior, with the end (winning) justifying the means (use of performance-enhancing drugs and supplements)."[72]

As discussed in the next section, it is likely to be difficult to discourage enhancement use that is internally motivated, as opposed to being forced on people by others. The EEOC can prohibit employers from punishing employees who refuse to use enhancements, but employers don't have to bother; they simply can refrain from interfering with an employee's own decision to get ahead. So long as the employee's increased productivity outweighs any adverse effects that might reduce the employee's value to the firm, such as by making them too sick to work, employers have no incentive to limit the use of enhancements in the workplace.

But maybe we need not worry about people who feel irresistible pressures to use enhancements, so long as they are not actually coerced. The literature on informed consent in medical care takes the position that the only thing that matters in terms of whether or not a patient's informed consent to treatment is voluntary is whether they are subjected to excessive *external* pressure. As Ruth Faden and Tom Beauchamp explain, "In circumstances of severe economic deprivation, a person might accept a job or sign a contract that a person would refuse under less stringent economic circumstances. The prospect of starvation if an objectionable job offer is rejected seems to 'coerce' no less than an intentional threat by an employer or businessman to fire an otherwise unemployable person unless the person agrees to be transferred to an objectionable job. The psychological *effect* on the person forced to choose may be identical." Nevertheless, Faden and Beauchamp insist, "It does not follow . . . that persons in such 'coercive situations' do not act *autonomously*." In Faden and Beauchamp's view, these people still can make voluntary decisions. The same is true, they believe, when a patient who is severely ill feels that she has no choice but to accept a physician's recommended course of treatment: "Natural, environmental, and circumstantial threats, such as those presented by disease, are not in the relevant sense *controlling*." In short, "in a true situation of coercion, what *controls*, and thus deprives one of autonomy, is the will of another person, substituted for one's own will or desire."[73]

The lack of choice presented by a patient's medical condition also is dismissed by the authors of a more recent volume on informed consent: "Being ill brings with it a multitude of pressures, and a patient suffering from a life-threatening disease may feel as though she has little choice regarding treatment. . . . However, consent to treatment under such circumstances should not be considered involuntary."[74]

It is understandable why bioethicists embrace this position. The question of when a choice is truly "free" has baffled philosophers for eons. No rational decision is without a reason. In many instances, the reason may be compelling. Elite athletes, who have trained all their lives for a shot at the Olympics, may feel an enormous compulsion to win, but that does not mean that we should regard their decision to use enhancements as involuntary. Philosopher Robert L. Simon observes: "We need to be careful about applying the notion of coercion too loosely.

After all, no one is forced to try to become a top athlete. The reason for saying top athletes are 'coerced' is that if they don't use performance-enhancing drugs, they may not get what they want. But they still have the choice of settling for less. Indeed, to take another position is to virtually deny the competence of top athletes to give consent in a variety of sports related areas including adoption of training regimens and scheduling. . . . I would suggest that talk of coercion is problematic as long as the athlete has an acceptable alternative to continued participation in a highly competitive sport."[75]

The view that decisions made in high-pressure situations are not voluntary, moreover, risks obliterating the principle of informed consent in medical care. As Faden and Beauchamp observe, "If we concluded that the 'threats' created or introduced by serious illness needing therapy were coercive, we would be forced to conclude that many patients who choose, after thorough deliberation, for or against therapies are not acting autonomously." Simply put, "to reach the conclusion that, as a general rule, substantial autonomy is not possible for persons beset by severe illness would be to eliminate the possibility of informed consent precisely where it is often most important." The alternative to regarding people as able to act freely even in high-pressure situations would be to impose on them someone else's notion of what was best for them. Philosopher W. M. Brown puts it succinctly in the context of athletes: "Ironically, in adopting such a paternalistic stance . . . we must deny in them the very attributes we claim to value: self-reliance, personal achievement, and autonomy."[76]

But some of these bioethicists go too far, or, rather, they sound like they may be forgetting another basic tenet of medical ethics. This tenet, which underlies the doctrine of medical malpractice, states that a physician should not provide a patient with a treatment that is "unreasonable." What is reasonable in turn depends on the patient's condition: a treatment that could cause death might be reasonable if the patient were terminally ill but not if the patient were only suffering from a minor ailment. Accordingly, if a patient makes a risky medical decision that no reasonable person would seem likely to make under the circumstances, we might well question whether the patient was capable of making a rational decision, was being coerced, or was responding to undue pressure. The same approach might apply to populations that would be tempted to use dangerous biomedical enhancements in high-pressure situations. At the point at which it could be said that no reasonable person in that situation would choose to use the enhancements in question, society might be justified in trying to stop them from doing so, although this leaves open the question of what methods society may use.

To summarize the discussion so far, many of the objections to enhancement use for self-satisfaction are unpersuasive. Some are simply impenetrable, such as that enhancements "deform the character of human desire." Other objections rest on false or improbable assumptions, such as that enhancements are unnatural, sinful, or unearned; that the accomplishments they facilitate are not real; or that those who use them are not self-directed. Nevertheless, those who assert these objections are themselves free to refuse to use enhancements and to try to persuade others not to use them. But these objections do not entitle them to make enhancement use for self-satisfaction illegal.

The use of biomedical enhancements to gain a competitive edge raises additional objections. Again, some are unconvincing, such as that enhancement use would be pointless because everyone would do it; that the social rewards that enhancements might engender are undeserved; that enhancement use would confound the comparison of achievement, such as in sports; and that enhancements would violate the "spirit" of competition.

But some of the objections to biomedical enhancements are not so easily dismissed. For example, it might be hard to tell if a given enhancement works, enabling unscrupulous or slipshod entrepreneurs to market unsafe and ineffective products and services to unwitting consumers. Although the health hazards of enhancements are often exaggerated, some enhancements are indeed dangerous, especially when they are obtained on the black market and administered without medical supervision, and especially when used by children. Enhancements may be unaffordable for large segments of society, including those who are the most disadvantaged by their lack of natural talent or luck. Finally, people may be coerced into using risky enhancements or might feel overwhelming pressure to do so by virtue of their circumstances.

Only this last group of concerns justifies some measure of societal control, including measures that substantially curtail personal freedom and economic enterprise. What steps can society legitimately take? How likely are they to succeed, and at what cost?

Chapter 7

Enhancements in Sports

LISTENING TO THE CRITICS, you would think that the use of biomedical enhancement in sports was a recent phenomenon. Before the development of synthetic steroids, you would be led to believe, sports were "natural" and "clean." As we saw in chapter 3, nowhere was this impression created more clearly than during the 2005 congressional hearings on steroid use in major league baseball, where Jim Bunning, Republican senator from Kentucky, was contemptuous of the current career-lengthening practices that players of earlier generations did not have access to. Another witness was North Dakota senator Byron Dorgan. "Tragically," he lamented, "what once was a 'field of dreams' may deteriorate into a quagmire of controlled substances."[1]

But Dorgan's "field of dreams" is a pipe dream. The history of sport is a chronicle of enhancement use. Greek athletes in the third century B.C. are reported to have taken mushrooms to enhance performance.[2] Philostratos describes how Olympic athletes ate bread laced with the juice of opium poppies. Pliny the Younger (61 B.C.–112 A.D.) mentions runners who swallow a decoction made from hippuris, which may be related to ephedrine.[3] Even the World Anti-Doping Agency acknowledges that Greek athletes at the ancient Olympics drank herbal beverages to give them energy.[4] A. J. Higgins, who heads the medical advisory group of the Fédération Equestre Internationale, tells of a first-century B.C. physician and pharmacologist named Pedanius Dioscorides who promoted an infusion of rosemary before exercise and reports that the ancients also used dog and sheep testicles, ginseng, hallucinogenic mushrooms, hemp, opioids, kava, plant seeds, and dried figs. "The swallowing of a stone taken from the stomach of a cockerel that had won a cock fight was said to be popular," Higgins continues, "although eating the cockerel itself in the hope of ingesting some of the bird's high levels of testosterone would probably have been more helpful. This same empirical aim may, at least in part, explain the penchant of some athletes for drinking urine collected from 'strong animals.'"[5] During the late nineteenth century, the substances of choice were narcotics, amphetamines, and various patent preparations.[6] (A number of sources claim that cyclist Arthur Linton died in 1886 from an overdose of a stimulant called trimethyl, and call this the first fatality from doping.[7] In fact, Linton died after winning the Paris-to-Bordeaux race in 1896, and his death was attributed to typhoid.) In a famous incident in 1904, a Stanley Steamer drove alongside Olympic marathoner Thomas Hicks, serving him egg whites, sponges of warm water, French brandy, and strychnine. (Hicks came in first.)[8] After winning the Tour de France in 1924, Henri Pélissier displayed to journalists the cocaine, chloroform, and various pills in his medicine bag.[9] Science journalist Karen Birchard claims that "amphetamines came into their own in the Berlin Olympics of 1936."[10]

From a historical standpoint, in fact, what is striking is not that athletes are using enhancements but that people are objecting to it.[11] There is no record of any objection to athletes' use of biomedical enhancements before the second decade of the twentieth century. Until then, the attitude seems to have been: if something allows you to perform better, go ahead and take advantage of it. And even though the attitude toward doping in sports began to change in the late 1920s, the change was slight, and no effective measures were taken to stop it for the next 40 years.

Only among horseracing enthusiasts was there opposition to doping before the 1920s. By 1912, Britain had made the doping of horses illegal, and all major countries had instituted saliva testing for drugs such as theobromine (a diuretic compound similar to caffeine and found in chocolate), caffeine, cocaine, morphine, and strychnine. When the United States in 1933 legalized parimutuel betting—which determines the amount of the winnings by the amount betted rather than by a system of fixed odds—doping became rampant and included stimulants, heroin, and local anesthetics. According to A. J. Higgins, it was estimated at the time that half of the horses racing in the United States had been given either stimulants or anesthetics.[12] This led to stringent testing standards.

When it came to enhancement by human athletes, the first stirrings of hostility did not appear until 1928, when the International Amateur Athletic Federation declared its opposition to doping in connection with the Amsterdam Olympic games of 1928. By that time, amphetamines had become the primary doping substance, replacing strychnine.[13] In 1933, Paul Rousseau, a member of the French National Olympic Committee, claimed in a statement to the International Olympic Committee (IOC) that doping was a violation of the spirit of the Olympics: "Injections are given and also oxygen inhalations. Are all these actions worthy for true athletes in the most elevated sense of the word? Is this what one has wanted? We do not think so."[14] Rousseau's report triggered an inquiry into doping, but no further action was taken.

In 1937, Lord David Burghley, a member of the British delegation to the IOC, raised the subject of doping again at a meeting in Moscow. Burghley himself had been an Olympic champion, winning the 400-meter hurdles at the 1928 Olympics, and he later served as president of the International Amateur Athletic Federation from 1946 until 1976. (One of his greatest claims to fame was his circumnavigation of the Great Court at Trinity College, Cambridge, during the time it took the Trinity College clock to chime the 12 o'clock hour. This feat was later missattributed to fellow Cambridge student Harold Abrahams in the film *Chariots of Fire*, as a result of which Burghley refused to see the film.) The minutes of the 1937 IOC meeting state that Burghley "gave his colleagues information on the practice, means and effects of doping."[15] A year later, the IOC endorsed a finding in a report from a committee appointed in Warsaw that stated: "The use of drugs or *artificial* stimulants of any kind must be condemned most strongly, and everyone who accepts or offers dope, no matter in what form, should not be allowed to participate in amateur meetings or the Olympic Games."[16] But there was no explanation of how to distinguish a natural from an artificial stimulant, and, more significantly, the IOC made no attempt at enforcement.

During World War II, concerns about doping in sports were shelved in favor of research projects to develop new types of amphetamines for military use and to explore the chemistry and activity of steroids. But the doping issue resurfaced in the 1950s, amid rumors that the Soviets were experimenting with testosterone as a means of improving athletic performance and reports that discarded syringes had been found strewn across locker room floors in the Olympic villages.[17] In 1954, an American physician, John Ziegler, accompanied the U.S. weightlifting team to the World Weightlifting Championships in Vienna. Supposedly, after a few too many glasses of wine, a Soviet team physician admitted to Ziegler that the Russian weightlifters had been given testosterone injections. (Ironically, Ziegler, convinced that he could develop a better oral testosterone derivative, returned to the United States and, in collaboration with the pharmaceutical company Ciba, invented Dianabol, the first anabolic steroid marketed in the United States and the most widely abused steroid of all time.)[18]

During the 1950s, attention also focused on amphetamines. Following a *New York Times* report in 1957 that Olympic and professional swimmers admitted that they were using "pep pills," the American College of Sports Medicine appointed a committee to study amphetamine use among American athletes.[19] Two years later, Henry K. Beecher, a Harvard Medical School professor best known for his work on the ethics of human subjects research, published a study in the *Journal of the American Medical Association* confirming that amphetamines enabled swimmers to beat their personal best times.[20] In 1960, 22-year-old Danish cyclist Knud Jensen collapsed from heatstroke approximately 13 miles from the finish line of the 100-kilometer team road race in the Rome Olympics and later died at the hospital.[21] Subsequently it was discovered that Jensen and two teammates had taken large doses of amphetamines.[22]

European governments and sports organizations slowly began to stir. In 1963, the Council of Europe set up a commission on drugs and doping, but the committee was unable to agree on a definition of doping.[23] In 1965, France and Belgium introduced antidoping laws, and in 1966, the international governing bodies of cycling (the UCI) and soccer (FIFA) introduced testing for athletes in championship competitions.[24]

The IOC, meanwhile, lagged behind. A year after Knud Jensen's death in 1960, it had begun discussions about the problem of doping with the Federation Internationale Medicine-Sportive (FIMS), an organization of sports physicians, and it now commissioned reports, including one in 1965. But not until after another death attributed to amphetamine use occurred in 1967 was the IOC moved to act.

This time, the death was not during the Olympics but rather the Tour de France; British cyclist Tom Simpson collapsed on an incredibly hot day after hours of physical exertion. His official cause of death was listed as "heart failure caused by exhaustion," but Simpson previously had admitted publicly to using amphetamines—likening them to a few extra cups of coffee—and the autopsy report found both amphetamine and methyl-amphetamine in his system.[25] Gradually it became clear that stimulant use was rife among elite cyclists. French cyclist Jacques Anquetil denied that anyone used "dope" but claimed that "stimulants were another thing. Everybody had to be hyped up to maintain the speeds demanded by the public."[26] (By this time, it was also clear that anabolic steroids were in widespread use. By 1968, more than a third of the American track-and-field team was reported to be using them.[27] However, there were no confirmed reports of deaths from steroids.)

The IOC decided that it could no longer content itself merely with uttering antidoping platitudes. It formed an Olympic Medical Commission, which promulgated a list of banned substances, and athletes were tested for the first time at the 1968 Summer Games in Mexico City. The initial list included only narcotics and analgesics, because those were the only substances that could be detected by available tests.[28] Thus began the cat-and-mouse game that has persisted ever since. A new doping substance is spotted or suspected, but there is no way to test athletes to determine if they have used it. Laboratories affiliated with the antidoping campaign eventually develop a test, and the substance is added to the prohibited list. Before long, a new substance turns up, and the process starts over. Erythropoietin, which increases the supply of oxygen to the tissues, was first synthesized in 1979, and athletes were believed to have begun using it in the early 1990s. But a valid and reliable test was not developed until 2000.[29] The first test for anabolic steroids wasn't available until 1976, almost 20 years after they first became commercially available in the United States.[30] Antidoping scientists not only have to keep up with doping methods but also must develop methods to detect substances that block tests from detecting doping substances. In 1985, the IOC prohibited the manipulation of urine samples, and it added probenecid and other masking agents to the prohibited list two years later. Chorionic gonadotropin, which reverses the testicular shrinking that is a telltale of anabolic steroid use, was added to the list in 1987.[31]

Despite its efforts, the IOC's record in catching athletes who doped remained poor. Although the East Germans' systematic doping program was in full swing at the time, no athletes tested positive at the Moscow Games in 1980.[32] From 1976 until 1994, only a dozen or so athletes tested positive for enhancement substances in any Olympic games, and in several Olympics there were no positive test results at all.[33] The perception began to grow that the IOC wasn't serious about stopping doping. A glaring example was the IOC's lax response to accusations that Chinese swimmers were using enhancement substances during the 1990s. Neither the IOC nor the international governing organization for swimming, FINA, acknowledged that anything untoward was taking place, and when Chinese swimmer Yuan Yuan was caught with 13 vials of human growth hormone (HGH) at the 1998 world championships in Perth, Australia, enough for the entire Chinese swimming team, only she was sanctioned.[34] Speculation had it that this was connected to the fact that China had nominated the president of the IOC, Juan Samaranch, for the Nobel Peace Prize in 1993.

Matters came to a head in 1998, when the Tour de France was discovered to be riddled with doping. An entire team, Italy's Festina, was disqualified. After Samaranch caused an outcry by telling a journalist that he thought the antidoping program was too strict, in that some of the substances that athletes were using were not particularly dangerous, the IOC held an emergency meeting and decided that it needed to take itself out of the front lines of the antidoping campaign.[35] In 1999, a new organization based in Lausanne, Switzerland, the World Anti-Doping Agency (WADA), was born. WADA is governed by a committee comprised of equal numbers of representatives from the IOC and world governments, with the latter participating on the basis of two international legal instruments, the International Convention against Doping in Sport and the Copenhagen Declaration. WADA is responsible for issuing and enforcing the World Anti-Doping Code, first applied at the 2000 Sydney Olympics, as well as the List of Prohibited Substances and Methods. WADA also certifies testing laboratories and funds antidoping research.

A similar series of events took place in the United States. Before 2000, the U.S. antidoping program was administered by the U.S. Olympic Committee. But, like the IOC, the USOC was criticized for not being serious enough about punishing doping. A USOC committee therefore recommended that an independent antidoping organization be established, and on October 1, 2000, the U.S. Anti-Doping Agency (USADA) came into existence. Like WADA, USADA conducts antidoping testing and research as well as administering the process of adjudicating charges against athletes. The organization is controlled by a ten-member board presently comprised of four physicians, a sports lawyer, a swim coach, four former Olympic athletes, and the former drug czar for the state of California.[36] In 2005, it conducted 8,175 tests and imposed sanctions on 20 athletes.[37]

WADA's authority extends well beyond the Olympics. For example, it regulates the Paralympics. In 2003, Chuck Lear, a paralympic archer who had lost a leg and arm in Vietnam, received a public warning for testing positive for the banned substance metoprolol. In 2004, wheelchair basketball player Paul Hill was banned from competing for two years for using the steroids 19-norandrosterone and 19-noretiocholanolone, and in April 2006, wheelchair basketball player Jermell Pennie was suspended for two years for using formestane, a treatment for postmenopausal breast cancer that reduces the production of estrogen.[38] (This is helpful to athletes who take anabolic steroids because elevated levels of male hormones like testosterone also cause elevated levels of the female hormone estrogen, which leads to gynecomastia, or growth of breast glands, increased fat deposits, and higher water retention.) During the 2004 Paralympic Games in Athens, an Estonian powerlifter was disqualified for using a diuretic agent; two powerlifters forfeited bronze metals after testing positive for steroids; and a visually impaired tandem cyclist lost his silver medal after his "pilot" tested positive for a glucocorticosteroid, an anti-inflammatory agent believed to enhance endurance.[39]

WADA also oversees the antidoping programs for the Commonwealth Games, the World Cup, Wimbledon, the French Open, the Australian Open, the U.S. Open, the Davis Cup, the Tour de France, the U.S. Tennis Association, the International Association of Athletics Federations (track-and-field), the International Basketball Federation, the International Gymnastics Federation, the International Hockey Federation, the International Triathlon Union, the International Swimming Federation, the International Table Tennis Federation, the World Taekwondo Federation, the World Bridge Federation, and the International Chess Federation.

That's right: bridge and chess. Both games hope to become recognized as Olympic events, and therefore their international governing bodies have embraced the Olympic antidoping program. The Spanish Chess Federation began an antidoping program in 1999, banning, among other things, the excessive use of caffeine.[40] In 2003, all international chess competitions subjected themselves to WADA, and antidoping testing was conducted when chess was played for the first time in the 2006 Asian Games.[41] Meanwhile, the World Bridge Federation implemented random drug testing at the 2000 world championships, and Disa Eythorsdottir was stripped of a silver medal for refusing to take a drug test at the world open bridge championships in Montreal in 2002.[42]

Typically, WADA tests the four highest-ranked athletes in a sport, plus other competitors chosen at random.[43] This amounted to 2,941 out-of-competition tests worldwide in 2006, yielding 57 adverse findings.[44] The test samples (blood or urine) usually are separated into two parts, vial A and vial B. If the A sample tests positive for a banned substance, the athlete may request an additional test on the B sample. Penalties for a first doping offense range from a warning to suspension from competition for a minimum of two years. Penalties for other offenses, such as a second instance of doping, use of a masking agent, refusing to undergo a drug test, or contaminating the results, can result in further fines of up to $100,000 or even a possible lifetime suspension.[45]

Given the high stakes for the athletes, who typically have invested many years to reach these elite levels of competition, it is not surprising that the WADA system has its detractors. After examining 250 cases in which competitors were penalized, *Los Angeles Times* Pulitzer Prize–winning reporter Michael Hiltzik complained in 2006 that WADA "imposes severe punishments for accidental or technical infractions, relies at times on disputed scientific evidence and resists outside scrutiny." Moreover, says Hiltzik, "elite athletes have been barred from the Olympics, forced to relinquish medals, titles or prize money and confronted with potentially career-ending suspensions after testing positive for a banned substance at such low concentrations it could have no detectable effect on performance."[46] Hiltzik cites several cases as examples. Alain Baxter, the first British Alpine skier to win an Olympic medal (placing third in the slalom at the 2002 Winter Games in Salt Lake City), was stripped of his medal after he tested positive for methamphetamine. It turned out that he had used a Vicks Vapor Inhaler to treat his chronic nasal congestion, just as he had back in Britain. But he bought the inhaler in Utah, and the U.S. product, unlike the British version, contained traces of a chemical structurally related to methamphetamine but without the stimulant effect. Nevertheless, the WADA arbitration panel let his conviction stand. In another case, the mother of a 17-year-old Italian swimmer bought an antibiotic cream to treat her daughter's foot infection, not realizing that the ingredients included a banned steroid. The daughter failed a urine test in 2004 after applying the cream between her toes. Although the arbitrators agreed that the cream had had no effect on her performance, they nevertheless suspended her for one year. A third case involved U.S. skeleton racer Zach Lund, who was banned from the 2006 Winter Games in Turin after testing positive for finasteride, a substance believed to be able to mask the use of steroids. The finasteride was an ingredient in the baldness remedy Propecia, which Lund had been using for several years. (Although Hiltzik did not mention it, there also was the case mentioned in chapter 3 of Andrea Raducan, the Romanian gymnast who lost her gold medal at the Sydney Olympics after testing positive for pseudoephedrine, an ingredient in nonprescription tablets she had taken for a cold.)

Hiltzik objects to a number of specific aspects of the WADA process. He does not think that athletes should be punished for inadvertently using tiny amounts of banned substances. And he views the entire system as biased against accused athletes. Cases are resolved by arbitration, and in many countries, including the United States, athletes do not have a right to obtain a judicial review of the arbitrators' decision. Hiltzik points out that "in the vast majority of cases, including every case heard in the U.S., the arbitrators have upheld the violation." Moreover, only WADA-certified laboratories can conduct doping tests, so athletes cannot have tests repeated at independent labs. Added to this are rules prohibiting WADA labs from performing tests in defense of an accused athlete and from allowing its experts to testify on behalf of an athlete in a doping case or in any other way criticizing the science behind any WADA test procedures.

Hiltzik has been vigorously attacked by Richard Pound, the former Olympic swimmer who was WADA's first chairman, for opposing penalties for trace amounts of substances taken inadvertently, WADA's so-called strict liability standard. "If you didn't know what was in there," said Pound, "it's your own damn fault."[47] But WADA's stance finally is changing a little. Numerous national Olympic organizations have criticized the strict liability standard, urging WADA to stop sanctioning athletes for trivial or accidental exposures. WADA wants to reclassify certain substances, mainly stimulants, so that a positive test result would not necessarily lead to a harsh penalty.[48] At the same time, however, WADA is proposing to increase the penalties for intentional doping, and Marion Jones's 2007 confession that she used steroids after all will strengthen the hand of the antidoping forces.

In the United States, college and professional sports are not under WADA's purview; instead they operate their own antidoping programs. The 1,200 institutions that belong to the National Collegiate Athletic Association require students to consent to be tested as a condition for participating in varsity sports. After being raked over the coals in congressional hearings, Major League Baseball began random testing of players for steroids in 2003. The National Football League, the National Basketball Association, and NASCAR have their own programs.[49] The PGA Tour announced that it will commence testing golfers in 2008.[50]

Numerous other sports and games perform drug testing. In 2001, the Australian Cricket Board banned a player for two years for using steroids. The British Darts Regulation Authority suspended a player for 58 days for testing positive for marijuana.[51] American school children also are being tested.

Although we now have a sense of the chronology and structure of the modern antidoping movement, we have not determined what gives it its strength, what sustains its momentum. Clearly many people are concerned about what they perceive to be the health risks of the enhancements used in sports, and many view the use of enhancements as unethical even if it is not prohibited by the rules of the game. But as we saw in chapter 3, the health risks tend to be greatly exaggerated by antidoping crusaders, and there is no convincing reason why the use of biomedical enhancements is inherently unethical. We see that the IOC began to test athletes in 1968 after an amphetamine-associated death in the Tour de France. But why did the IOC act then and not earlier? After all, there had been an amphetamine-related death at the Olympic Games themselves in 1960. Reports of widespread doping in cycling and disenchantment with Juan Samaranch propelled the IOC to create WADA in 1999. But why was it only then that the sports world began to take serious action, when Lord Burghley was sounding the alarm way back in 1937? And what continues to fuel rabid antidoping sentiment, like this rant from *Chicago Sun-Times* sports columnist Jay Mariotti: "Do you like being ripped off and bamboozled by those you entrust with your daily entertainment? Didn't think so. So where is the outrage among the paying customers, the consumers directly affected? Where are the demands for reform? Congress cares. Anti-doping crusaders such as Dick Pound care. Do you care?"[52] Finally, why did George W. Bush feel it necessary to take time out of his second State of the Union message to urge the country to "get tough, and to get rid of steroids now"?[53]

To explain what is happening, the current antidoping crusade must be placed in a broader historical context. The first thing to realize is that the antidoping war is part of the larger War on Drugs. The first rumblings about the use of biomedical enhancements occurred around the same time that the first U.S. drug abuse laws were being enacted in the early twentieth century. Fueled by prejudice against Chinese immigrants, the puritanical streak of the Progressive movement, and the economic self-interest of physicians in blocking sales of opiate-containing patent medicines by pharmacists, Congress passed the Harrison Act, restricting the sale of narcotics, and the Volstead Act, prohibiting the sale of alcoholic beverages.[54] Other substance control laws followed: the Narcotic Drug Import/Export Act in 1922, which increased penalties for drug violations and further restricted the importation of opium and coca, and the Heroin Act of 1924, which made the domestic manufacture and possession of heroin illegal.[55]

Nor is it a coincidence that the Olympic drug testing program began in 1968, the same year that Richard Nixon became president with a pledge to suppress the youth-oriented drug culture. The antidoping war in fact can be seen as an extension of the culture clash between "jocks" and "hippies" that started during the 1960s, immortalized in films such as *Animal House*. Nothing threatened the "straight," patriotic, all-American athlete like the prospect of sports being infiltrated and overrun by drug-crazed "freaks." This also may help explain why antidoping bans are so arbitrary—permitting some forms of enhancement such as improved equipment and dietary modification but not others—because many of the same college athletes who taunted the hippies for smoking pot and taking LSD thought nothing about drinking themselves into oblivion every chance they got.

The link between the war against doping and the War on Drugs is plain today in the fact that sports tests not only for performance-enhancing substances, but also for recreational drugs. British Olympic gold medalist Mark Lewis-Francis lost his silver medal from the 2005 European Indoor Track-and-Field Championships, for example, after he tested positive for marijuana. A runner with a positive marijuana test was disqualified from the U.S. 400-meter relay team at the Athens Olympics. After testing positive for THC (the active ingredient in pot), Canadian snowboarder Ross Rebagliati lost his gold medal in snowboarding at the 1998 Nagano Olympics. (It later was restored to him after arbitrators ruled that the IOC did not have a formal agreement with the International Ski Federation to ban the substance.)[56]

The war against doping also was the wedge that the conservatives on the U.S. Supreme Court used to pry open the Constitution's protections against unreasonable search and seizure in order to uphold random recreational drug testing of school children. The Court's slide into this constitutional cesspool began in 1991, when James Acton, a seventh-grader at the Washington Grade School in the tiny logging town of Vernonia, Oregon, decided he wanted to play football. To his and his parents' surprise, he was told that he could do so only if he underwent drug testing. He would be tested at the beginning of the season and at random times thereafter. Upon being notified that a test was taking place, James would have to produce a urine specimen at a urinal in the presence of an adult monitor, who would watch and listen for the normal sounds of urination. (Girls were allowed to use a closed stall while the monitor listened outside, then checked to see that the sample was at body temperature.) The striking fact was that the tests were not for steroids and other performance-enhancing drugs but for marijuana and cocaine. (The school also tested for amphetamines, which are used for performance enhancement, but which were targeted by the school because of their recreational use.)

James and his parents sued the school district to block the testing program. In previous cases, they argued, the United States Supreme Court had made it clear that government entities, including public schools, could not conduct random drug testing. A federal court of appeals sided with the parents, but the Supreme Court disagreed, holding that random testing was permissible so long as the students who were tested were athletes.[57]

How did the fact that the students being tested played sports justify testing them for non-performance-enhancing drugs? According to the six justices who joined in the majority opinion, the testing was necessary to ensure the safety of student athletes, because "the risk of immediate physical harm to the drug user or those with whom he is playing his sport is particularly high." The justices were concerned that illicit drugs could impair the students' judgment, slow their reaction time, and lessen the perception of pain. They also asserted that the drugs being tested for were particularly dangerous when used during exercise. Citing a single article, the Court claimed that marijuana, as well as amphetamines and cocaine, created significant cardiovascular risks during exercise. The majority also expressed the concern that student athletes were role models for other students and could therefore induce other students to use illegal drugs. Yet in a dissent in which she was joined by Stevens and Souter, Justice Ginsburg argued convincingly that rationalizing the testing by invoking the dangers of recreational drugs during school athletics was nonsense. School officials had instituted suspicionless drug testing because of a perceived recreational drug problem at the school, not because of any drug-related sports injuries, and the real reason that they had proposed to test only student athletes was that they thought (correctly, it turned out) that this would help the testing program pass constitutional muster. Sure enough, in 2002, the Court abandoned all pretense of linking drug tests to school sports and upheld suspicionless drug testing for all children involved in any extracurricular activity.[58]

WADA's inclusion of tests for marijuana has provoked strong opposition from other antidoping bodies. The British minister for sport, for example, objected that, because WADA was not in the business of "policing society," "social drugs" that do not enhance performance should be removed from WADA's list of prohibited substances.[59] WADA's chairman Dick Pound responded: "Who's to say that by taking cannabis in a sport like gymnastics, where there is a fear element, you are not giving yourself an advantage by being more relaxed?"[60] Pound later conceded that he couldn't think of a sport in which marijuana would improve performance.[61] But marijuana had to remain on the WADA list, explained Pound, to avoid upsetting the U.S. government, which contributes more than any other country to WADA's budget, and whose deputy director of national drug control policy at the White House sits on WADA's board.

The second historical phenomenon that has given the antidoping movement its strength is the Cold War. International sports competitions, and the Olympics in particular, often reflect ideological rivalries and serve national political objectives. The 1936 Berlin Olympics were orchestrated by Adolf Hitler to showcase the Nazi worldview, and African-American Jesse Owens's four gold medals were seen by many as a blunt refutation of German racial stereotyping. A few weeks after the Russians crushed the Hungarian uprising in 1956, the two countries literally slugged it out at the Melbourne Olympics in a game of water polo. In what became known as the "Blood in the Water" match, the Hungarians were awarded the victory when the judges stopped the game after the Russian captain punched a Hungarian player in the eye. (After going on to win the gold medal, half the Hungarian water polo team defected to the West.) Then there was the breathtaking U.S. defeat of the Soviet ice hockey team at the 1980 Winter Games at Lake Placid. For the United States, this had been a winter of deep discontent. The Iranians were still holding 52 American hostages, and a month earlier, the Soviets had invaded Afghanistan. No one expected the American team to do well, but it fooled everyone, bested the Russians, and went on to beat Finland for the gold medal. After ABC sportscaster Al Michaels ticked off the final seconds of the U.S.-Russian game with the words: "Eleven seconds, you got ten seconds, the countdown going on right now . . . Morrow up to Silk . . . five seconds left in the game! Do you believe in miracles? Yes!" the incident became known as the "Miracle on Ice."

The Cold War permeated not only sports but also the campaign against doping. Opposition to steroids was in part a response by the West to the success of Warsaw Pact doping programs in winning Olympic medals. Nationalism and anticommunism also help explain the vigor of the attacks on China following revelations at the 1998 World Swimming Championships of widespread doping among members of its swim team. In effect, China has replaced East Germany as the target of Western condemnation of state-sponsored doping. As one sports anthropologist observed, "When China became a 'world sports power,' American journalists found it all too easy to slip China into the slot of the 'Big Red Machine' formerly occupied by Eastern Bloc sports teams."[62]

The war against doping undoubtedly also is stimulated by a fear of new biomedical technologies and their infiltration into new spheres of human activity. Medical advances produce unease as well as awe. We marvel at the artificial tissues, joints, and organs developed by biomedical engineers, but we worry about where to draw the line between the "human" and the "robotic." New reproductive technologies like surrogate wombs, in vitro fertilization, and preimplantation genetic diagnosis can reduce the frequency of birth defects and allow infertile couples to have children, but we fret over whether they will replace old-fashioned sex. We hear claims that our growing skill at tinkering with DNA may enable us to reverse the aging process, but our hope at the prospect of postponing death is mixed with trepidation about the impact on the family and the workforce. Transhumanists offer us a vision of a posthuman utopia, but Cassandras like Michael Crichton warn us about genetic monstrosities and nanotechnology run amok.

The nostalgia manifested by opponents of doping likewise is in part resistance to the "brave new world" of modern science. One can hardly open the sports pages without hearing about new enhancement techniques. The Balco investigation introduced us to "designer" steroids. The 2008 WADA list of prohibited substances includes for the first time "selective androgen receptor modulators" and "myostatin inhibitors."[63] WADA is still unsure about whether or not to ban the use of "nitrogen houses." Sportswriter Steve Kelley naïvely laments that "the great professional athletes of the 1960s and '70s certainly were genetically endowed, but their performances, their statistics, their greatest moments weren't artificially enhanced." The old-fashioned amphetamines, steroids, and blood transfusions of yore have been joined by beta blockers and recombinant DNA-manufactured synthetic hormones.[64]

Finally, doping produces a feeling of visceral distaste in some people, an emotional reaction that bioethicist Leon Kass and others call the "yuck factor." As we have seen, Kass places great stock in the ability of this aesthetic/moral sixth sense to identify inappropriate behavior, as he explains in an article in *The New Republic*: "In crucial cases . . . repugnance is the emotional expression of deep wisdom, beyond reason's power to fully articulate it."[65] The initial crackdown on steroids, for example, was motivated in part by the ugly images of syringes littering locker room floors. The East German doping program was vilified not only because of the damage it caused athletes' health and its role in the Cold War but also because of the unsightly, masculine appearance of the East German female athletes. Charlie Francis, the Canadian running coach, relates how one evening "I spied two of the G.D.R.'s female throwers on their way to the cafeteria for dinner. They were gotten up in frilly dresses with matching purses, and were perched on improbably flimsy heels. In between the dresses and the shoes, one was reminded of why these women were here: their calves were like tree trunks, their Achilles tendons like bridge cables. A childhood memory flashed before me: dancing hippos from *Fantasia*."[66] In response to a complaint by an

American swimmer at the 1976 Olympics that the East German women had "manly frames and deep voices," an East German official responded that they "came to swim, not to sing."[67]

The link to the Cold War and the War on Drugs, the fear of being at the mercy of powerful new technologies, and the revulsion engendered by some of the effects of doping certainly go a long way toward explaining the vigor of the antidoping movement. But they are explanations, not justifications. The War on Drugs is no less a social disaster as its predecessor, Prohibition. It has wasted billions of dollars, jammed millions of people into overcrowded and ineffective jail systems, provided an excuse for violating civil liberties, and taught generations of youths to flaunt the law. Modeling a war against doping on the War on Drugs is like encouraging modern shipyards to mass-produce Titanics. The other factors are likewise weak rationales for banning biomedical enhancements in sports. Fear of the future also is no excuse for repeating the mistakes of the past. Liberal societies must be wary of punishing their citizens because they offend other citizens' aesthetic sensibilities; this is permissible, if at all, only under exceptional circumstances, and it is dubious that doping in sports qualifies. And finally, the Cold War is over.

But here's the important thing: the lack of a strong ethical or policy rationale for opposing doping in sports, the sense that a ban on doping is arbitrary, is perfectly OK. The rules of sport *can* be arbitrary. Why else are there nine players on a baseball field rather than eight, and batters get only three strikes instead of four? The first rules for basketball apparently called for nine players on a team because the originator of the game happened to have 18 players handy. Occasionally there is a rebellion against the arbitrariness of the rules; as mentioned earlier, WADA is in the process of relaxing its antidoping rules to reduce the penalties for athletes who inadvertently use small amounts of banned stimulants, such as those found in over-the-counter cold medicines.[68] But for the most part, participants and fans don't care that the rules are arbitrary so long as the game is played according to the arbitrary rules that everyone is used to.

In short, a sport is entitled to adopt pretty much any rules it wishes. Of course there are limits to what can be permitted. The rules may not call for behaviors that violate provisions of the law that govern society in general outside of sports. A sport cannot discriminate on the basis of race, religion, or national origin. Nor can it require athletes to kill each other. But otherwise, a sport is free to stipulate how it must be played, no matter how arbitrary: with one hand tied behind your back, standing on your head, blindfolded. Some nostalgia buffs, for example, enjoy shooting at targets with black powder muskets of the type used in the Civil War. They are perfectly entitled to do so as well as to insist that anyone who wants to compete in their events must restrict themselves to the same equipment.

The problem comes when the advocates of a particular set of rules in sports come to believe that their rules are not only not arbitrary but also *morally correct*; for example, when they think that there is something wrong about using a modern rifle, even outside a "black powder" match. This attitude was illustrated by the president of the Federal Republic of Germany, when he told the West German National Olympic Committee that "we can already see on the horizon the danger that specific athletic types will be bred by means of more or less concealed chemical or even genetic manipulation. . . . In the long run, [sport] will master this situation only if it recognizes it as an existential issue rooted in moral premises."[69] This air of moral superiority is also reflected in an editorial in the journal of the Royal Institute of Philosophy, which asks: "Do not most of us feel that there would be something tarnished and corrupt about a sport where ultimate success depends on the use of drugs? Is there not a tinge of special pleading about calling dedicated fitness training artificial in the same way as injecting extra testosterone? . . . And is there not something right about the deep-rooted intuition that the achievement of even the most highly coached and fanatically fit athlete is real in a way a drug induced performance is not . . . ?" The essay concludes that "the real challenge is to articulate and elaborate the anti-drugs case so as to reveal the pro-drugs arguments for the sophistries they are."[70]

Yet even the tendency to confuse arbitrary rules with moral imperatives would not be a serious problem if sports merely went about enforcing the rules on its own. The real problem arises when doping opponents enlist the aid of the government to enforce rules that are arbitrary, that is to say, when the government makes the violation of arbitrary rules a crime.

In the United States, at least, this may be unconstitutional. As the Supreme Court emphatically proclaims: "Over and over again we have stressed that 'the nature and the theory of our institutions of government, the principles upon which they are supposed to rest . . . do not mean to leave room for the play and action of purely personal and arbitrary power' . . . and that the essence of due process is 'the protection of the individual against arbitrary action.'"[71] There are only three circumstances in which the government can enforce arbitrary rules, and none of them apply here. One is when the government creates what is known as an "irrebuttable presumption" to avoid incurring enormous administrative costs. The prime example is age limits on activities like driving, drinking, and voting. The age cutoffs are admittedly arbitrary: there are undoubtedly teenagers who are mature enough to engage in these activities before they reach the minimum age (and certainly there are adults who can't handle alcohol, shouldn't be behind the wheel, and cannot make an informed choice among the candidates on a ballot). It would be fairer, therefore, if teens were allowed to try to prove that they should be allowed to drink, drive, or vote through some sort of hearing process rather than be subject to a blanket approach. But the Supreme Court has upheld the use of irrebuttable presumptions like these because the cost of holding individualized hearings would be prohibitive. This rationale obviously does not apply to the rules against doping, however, because the testing programs increase rather than decrease administrative costs.

Arbitrary action by the government also is permissible when the government wants to attack a problem but does not have the resources to attack all of it. When a traffic cop stops you to give you a ticket for speeding, for example, you won't get anywhere by complaining that lots of other people were speeding as well. This exception also does not fit the antidoping campaign. Presumably you did deserve to get a ticket. But the antidoping campaign arbitrarily punishes people for doing things for which they should not be punished. If anything, it tickets too many "drivers," not too few.

Finally, the government can apportion benefits and burdens by methods that are arbitrary. As we saw in chapter 3, courts have approved the use of lotteries for deciding which people in an overcrowded lifeboat should be kept alive and which should drown. Lotteries also are used to determine who should be drafted into the military. A lottery is completely arbitrary; no one wins (or loses) because they deserve to. But the reason the rules against doping are arbitrary is not because there is no better way to distribute benefits and burdens.

Nevertheless, antidoping advocates enlist the aid of the government in making the use of biomedical enhancements illegal whenever they can. For the most part, the federal government stayed out of Olympic sports until 1978, when Congress passed the Ted Stevens Olympic and Amateur Sports Act.[72] Even then, all Congress did was to establish and charter the U.S. Olympic Committee and require the creation of national governing bodies for each Olympic sport. Far from asserting government control, the act granted the USOC exclusive authority over "all matters pertaining to United States participation in the Olympic Games."[73]

Beginning in the late 1980s, however, the use of drugs in sports, and steroids in particular, began to attract Congress's attention. Before 1988, steroids were regulated like any other prescription drugs by the Food and Drug Administration. But in 1988, Congress passed the Anti-Drug Abuse Act, which amended the food and drug laws to make it a felony to distribute steroids for nonmedical purposes.[74] The crime was punishable by up to three years in prison and by up to six years if it involved a minor. In 1990, Congress enacted the Crime Control Act of 1990, which categorized steroids as a "schedule III" controlled substance, placing them under the jurisdiction of the Drug Enforcement Administration (DEA).[75] Legislators had sought first to designate steroids as a Schedule II controlled substance, the class reserved for the most dangerous drugs that have some legitimate medical use, such as cocaine and morphine. But the congressmen desisted after one pointed out that, under schedule II, adolescents who shared steroids with each other, and who therefore would be guilty of "distributing," could be sentenced to up to 20 years in prison. (The House of Representatives also had wanted to include a penalty of up to two years in prison for personal trainers and coaches who "attempted to induce or persuade athletes to use or possess anabolic steroids," with the prison term increasing to up to five years if the athlete was a minor, but this provision was dropped before President George H. W. Bush signed the bill into law.)

Yet even a schedule III classification for steroids is dubious under the Controlled Substances Act. That act requires that substances placed in schedule III, in addition to having a potential for abuse (albeit less than substances in schedules I and II) and a currently accepted medical use, must also be shown to lead to moderate or low physical dependence or high psychological dependence.[76] According to a report by the U.S. Sentencing Commission, which is charged with reviewing the enforcement of the antisteroid laws, Congress thought that steroids met the last requirement because "many medical and public health experts concluded that steroids can lead to psychological addiction, and a small number of studies indicated that steroid abuse leads to physical dependence." But the Commission reported that "information provided by DEA, reflecting then current knowledge, indicated that steroids were not physically or psychologically addicting."[77]

The legal significance of Congress's placing steroids under the Controlled Substances Act cannot be overstated. The Federal Food, Drug, and Cosmetic Act, the law enforced by the FDA under which steroids had been regulated before 1990, punished only the *distribution* of steroids for a nonmedical use. But the Controlled Substances Act also punishes *possession*. This still doesn't go far enough for governmental action to be capable of dealing with the doping problem in sports, because athletes must be prevented not only from possessing prohibited substances but also from *using* them in such a way as to improve their performance. Under the Controlled Substances Act, the government could not convict someone merely for testing positive for having a controlled substance in his or her system. In 2003, Senator John McCain introduced a bill that would have directed the National Institute of Standards and Technology to establish a program actually to detect illegal steroids in athletes, but the bill did not pass.[78]

But Congress wasn't finished. In June 2003, a track coach named Trevor Graham sent a syringe containing an unknown chemical to the U.S. Anti-Doping Agency, which in turn sent it to the premier Olympic testing lab run by Don Caitlin at UCLA. The substance turned out to be tetrahydrogestrinone or THG, a steroid that had been developed expressly to defeat antidoping tests by being detectable in the body for only a short time and destroyed by standard detection tests. The syringe in turn was traced to a Burlingame, California, dietary supplement manufacturer, BALCO, which was associated with a group of athletes who were rivals of the ones that Graham coached. In February 2004 four men were indicted on charges of illegally distributing steroids and other performance-enhancing drugs to athletes and making a concerted effort to conceal the distribution by using code words to refer to the drugs in communications with athletes. The indictments named not only two BALCO executives but also the personal trainer for baseball player Barry Bonds and a prominent coach of several Olympic track-and-field athletes.[79]

The BALCO case revealed that the sports world had been infiltrated by so-called designer steroids—drugs specially produced so as to be undetectable by current tests. It grabbed the attention of President Bush, who, as noted earlier, had challenged the country "to get tough, and to get rid of steroids now" in his second State of the Union address.[80] And it persuaded Congress to amend the Controlled Substances Act to crack down on designer steroids. The Steroid Control Act of 2004 added 26 specific steroids to schedule III.[81] It also eliminated a requirement in the 1990 law that the DEA had to prove that a steroid compound was anabolic (that is, actually promoted muscle growth) before the compound could be listed in schedule III. This had hamstrung the DEA because there was no accepted test method to establish this.

But let's go back to the 1990 legislation. At the time, Congress had taken aim not only at steroids but also at another drug that athletes were using to enhance performance, human growth hormone. And what Congress had done here was truly extraordinary. After moving steroids from the jurisdiction of the Federal Food, Drug, and Cosmetic Act to the Controlled Substances Act by placing them in schedule III, Congress substituted HGH in the provision of the Federal Food, Drug, and Cosmetic Act that had applied to steroids. But it made a subtle but far-reaching change in the language of that provision. To appreciate what happened, one must understand the way in which the FDA regulates drugs.

A manufacturer who wants to obtain FDA approval for a drug must identify one or more medical uses for the drug, called "indications," and must submit the results of large-scale studies in humans that convince the FDA that the drug is safe and effective for those specific uses. Once the FDA approves the drug, the manufacturer is permitted to market the drug, that is, to advertise it and have the company's sales force extol its virtues to health care practitioners, but only for the specific indications that were approved. However, a physician (or other practitioner who is allowed to prescribe drugs, such as physician assistants and nurse practitioners in many states) retains the legal authority to prescribe the drug to a patient for any purpose that the practitioner deems appropriate, even though the drug has not been tested or approved for that indication. This is known as "off-label" or "unapproved use" prescribing, and the physician's authority to engage in the practice dates back to the beginning of the federal regulation of the pharmaceutical industry, when the American Medical Association and other powerful medical groups insisted on it to preserve the physicians' clinical autonomy. When Congress added the provision about steroids in the Federal Food, Drug, and Cosmetic Act in 1988, it was careful to preserve this clinical autonomy by making it illegal to distribute steroids, but not if the steroids were prescribed by a physician, and under the law, a physician could prescribe them for any purpose, including for use as an enhancement. But when Congress passed the Crime Control Act of 1990 and substituted HGH for steroids in the food and drug law, it made it a felony to distribute HGH "for any use in humans other than the treatment of disease or other recognized medical condition, where such use has been authorized by the Secretary of Health and Human Services under section 505 and pursuant to the order of a physician."[82] The language is drafted so badly that it is difficult to be sure what it means, but the phrase "where such use has been authorized by the Secretary of Health and Human Services under section 505" has been interpreted to mean that physicians violate the law if they prescribe the drug for a purpose that has not been approved by the FDA, in other words for an off-label use. What is especially noteworthy is that this is the only occasion on which Congress has placed such a limit on a physician's prescribing authority under the food and drug law. It thus represents an unprecedented invasion of physician autonomy.

After the 2004 crackdown on designer steroids, Congress returned to the doping issue in the winter of 2005 and held hearings to investigate the use of steroids in Major League Baseball. Calling the hearings "Restoring Faith in America's Pastime," it subpoenaed players and executives and also heard from a line of witnesses who condemned steroids.[83] The most poignant witness was the parent mentioned in chapter 3 who claimed that steroids made his son commit suicide, and his account, as well as his heart-wrenching appeal to "please help us to see that our children's lives were not lost in vain," attracted huge media attention. Senator John McCain threatened to revoke baseball's exemption from federal antitrust laws if it did not clean up its players.[84] Later hearings targeted professional basketball and football.[85] In November 2005, McCain and former pitcher Jim Bunning introduced a bill called the Integrity in Professional Sports Act that would have imposed an Olympic-like antidoping program on professional athletes. The bill called for players to be tested without advanced notice at least five times a year. A positive result would lead to a two-year suspension without pay. A second offense would result in a lifetime ban. The bill stalled when Major League Baseball and the players' union agreed to a program that would suspend a player for 50 games after one positive test, 100 games after two tests, and ban the player for life after a third positive result.[86] (Baseball now tests the 40-man team roster once during spring training and at least once more during the season. It also conducts 600 random tests, with as many as 60 during the off-season. Between 2005 and April 1, 2007, a total of 14 players have tested positive.)[87]

Most states have updated their own controlled substance acts to include anabolic steroids. They have also made efforts to regulate steroids in schools and to conduct public education campaigns about the risks. A survey conducted by the National Federation of State High School Associations found that almost 4 percent of high schools test for steroids. In 2006, New Jersey became the first state to require steroid testing of high school athletes. Students who test positive are banned from competition for one year. The first round of random testing of top athletes, involving 150 students, produced no positive results.[88]

Antidoping advocates have important reasons for wanting to involve the government in their campaign. In the first place, it is about money: most of USADA's budget, $12 million in 2005, is funded by Congress.[89] Second, the government wields the power of the law. This enables it to do things that the sports organizations themselves cannot: issue subpoenas, seize materials, and arrest and incarcerate offenders. As WADA chairman Pound observed in promoting collaboration between WADA and criminal investigators, "The next generation of breakthroughs in the fight against doping in sport will be sport authorities working with public authorities who have the power to investigate and seize evidence the sport authorities don't have."[90] Third, by enlisting law enforcement officials in their fight, antidoping forces can divide the targets. As the director-general of WADA, David Howman, explains, "They're interested in traffickers and we're interested in users." Howman describes how WADA has been cooperating with investigators in the BALCO investigation as well as in a probe of Internet steroid sales being spearheaded by the district attorney of Albany County in New York.

The United States is not the only nation in which the government has joined sports organizations in attempting to stop doping. WADA has assisted Spanish authorities in an investigation known as Operation Puerto, which has led to the arrests of several individuals for blood doping, including in connection with the 2006 Tour de France.[91] Both France and Italy have criminalized doping in sports. During the 2006 Turin Winter Olympics, after receiving a tip from WADA via the International Olympic Committee, the Italian police raided the house where the Austrian biathlon and cross-country skiers were staying. They were looking not only for evidence of doping but also for a former team coach named Walter Mayer, who had been banned from the 2006 and 2010 Winter Games for using blood doping on athletes in 2002.[92] At some point around the time of the raid, Mayer jumped in his car, took off north, and crossed into Austria. After driving for about 250 miles, he pulled over to take a nap, but fled when an Austrian police car stopped to check. After a 15-mile chase, he rammed his car into a police barricade and was taken to a psychiatric hospital.[93]

All this shows that, having gotten much of its initial energy from the War on Drugs, the war against doping and the War on Drugs have merged. Sports organizations are punishing athletes for using non-performance-enhancing recreational drugs, while steroids and HGH have joined the growing list of substances that governments feel must be kept out of the hands of citizens when used for nonmedicinal purposes. The ultimate irony is that a recent survey revealed that most people in the United States who use steroids do so for physical self-improvement rather than to compete in sports.[94] In other words, a drug that is condemned to preserve competition in sports is being used predominantly for self-satisfaction, rather than to obtain a competitive edge.

Chapter 8

The Lessons from Sports

THE HISTORY OF the antidoping war in sports and its link to the wider War on Drugs leads to the question of whether the antidoping policy in sports is the correct approach to take in controlling the use of biomedical enhancements outside of sports. If it is, then we should expect a full-fledged partnership of government and private entities aimed at preventing the use of a broad set of prohibited interventions. If the unjustified approach taken by elite sports is not appropriate outside of sports, then we need to identify better ways to minimize the potential harms from biomedical enhancements.

Imposing a Ban

The experience of sports and other gamelike competitions makes several things clear. One is that a ban on biomedical enhancements would be exceedingly difficult to enforce. In the first place, we would have to decide what counted as a prohibited enhancement. It is hard to believe that cosmetic surgery would be included, for example, at least outside of beauty contests. Imagine the outcry from surgeons and their patients. Suppose we adopted the WADA criteria for deciding what substances to place on the prohibited list and banned anything that (1) enhanced performance; (2) was a health risk; and (3) was "against the spirit" of the endeavor in question.[1] Because virtually anything taken into the body poses some health risk, we would have to determine how much risk was acceptable, presumably after balancing it against the benefit to be gained in terms of improved performance. This is something the FDA does all the time in regard to medical interventions, but there is little reason to expect that the FDA (or, in many cases, any expert body) has sufficient expertise to make valid comparisons in the case of biomedical enhancements. Congress might seek to amend the Federal Food, Drug, and Cosmetic Act to furnish the FDA with the necessary expertise, but where would it come from? With due respect to Leon Kass and Michael Sandel, what training prepares one to decide that the risk from an enhancement so clearly outweighs the benefit that competent adults should not be allowed to use it? Francis Fukuyama and colleague Franco Furger suggest that an expert government body be established to make decisions about what technologies should be permitted.[2] But then the decision about what enhancements to ban might depend less on scientific data about risks and benefits and more on the ideological views of the members; a conservative group such as President Bush's bioethics advisory council would be bound to be far more prohibitive than a more liberal body. Perhaps Congress would make its own risk-benefit assessments, as it did when it placed steroids in schedule III on the Controlled Substances List and made it a felony to prescribe human growth hormone for off-label purposes. But then the decisions might be political rather than scientific.

Even if we could agree on the criteria to be used in deciding what should be banned, there would be borderline cases that would defy ready classification. As noted above, many technologies straddle the border between enhancements and medical therapies. Consider what might be called "non-health-oriented injury prevention." A good example is the biomedical enhancement research program of the Department of Defense described in chapter 1. The objective of this program, as we saw, is to protect soldiers from battlefield injuries by giving them greater energy and cognitive abilities, enabling them to go without sleep and normal food for longer periods, and providing them with tougher bodies. If successful, this research would lead to capabilities that exceeded species norms, and perhaps even species limits. In one sense, these interventions resemble preventive medicine in that they aim to preserve health. But in the case of preventive medicine, the goal simply is to preserve health, whereas in the military program, the goal is to promote health so that the soldiers can complete their specific missions. In that sense, non-health-oriented injury prevention is more like enhancement, because it is intended to improve performance. If society decided to ban biomedical enhancements, should it place non-health-oriented injury preventive measures on the prohibited list? Or should it classify them the same as immunizations, which, although they give a person a greater-than-normal immune response, would be regarded as permissible preventive medicine rather than enhancement? Of course, that the ultimate objective of military research is presumably to promote national security is likely to tip the scales in favor of permitting soldiers to use the interventions. But as Lasik surgery illustrates, the fruits of military research can make their way into civilian life.

If this means that we would be willing to prevent soldiers from being hurt so they can better do their jobs, what about firefighters, or rescue workers, or anyone in a dangerous occupation? Indeed, what about athletes? As we saw in chapter 3, steroids enhance athletic performance most directly by reducing muscle injury during exercise. This makes steroids too a type of non-health-oriented injury prevention. Would we allow people to use steroids to avoid injury when performing physical labor? If so, can we justify denying steroids to athletes? Of course, as we said before, because sports are free to adopt their own rules, they are free to decide which enhancements, if any, they will allow athletes to employ. But when the government is making the decision and the result determines whether or not someone is guilty of a felony, arbitrariness is not a constitutional option.

Enforcing the Ban

Let's assume for the sake of argument that we were somehow able to agree on a list of prohibited enhancements. To interdict them, the government would have to erode physicians' clinical autonomy by preventing them from prescribing approved drugs for off-label uses. As noted in chapter 7, the only precedent for this is the case of human growth hormone. Even the laws that regulate controlled substances, which permit physicians to give them to patients only for legitimate medical purposes, give physicians the discretion to prescribe them for off-label uses.

When we consider enhancing future rather than existing persons, a ban on enhancements would not only interfere with physician autonomy but also intrude on parents' constitutionally protected reproductive freedom. A number of the enhancements targeted by opponents, particularly those involving genetic technologies, would be employed in the course of reproduction, including the selection of desirable donor eggs and sperm, the implantation of desirable embryos following preimplantation genetic testing, and fetal testing for nondisease characteristics followed by abortion. In a long line of cases, including *Roe v. Wade,* the Supreme Court has recognized a right of privacy or liberty in connection with reproductive decisions about whether or not to have a child. Because under *Roe,* parents have the right to abort a fetus for whatever reason during the first trimester, it follows that they have the right to abort a fetus based on its nondisease characteristics. Furthermore, although the Supreme Court has not considered whether the rights associated with procreation extend to assisted reproductive techniques such as egg and sperm donation, in vitro fertilization, and preimplantation genetic testing, the increasing prevalence of these practices suggests that they too may be protected under the umbrella of reproductive freedom. In that case, any attempt by Congress or state legislatures to enact a law that interfered with a fundamental right of this nature therefore would be unconstitutional unless it passed an extremely stringent test; the courts would have to be persuaded that the law was the "least intrusive means" of furthering "a compelling state interest."

Could a law preventing the birth of an enhanced child be said to fulfill a compelling state interest? Would the threats posed by genetic enhancement be sufficiently dire to satisfy this standard? The answer is uncertain, depending in great measure on how persuasively opponents could show that genetic enhancement posed a direct threat to the enhanced child. Law professor John Robertson maintains that, in selecting which of the dozen or so embryos fertilized in vitro to implant in the womb, parents are entitled to identify the most desirable embryos in terms of nondisease as well as disease characteristics, particularly if, as Robertson notes, the parents can show that they would not want to have children at all unless they could make these choices. "A consistent commitment to procreative liberty," Robertson argues, "necessarily leaves parents wide prebirth discretion to select—or not—the characteristics of their offspring."[3] Dartmouth bioethicist Ronald M. Green agrees as a matter of ethics: "Parents are best suited to understand and shape the lives of their offspring. Their freedom of decision in this area should have presumptive priority in our moral and legal thinking. Only in extreme cases are we warranted as a society in denying them access to the professional services they need to realize their choices or in preventing them from exercising those choices."[4]

Only two legal cases have addressed the constitutionality of government interference with assisted reproduction. In the first, a federal court invalidated an Illinois law that made it illegal to experiment on a fetus. The court held that, in addition to being impermissibly vague, the law could be interpreted to prohibit embryo transfer—the process by which an embryo fertilized in the laboratory is implanted in the womb—and this would unconstitutionally restrict "a woman's fundamental right of privacy, in particular, her right to make reproductive choices free of governmental interference with those choices."[5] The second case involved a teacher who alleged that she had been fired by an Ohio public school board because she was an unwed mother who had become pregnant with the aid of artificial insemination. The court held that "a woman has a constitutional privacy right to control her reproductive functions. Consequently, a woman possesses the right to become pregnant by artificial insemination."[6] Although neither case directly addresses government regulation of genetic enhancement, they seem to support Robertson's and Green's position. Laws preventing the birth of enhanced children would be tough to sustain constitutionally without a strong showing of potential harm to the child.

At present, there is little government regulation of the U.S. assisted reproduction industry. After the Federal Trade Commission in the late 1980s found that infertility clinics were exaggerating their success at producing live births with IVF, Congress in 1992 enacted the Fertility Clinic Success Rate and Certification Act, but all this requires is that the clinics report their success rates to the federal Centers for Disease Control and Prevention (CDC) so that the CDC can standardize their results.[7] There is little state regulation of IVF clinics, and virtually no controls on the donor egg and sperm industry or on preimplantation or prenatal genetic testing. While the federal Clinical Laboratories Improvement Act and amendments give the government the authority to impose special standards on laboratories conducting genetic testing, oversight is divided among the FDA, CDC, and the Centers for Medicare and Medicaid Services (CMS) within the U.S. Department of Health and Human Services, and none of these agencies has seen fit to do much to assure that the tests are accurate, much less to control which tests may be offered. In fact, CMS recently declared that, due to the cost, it would not strengthen its standards for genetic testing laboratories.

Assuming that a new regulatory regime would be needed to regulate reproductive enhancement, one model would be the Human Fertilisation and Embryology Authority established in Great Britain in 1991 under the Human Fertilisation and Embryology Act of 1990. This agency not only licenses IVF clinics, it also controls the preimplantation genetic testing that they can perform, and, under its guidelines, it considers permitting new tests "only where there is a significant risk of a serious genetic condition being present in the embryo."[8] This suggests that the authority would not approve tests for nondisease characteristics. But the British do not have the same constitutional framework of individual rights as in the United States, and it is unclear if similar restrictions on testing in the United States would survive constitutional challenge in the courts.

The issues raised by reproductive technologies, however, are among the least of the enforcement problems that would be created by an attempt to ban biomedical enhancement. Curbs on preimplantation testing like the ones imposed in Britain would target health care professionals and the hospitals and clinics where they work. They thus resemble the many other legal requirements and restrictions to which these providers are subjected, such as the prerequisites for obtaining individual and organizational licenses and certifications, public health reporting obligations, and limitations on the scope of practice. But a prohibition against biomedical enhancements would have to stretch well beyond legitimate health care providers to reach commercial purveyors, such as the chemists and entrepreneurs who once manufactured and distributed enhancements to athletes. There also would need to be penalties for possession to discourage people from obtaining enhancements on the black market. The War on Enhancements therefore would become a subset of the War on Drugs. Whenever the police conducted a search for illegal drugs of abuse, they also would be on the lookout for illegal biomedical enhancements.

But a war against enhancement would have to go beyond even the War on Drugs. For one thing, there would need to be new rules telling the authorities when they would be entitled to conduct a search of one's home, automobile, or person. Under the Fourth Amendment to the Constitution, searches are permitted when the police have probable cause to link a person to a crime. The question is what constitutes probable cause to conduct a search for illegal enhancements. Although it can be information from a reliable third-party informant, probable cause often is created by the individual's own behavior, such as driving erratically or fleeing from the scene of a crime. Conceivably, then, the police would have probable cause to search for illegal enhancements whenever they reasonably suspected that a person had been enhanced—that is, when they performed better than expected. Every time college students of average ability unpredictably aced an exam, for instance, the police would be authorized to search their lockers, cars, and dorm rooms. A ban on enhancement also would have to punish people for lawfully possessing enhancement substances with legitimate medical uses and then employing them for enhancement purposes. But even that degree of government intrusiveness would not be sufficient. A ban on enhancements also would have to catch people who purchased enhancement drugs illegally, ingested or injected them to obtain the enhancement benefit, and were no longer in possession of the substances when confronted by law enforcement personnel. The prohibition therefore would have to target not only the manufacture, distribution, and possession of the illegal enhancements but also their use. And it is crucial to realize that the War on Drugs doesn't go nearly this far. True, the police subject drivers to sobriety tests to determine if they have used alcohol, but it is not the "use" of alcohol that is illegal but the act of being under the influence to a degree that impairs ability to drive safely. In a War on Enhancement, "sobriety tests" would have to be performed, not just when enhancements led people to behave dangerously but also whenever there was an advantage to be gained by enhancement—which is effectively at any time.

It turns out that we do have a model for this type of regime. This is precisely what sports organizations do in seeking to prevent doping. When Olympic athletes forfeit their medals or are suspended from competition, it is typically because they have been caught *using* prohibited substances, not just possessing or distributing them. The rules of baseball, for example, prohibit players from "*using*, possessing, selling, facilitating the sale of, distributing, or facilitating the distribution of any Drug of Abuse and/or Steroid."[9]

That a ban on enhancements would have to interdict use may be obvious. What may not be so obvious, though, is what this would look like. To get an idea, consider the life of Mari Holden. She must disclose her whereabouts to the authorities at all times. She files written reports detailing her daily routines—when she leaves her home, where she goes, how long she stays. If she interrupts her routine for a single day for any reason—to take a class, attend graduation, get married—she must fax the authorities an updated schedule. Armed with knowledge of her location, a stranger is entitled to show up without warning at any time and force her to urinate while they watch. The only concession to modesty is that, like Holden, the watcher is a woman.

Consider: What exactly has Mari Holden done to deserve such an invasion of her privacy? She is not a convicted criminal. She is not under house arrest or on parole. Instead, Holden is a top cyclist, an Olympic athlete. In 2000, Holden won the silver medal in the times trials at the Sydney Olympics. That same year, she also won the world time trial championship. She was a U.S. cycling champion six times. The regime described above is how the U.S. Anti-Doping Agency conducts its "out-of-competition" antidoping testing program. (During competition, Holden and her fellow athletes are notified and given 60 minutes to present themselves for testing at a Doping Control Station.) If Holden had won gold instead of silver at the Sydney Olympics, she would be tested even more often; the higher the athlete's ranking, the more frequent the tests.

Imagine what it would be like if a similar regime were imposed outside of sports. We would have to endure testing whenever we competed—at school, at work, and, since so many of us work at least in part where we live, at home. Moreover, because the positive effects of enhancements might persist after the use of enhancements ceases, the way the performance benefits provided by certain forms of enhancements in sports do, testing would have to take place on some schedule "outside of competition"—in other words, during our private lives. Moreover, to prevent people from masking the enhancement or otherwise thwarting the analyses, the tests would have to be conducted without forewarning, which means that, as we go about our lives, the authorities would have to know where we are at all times. And remember: so long as the tests continue to employ urinalysis, which is currently the cheapest test method, it would be necessary for the specimen to be obtained under observation.

When Major League Baseball got religion and began a serious antidoping program after being threatened with severe sanctions during the 2005 Senate hearings on steroids, it quietly assigned people to watch players covertly from the time they are notified that they are to be tested until they produce a urine sample, in order to detect efforts to defeat the tests, such as by consuming large amounts of liquids to dilute the concentrations of substances in the urine. The secret surveillance sometimes lasts for hours. Yet even this doesn't satisfy WADA member Dr. Gary Wadler, who criticizes the practice of allowing a player who can't produce a sample to try again an hour later, and if not successful, to continue trying until an hour after a game. Scoffs Wadler: "If a guy can't do it, he comes back in an hour? Give me a break. They should say that he will be chaperoned from the moment of notification. It shouldn't even be 30 seconds later."[10]

How would you like to be subjected to this kind of testing?

But we still have not appreciated what a full-blown war against biomedical enhancement would be like. For a ban to be complete, it would have to be illegal not only to use an enhancement drug but also to manipulate a person's genes to produce an enhancement effect. If a genetic enhancement enabled the body to produce more of a substance like EPO or HGH than the body produces naturally, it may be difficult to distinguish the added from the naturally occurring material. For one thing, exercise alone may stimulate the body to produce more of certain performance-enhancing chemicals. WADA has developed what it claims is a valid and reliable test for "exogenous" EPO—that is, EPO that is injected from outside the body—but it is not clear that the test can identify extra amounts of endogenously produced EPO, and the WADA test has been criticized as being inaccurate even for detecting EPO that is exogenous.[11]

According to geneticists, the ability to detect a genetic modification may depend on whether the resulting product—EPO, for example—functions within the cells that have had their DNA modified to produce it or instead is secreted by these reprogrammed factory cells and then travels in the body to function elsewhere. The latter would be easier to spot through direct testing, because secreted substances would be more likely to show up in samples of blood or urine. But to develop a test for the substance, we would need to know what we are looking for. Don Caitlin's Olympic testing lab at UCLA was able to develop an assay for the designer steroid produced by BALCO, it will be recalled, because Caitlin had received a syringe containing the chemical and therefore knew what the test needed to find. But there won't always be a sample of a genetic enhancement to design a test around. Nor can we hope to be able to determine when genetic enhancement has taken place by identifying the vehicles, or "vectors," that are used to carry the modified genes to their intended destinations in the body. This isn't possible because the vectors, which might be common viruses, do not survive for long before being destroyed by the body's immune system. Moreover, although the immune response would produce antibodies with which to combat the viral vector, it would be difficult to distinguish them from the antibodies that the body produces in response to the same viruses that were present in the natural environment.

When an enhancement substance produces its enhancement effect by acting directly on the cells that manufactured it, the only direct way to test for it is to examine the cells themselves to ascertain if they have been genetically reprogrammed. But this would entail performing a biopsy—essentially punching out a piece of tissue where the cell was believed to be located. This is a far more invasive procedure than simply asking someone to provide a urine sample or even drawing a sample of their blood. It might be possible instead to figure out what happens to the enhancement substance once it is employed (metabolized) by the body, that is, to test for its metabolites, but that also would not be easy, at least without knowing in advance what metabolites you are looking for. Another alternative would be to discern the changes in body function that would indicate that the enhancement had altered the body's normal physiological processes or "homeostasis." But this too may be extremely difficult, particularly if the changes are subtle.

One approach that has been suggested is to establish some sort of "baseline" profile for people against which later test results can be compared. Authorities in Australia, for example, have proposed that Olympic athletes be required to compete internationally in the year before an Olympiad so that antidoping officials can determine if their subsequent Olympic performance is so much better that doping should be suspected.[12] Similarly, WADA is considering creating a biological "passport" for each Olympian that would keep track of their blood and urine values at set points during their careers so that variations due to doping could be detected, and a report by a committee of the British House of Commons has recommended that the United Kingdom experiment with such a passport system before the 2012 Olympics.[13]

In my book *Wondergenes,* I proposed a similar approach, in which a person's genetic profile would be analyzed and stored at birth, to determine whether their genes had been altered for enhancement purposes by comparing the original profile with the results of later genetic tests. More important, by comparing a parent's genetic profile with that of their offspring, such a "genetic passport" might be able to indicate if parents had enhanced their children's genes before birth. Still, none of these techniques would reveal whether parents had employed preimplantation genetic testing and selected embryos for implantation based on nondisease characteristics, which some might object to as a form of enhancement. Moreover, the idea that the government would have access to everyone's personal genetic information might strike many people as an impermissible invasion of privacy. (As it turns out, the government already has access to this information for many people, in the form of "Guthrie cards"—the cards on which are stored the blood samples taken from everyone at birth under state newborn screening programs. Some states preserve these records for many years; since they contain spots of actual blood, complete with copies of the newborn's DNA, the government could, if it wanted, retrieve the cards and analyze the DNA.)

Enforcing the Ban Overseas

If enhancements were illegal, there would be a black market not only in the United States but also abroad. Obviously the United States would be concerned about shipments of illegal enhancements being smuggled into the country. U.S. authorities already have their hands full trying to stop the influx of illegal aliens and drugs along the six thousand miles of land borders with Canada and Mexico as well as the more than twelve thousand miles of coastline. How much extra effort would be required to block the importation of illicit enhancement products attracted to our shores by the high prices driven by the demand? Would we be willing to pay for the additional enforcement personnel and checkpoints? Just think of how difficult it would be to intercept Internet sales of enhancement products from abroad. Currently it is possible to purchase prescription drugs over the Internet after paying for an electronic physician "consultation."[14] In 2000, one reporter used the Internet for two months to amass 30 capsules of Xenical, 30 tablets of Prozac, 100 Ultrams, 100 penicillin, a kit with four birth control pills, and five bottles of injectable Xylocaine, and he was awaiting shipments of Valium and fen-phen, this last a combination drug withdrawn from the U.S. market in 1997.[15]

Instead of bringing illegal enhancements into the country, people might get themselves enhanced abroad. When abortions were illegal in the United States, Americans got them in Mexico. Currently travelers go overseas to obtain organ transplants, especially to countries where organs can be purchased, a practice that is illegal in the United States.[16] There also is a thriving market abroad for cosmetic surgery, which can be bought more cheaply in many other countries. Companies advertise "cosmetic surgery holidays," which combine sightseeing or a stay at a spa with a facelift or breast augmentation.[17] One company arranges cosmetic surgeries in 37 countries, from Argentina to the Ukraine.[18]

Clearly the availability of highly effective enhancements abroad would attract large numbers of these "enhancement tourists." If the United States were serious about such a ban, it would have to take steps to prevent people from using enhancements abroad and then returning home to take advantage of the enhancement effects. The United States would have to persuade other countries to adopt similar restrictive policies on the manufacture, distribution, possession, and use of enhancement products and services. Some nations, especially those in Western Europe, might follow the lead of the United States. In some respects, they already have taken more comprehensive steps to control biomedical enhancement. As noted earlier, the United Kingdom regulates IVF practices more thoroughly than the United States, and the Council of Europe adopted a convention against genetic enhancement in 1997, declaring that "an intervention seeking to modify the human genome may only be undertaken for preventive, diagnostic or therapeutic purposes and only if its aim is not to introduce any modification in the genome of any descendants."[19]

Efforts to ban human cloning serve as a precedent for trying to secure a uniform and mandatory international stance against a particular type of biotechnology. In a 1997 joint communiqué, the Group of Eight (G8)—the United States, Britain, Germany, France, Italy, Japan, Canada, and Russia—stated that it had agreed on "the need for appropriate domestic measures and close international cooperation to prohibit the use of somatic cell nuclear transfer to create a child."[20] The Council of Europe established a convention that same year containing a separate protocol prohibiting human cloning, followed by a similar resolution in 2000 by the European Parliament.[21] In 2001, law professor and bioethicist George Annas urged the international community to adopt a "Convention of the Preservation of the Human Species" to prohibit reproductive cloning and germline genetic engineering.[22] In the United Nations, action began in 2001 in the General Assembly to pass a nonbinding resolution to begin a process of establishing a treaty to ban cloning, but it was stalled when members could not agree on whether to ban cloning for therapeutic as well as reproductive purposes, as the United States and Costa Rica had urged. The World Health Organization's World Health Assembly in 1997 passed a resolution against reproductive cloning, as did UNESCO the same year in its Universal Declaration on the Human Genome and Human Rights. The Human Genome Organization (HUGO), an international group of genetic researchers, came out against reproductive cloning in 1999.[23] (Ironically, it has never been illegal to clone a human being in the United States.)

An effective international ban on biomedical enhancement would be extremely difficult to achieve, however, unless it received the active support of all nations. The U.N. Security Council has the legal authority to compel a country to submit to its will by using or threatening to use armed force or economic sanctions, but only when the target country has been found to have violated Article VII of the U.N. Charter by posing a "threat to the peace, a breach of the peace, or an act of aggression"—provided that none of the five permanent members of the Security Council (China, France, Russia, Britain, and the United States) blocks U.N. action by exercising its veto power. It is extremely unlikely that the use of biomedical enhancement would be found to violate Article VII of the U.N. Charter. Even if an international ban were adopted by treaty, convention, or resolution, these would not have a binding effect on a country unless it ratified the treaty or convention or agreed to abide by the resolution and then enacted legislation to make the international obligation part of its domestic law. The International Court of Justice can impose binding judgments on nations, but only if they consent to the court's jurisdiction in the particular matter. Even if countries did endorse an international agreement to ban biomedical enhancement, they can withdraw simply by giving the applicable international governmental body notice (generally six months).

If a country chose not to abide by a worldwide prohibition against enhancement, the nations supporting a ban would have to try to pressure the country to comply. One option would be economic sanctions, including a reduction in foreign aid, trade restrictions, limitations on travel by its citizens, the seizure of assets held abroad, or the refusal to recognize intellectual property rights, such as patents, in objectionable enhancements. The International Emergency Economic Powers Act, for example, gives the president the authority to "deal with any unusual and extraordinary threat, which has its source in whole or substantial part outside the United States, to the national security, foreign policy, or economy of the United States." If the president declares that a threat from a nation creates a "national emergency," the act gives him the power to regulate or prohibit foreign financial transactions, except for postal, telegraphic, or telephonic communications that do not involve transfers of value and donations for humanitarian aid.[24] U.S. presidents have made extensive use of this authority. Between 1976 and 2006, presidents declared 39 "national emergencies" to restrict trade with certain countries; as a result, in 1998, 3 billion people in 29 countries were prevented from trading with the United States.[25] Trade restrictions also could be adopted under international trade agreements. The main agreement is GATT, the General Agreement on Tariffs and Trade, which is administered by the World Trade Organization (WTO).

An alternative to levying negative economic sanctions on countries that refuse to ban biomedical enhancements would be to offer them economic incentives. They could be given foreign aid or relieved of some or all of their international debt. This would be especially attractive to poor and developing countries.

Economic realities may limit the feasibility of some of these approaches. Trade sanctions, for instance, are double-edged. Applied against countries with needed resources or markets, they could hurt the sanctioning nations as much or more than the ones that were sanctioned. Because of its importance as a world market and as a source of cheap labor, for example, China in 2001 was admitted to membership in the WTO, thus gaining the benefits of most-favored-nation status, despite criticism of its record on human rights.

The question is whether all countries would endorse an enhancement ban, be it willingly or as a result of international pressure. There certainly could be good reasons for countries to refuse to jump on the antienhancement bandwagon. Enhancements that significantly increased the productivity of workers could accelerate the economies of both advanced and developing countries. Recall the prediction of James Canton of the Institute for Global Futures that the use of biomedical enhancements in the workplace is the key to being globally competitive in the future.[26] Nations extending hospitality to enhancement providers catering to foreigners also would gain the economic benefit of an international enhancement business. The resulting foreign exchange would be especially desirable for poorer countries with little strategic or military value and limited natural resources.

Could countries with small economies and scientific infrastructures gain the biomedical know-how and financial resources to produce sophisticated enhancement products and offer alluring enhancement services? Certainly. They would attract disgruntled researchers, physicians, technicians, and investors from countries that blocked them from pursuing their scientific, social, or entrepreneurial interests in enhancement medicine. Lucrative enhancement markets would draw foreign investment. Sufficient funds even might be forthcoming from wealthy government leaders and other members of indigenous elites.

There is plenty of precedent for scientists to emigrate abroad to avoid local restrictions on research and practice. In 1980, Martin Cline, a researcher and Chief of Hematology/Oncology at the UCLA Medical Center, wanted to try a novel treatment for an hereditary blood disorder called beta thalassemia that reduces the production of red blood cells, thereby depriving the tissues of oxygen and causing life-threatening anemia. Cline wanted to see if he could treat the disease with gene therapy by inserting genes into the patient's bone marrow that were programmed to manufacture the proper amount of red blood cells. He submitted an experimental protocol to UCLA's institutional review board (IRB), the group of in-house experts required to review proposed human experiments to determine if they fall within ethical and regulatory guidelines. But he grew frustrated at the delay, so he flew to Italy and Israel, where he performed his experiment on one patient in each country. The IRB eventually rejected Cline's protocol because he had not performed enough studies in animals. When a reporter for the *Los Angeles Times* discovered what Cline had done, he was stripped of his department chair at UCLA and disqualified from receiving future research funding from the National Institutes of Health.[27]

The effort to block human cloning has also led some Americans to announce their intent to move their cloning activities offshore. In 1998, maverick physicist Richard Seed declared that he would clone his third wife at a new facility he was building in Hokkaido, Japan, and that he already had raised $15 million of investment capital with the help of Tokyo-based businessman James Ryan. In 1999, Japan was reported to have denied Seed a license to operate his facility.[28] American fertility doctor Panayiotos Zavos and his Italian collaborator Severino Antinori announced that they would attempt to clone a human being in Israel, Cyprus, or one of the former members of the Soviet Union and that, if denied permission, they might even set up their laboratory on a boat in international waters.[29] (In 1994, Antinori was credited with enabling Rosanna Della Corte, at age 62, to become the oldest woman to bear a child, produced with a donated egg fertilized with her husband's sperm. In 2003, Della Corte lost her title to a 65-year-old Indian woman. Following pressure from the Vatican, Italian lawmakers that year enacted a law banning assisted reproduction for women beyond normal child-bearing age.)[30] Then there were the Raelians, a cult founded by former sportscar enthusiast Claude Vorilhon that believes that aliens founded life on earth by cloning themselves. In 2002, the Raelians claimed that their startup company Clonaid had successfully cloned a baby named Eve from an American mother somewhere else in the world. The claim was dismissed when the company refused to produce the child and mother for comparative DNA testing.

Human and economic capital are not the only resources that could flow across borders to create and sustain enhancement industries in willing countries. It would be hard to keep a lid on information about how to produce and obtain enhancements, which could be exchanged in scientific journals, at conferences, and electronically. For years, there has been a set of instructions on the Internet purportedly showing how to build an atomic bomb.[31] Apparently it was a spoof produced by the staff of a newsletter called the Annals of Improbable Research, but it reportedly fooled the Taliban, which kept the instructions in a Kabul home where they were found after the 2001 U.S.-led invasion of Afghanistan.[32] In 2006, the *New York Times* reported that a web archive established by the U.S. government included papers from Iraq's pre-1991 program on how to build a nuclear device for real.[33] Even general scientific information might be useful to offshore researchers. For example, the NIH requires that genetic researchers it funds make their findings public, such as by posting new discoveries about the structure and function of the human genome on government websites. This could aid researchers searching for ways to enhance people using genetic technology. In 2003, at the request of the National Science Foundation, the NIH, the CIA, and the Department of Homeland Security, the National Academy of Sciences created a blue-ribbon committee to consider how to limit access to genetic information that could aid would-be terrorists in building biological weapons. After almost a year of discussion, the committee sided with advocates of open scientific exchange and recommended against any attempt to classify the information in the interest of national security. If scientists are unwilling to restrict knowledge that could be used to attack the United States, it is unlikely they would take kindly to restrictions on communication about biomedical enhancements.

Finally, even if all countries paid lip service to a prohibition, their efforts might be undercut by government corruption. Take the War on Drugs in Mexico. In 1997, the head of its National Institute for the Combat of Drugs was arrested for collaborating with a drug cartel. The press linked President Carlos Salinas de Gortari's chief of staff and brother to drug trafficking. Accusations also were made against officials in the administration of Ernesto Zedillo, who succeeded Salinas, including the secretaries of defense and interior and the president's private secretary. In 2001, drug kingpin Joaquin Guzmán's escape from a maximum security prison took place with help from prison officials.[34]

The picture was not any brighter in a report prepared for Congress by the Congressional Research Service in 2007. Agents of the Mexican FBI (known as the AFI) and local police are described as enforcers for the drug lords, including kidnapping competitors and handing them over to cartels for ransom or torture. In 2005, 1,500 of the 7,000 AFI agents and one-fifth of the members of the Mexican attorney general's office were under investigation for corruption. When the administration of Vicente Fox sent federal agents to the town of Nuevo Laredo to crack down on drug trafficking, they were fired on by municipal police. In 2007, the Mexican government removed 284 federal police commanders for corruption, including federal commanders of all 31 states and the federal district.[35]

In short, the United States and its allies in the War on Enhancements are unlikely to be capable of preventing the enhancement industry from taking root in foreign countries. There simply is too much money to be made by welcoming enhancement tourists. Even if foreign governments made a show of cooperation, corruption would undercut their efforts.

In that case, the only recourse would be to attempt to prevent citizens from traveling abroad to avail themselves of banned enhancements. One approach would be to stop them physically. The U.S. government can restrict American citizens from traveling to certain foreign countries without specific government approval. For example, American citizens are forbidden to visit Cuba except for certain limited purposes. If the government finds that a trip abroad is "substantially likely" to seriously damage national security or foreign policy, it can revoke a person's passport, preventing them from traveling out of the country to any place that requires a valid passport for entry.[36]

Citizens who returned from abroad might be detained at CDC-run quarantine stations if they were thought to have been enhanced. Currently, quarantine is authorized for people suspected of having cholera, diphtheria, infectious tuberculosis, plague, smallpox, yellow fever, viral hemorrhagic fevers, SARS, and pandemic flu. In 2007, Andrew Speaker, a Georgia attorney diagnosed with infectious TB, was the first person ordered quarantined since a patient with smallpox in 1963.[37] Would-be immigrants seeking visas to reside permanently in the United States are required to undergo testing for 18 diseases and conditions, including venereal disease, tuberculosis, mental "defect" and retardation, "sexual deviation," and narcotic drug addiction.[38]

Another approach to stop U.S. citizens from obtaining enhancements abroad would be to make it a crime to do so. Presumably possession or use of enhancements would already be against the law, so anyone who returned enhanced to the United States could be punished just for *being* enhanced. But the law could sanction people in addition for the specific act of becoming enhanced in a foreign country, thereby adding to their fine or sentence. For example, the Protection of Children against Sexual Exploitation Act punishes American citizens who return to the United States after committing sex crimes against children in foreign countries.[39] When a defendant named Harvey who had photographed and sexually abused children in the Philippines challenged his conviction under this law on the ground that his conduct occurred abroad, a federal appeals court upheld the statute, stating that "no tenet of international law prohibits Congress from punishing the wrongful conduct of its citizens, even if some of that conduct occurs abroad."[40]

Punishing people for crimes committed in foreign countries runs into a number of practical problems, however. In the case just mentioned, the defendant admitted that he had taken photographs in the Philippines that police found in his house in Pennsylvania. But it can be difficult for U.S. law enforcement personnel to conduct an investigation of illegal conduct abroad, because they must rely on cooperation from their foreign counterparts. It also may be hard to bring the defendant into U.S. custody and to obtain the presence of foreign nationals to serve as witnesses in U.S. proceedings.

A final approach would be to try to prevent Americans from paying for enhancements in other countries. There are a host of laws and regulations governing the transfer of money abroad, and these have been strengthened as part of the war on terror. Anyone who transports more than $10,000 overseas must file a report with the Treasury Department.[41] There are special requirements for doing business with foreign banks and other financial institutions.[42] Taxpayers must report any foreign financial holdings, including bank accounts, on their federal tax returns.[43] These restrictions may not only limit the ability to move funds abroad to finance enhancement purchases but also interfere with attempts to invest in offshore enhancement enterprises.

Punishing Offenders

In the war against doping in sports, the primary punishment for an athlete who gets caught is forfeiting the competition and potentially being prevented from competing in the future. In egregious cases, athletes can be suspended for life. Purveyors of illegal doping substances, such as physicians who prescribe controlled substances for enhancement purposes, can be fined, imprisoned, deprived of the power to prescribe controlled substances, and stripped of their license to practice medicine. Manufacturers who sell drugs and other FDA-regulated products for use as doping agents could be found guilty of misbranding and fined. In rare cases, their senior executives could be imprisoned.

How should enhancement users be punished outside of sports? They too could be fined, put in jail, or denied the opportunity to compete. A student who tried to take an exam with the aid of a cognition-enhancing drug could be flunked; an employee who came to work under the influence of a performance-enhancer could be fired. But what if the enhancement produced a long-lasting effect? Would the culprit be barred from competing for as long as the effect lasted? What if, as is the case with cosmetic surgery and might be the case with certain forms of genetic enhancement, the effect was permanent? Would the person be banned for life?

An alternative might be to reverse the enhancement effect, if possible. A beauty contestant who had had an illegal nose job could be forced to undergo surgery to restore her nose to its original appearance. Genes to counteract an enhancement effect could be introduced into a person who had been genetically enhanced. Perhaps reversal would be offered as an alternative to other punishment.

Instead of preventing someone from competing or biologically reversing the enhancement effect, illegally enhanced persons could be handicapped, so that their enhancement advantage was negated. In *Wondergenes,* I explored this possibility at some length. To produce a more level playing field, some sports do practice some degree of handicapping. Amateur golfers calculate their handicaps and permit poorer players to use more strokes for a given hole, so that players of different abilities can compete more evenly. In boxing as well as Olympic wrestling, contestants are grouped according to weight. In races called "handicaps," horses are assigned weights known as "imposts"; better horses are given higher weights so that other horses have a chance to win; if a horse and jockey together weigh less than the assigned impost, the horse must reach the impost by carrying lead pads in pouches under the saddle. Similarly, to negate the effect of an illegal enhancement, an enhanced marathoner could be required to run an extra distance. A student who had tested positive for Adderall before an exam could be allowed to take the exam but given less time.

Another important measure might be to require individuals to divulge that they are enhanced to persons with whom they interact. In relationships in which one person invariably possesses greater knowledge or bargaining power than another, the law often requires the stronger party to disclose a conflict of interest to the weaker party. A law firm must notify a client when the firm has been asked to represent someone else whose interests compete with the client's, and cannot proceed to represent both parties without their mutual consent. Before enrolling human subjects in a medical experiment, researchers must disclose if they own stock in the company that makes the product. Requiring people to reveal that they were enhanced could be especially critical in the business world, where it would reduce the advantage that enhanced traits could give people in negotiations and other economic transactions. Ted Turner, who has bipolar disorder, is said to have stopped taking lithium, the drug he uses to calm the frenetic highs during which his mind races at fantastic speed, before the mammoth negotiations leading to the merger of Turner Broadcasting and Time Warner.[44] If his superior cognitive ability were attributable to an enhancement rather than the manic phase of his bipolar disease, he might be required to disclose that fact to his competitors.

In *Wondergenes,* I also suggested that the legal rules that govern business transactions might be changed so that interactions between enhanced and unenhanced persons were no longer "at arm's length."

Under the law as it now stands, the parties in ordinary business dealings are deemed to be at arm's length in the sense that they are expected to look out for themselves, rather than to look out for the other person's welfare. A buyer is supposed to have researched a product or service to determine if it is worth the price, rather than rely on the seller to disclose any shortcomings or flaws. This rule of self-protection is known by the Latin phrase *caveat emptor,* or "let the buyer beware." (Note that this rule has been changed in some cases by state or federal law; used car sellers in some states, for example, are required to inform a prospective purchaser if a car has been in an accident.) In certain instances, however, the law does not treat business relationships as being at arm's length. These are relationships in which one party invariably is in a superior bargaining position, for example, by possessing greater knowledge or expertise, but society does not want the weaker parties to expend the resources and effort necessary to protect themselves, such as by gaining a comparable degree of knowledge or hiring an expert advisor. These relationships are called "fiduciary" relationships. They include the relationship between lawyers and clients and between doctors and patients. In these cases, the law requires the stronger party to act in the weaker party's best interests instead of taking advantage of them, as someone might try to do in a relationship that was at arm's length. In *Wondergenes,* I suggested that the law might make enhanced individuals fiduciaries for unenhanced persons with whom they transact business. If unenhanced persons feel that they have been cheated by enhanced persons, the victims could ask the courts to cancel the transactions and require the enhanced persons to restore any money or other things of value that they had extracted.

But how far would this handicapping approach extend? Would only certain types or degrees of enhancement have to be disclosed, or would we have to tell each other, for example, how many cups of coffee we had consumed that morning? Would people who had used enhancements, say, to increase muscle mass be required to act as fiduciaries in transactions in which their strength gave them no special advantage, such as in ordinary business dealings? Would businesses be prohibited from hiring enhanced employees? Would colleges be expected to refuse to admit applicants who had been enhanced genetically by their parents? If handicapping were undertaken zealously in response to biomedical enhancement, moreover, why focus only on enhancements? Why not treat society as one massive playing field and extend handicapping to those who enjoy natural advantages? If this were taken far enough, we could find ourselves in the absurd situation that Kurt Vonnegut described in his futuristic short story *Harrison Bergeron*: "The year was 2081, and everybody was finally equal. They weren't only equal before God and the law. They were equal every which way. Nobody was smarter than anybody else. Nobody was stronger or quicker than anybody else. All this equality was due to the 211th, 212th, and 213th Amendments to the Constitution, and to the unceasing vigilance of the United States Handicapper General." Handicapping may sound intriguing, but to approach comprehensiveness, it would be highly impractical.

The Costs of Enforcement

Speaking of practicalities, how much would an all-out War on Enhancements cost? Think of the massive testing program that would have to be conducted. In 2006, the U.S. Anti-Doping Agency conducted 7,856 tests for prohibited substances.[45] There are only two laboratories accredited by USADA to perform these tests in the United States; until 2006, there was only one—the lab at UCLA run by Don Caitlin. How many more laboratories would be needed to test the entire population for traces of banned enhancements on an ongoing basis?

There would need to be not only testing for drugs but also DNA tests to detect gene doping. This would tax the available testing resources even further. In 1985, British geneticists first employed the results of DNA testing to solve a crime; an analysis of sperm left at the crime scene of a double rape / homicide enabled police to exonerate one suspect and helped convict another. Crime solvers have made increasing use of the technique ever since. Beginning in 1998, the FBI has maintained a database called CODIS (for "Combined DNA Indexing System) that contains the results of DNA analyses performed by state and federal crime labs on blood samples obtained from crime scenes, victims, and arrestees. CODIS now has about 5 million entries and has helped secure the convictions of more than fifty thousand criminals. But there is an enormous backlog of samples waiting to be tested so that the results can be entered into the database. The FBI alone has a waiting list of almost two hundred thousand samples—85 percent of all of the samples it has collected since 2001. The situation is only going to get worse, because Congress keeps expanding the categories of persons from whom DNA must be collected. In 2006, Congress mandated that the FBI test DNA obtained from all persons convicted of federal crimes, not just those convicted of a felony. This added eighty thousand more samples to the waiting list. A new law requires samples to be taken from all persons arrested or detained on suspicion of violating federal law, including illegal immigrants, which could increase the number of samples awaiting testing by as much as one million. The backlog at the state level is so bad that Congress since 1999 has appropriated more than half a billion dollars to increase laboratory capacity.[46] Now consider how much Congress would have to spend to provide enough laboratory capacity if it mandated repeated DNA testing for genetic enhancements, not just for people arrested for crimes but for everybody else too.

Laboratory resources are only a small part of the total manpower and infrastructure that would be needed to fight a War on Enhancements. Additional resources would be required to catch people who manufacture, distribute, possess, and use enhancements. Think of what it would take just to stop enhancement tourists from reentering the country. Each year, about 120 million people enter and leave the United States through 474 airports, seaports, and land border crossings.[47] Returnees suspected of having been enhanced abroad would have to be sequestered pending the results of testing. Currently only 83 employees of the U.S. Public Health Service operate quarantine stations at entry points.

Penn State sports science professor Charles Yesalis, a leading expert on the war against doping in sports, tellingly pointed out the resource problem in testimony before Congress in 2005:

> Even though the legal apparatus to control steroid trafficking exists, enforcement agents already are struggling to handle the problems of importation, distribution, sales, and use of other illicit drugs such as cocaine and heroin. Thus, the availability of performance-enhancing drugs in this country suggests there is reason to believe the United States may simply not have the law enforcement manpower to deal with apprehending and punishing sellers of performance-enhancing drugs. . . . The outlook that limited resources can be stretched to cover yet other drugs is not optimistic, especially given the increase in recreational drug use among adolescents and in light of the demands placed on all levels of law enforcement regarding homeland security.[48]

Now consider that, according to the National Center for Health Statistics at the CDC, about 8 percent of the population over the age of 12 uses an illicit drug in any given month.[49] To try to prevent this, the

United States spends somewhere between $35 billion and $50 billion a year. How many Americans would use illegal biomedical enhancements? Undoubtedly many, many more, if the list of prohibited substances and practices were as extensive as some antienhancement militants might like. But let's assume that only four times as many people would use enhancements as take illegal drugs, or about 30 percent of the population. If the costs of enforcement were proportional to the number of users, it would cost four times as much to stop them as we are spending on the War on Drugs. This is about $200 billion a year. To put this figure in perspective, it is roughly four times the annual budget for homeland security.

Even if we were willing to devote these kinds of government resources, what programs would have to be sacrificed to come up with the cash? Would we cut back on education? Welfare? Medicare? Defense spending? The war on terror? Would a War on Enhancement divert resources from the War on Drugs itself? If so, then as Charles Yesalis emphasized to Congress, the result would be unconscionable: "Based on what we know about the physical, psychological, and social effects of performance-enhancing drugs, it is neither realistic nor prudent that enforcement efforts for performance-enhancing drugs should take precedence over those for more harmful drugs."[50]

What's more, who would want to live in such a society? A ban on biomedical enhancement would require the government to conduct a highly intrusive campaign in which everyone is subjected to testing whenever they "compete" as well as randomly at all other times. The tests would look for evidence that a person has used illegal enhancements, including enhancements that altered his or her genes. Children would be tested to see if their parents have manipulated their genes before birth. Anyone with a positive test result would face penalties.

You can get an idea of what such a regime would look like in the film *Gattaca,* where the world is run according to a system in which people with enhanced genetic endowments reserve for themselves a monopoly on societal benefits, including the best occupations.[51] The hero, who is not enhanced, attempts to thwart the system by fooling the DNA tests that repeatedly are being performed on skin samples and on the cells that the body is constantly sloughing off. The effect that the film produces is chilling, as we see workers being tested as they enter their office buildings and watch the floor sweepings being analyzed for DNA at the end of the day to make sure that no one has slipped through the net.

To be sure, the society portrayed in *Gattaca* is one that is dominated by enhanced individuals, while the ban that we have been discussing would have the opposite goal of preserving the interests of those persons who were not enhanced. But the totalitarian tactics and the resulting atmosphere of fear, distrust, and recrimination would look the same. So imagine being forced to deliver a biological sample before being allowed to go to work or to school as well as being subject to random testing at any other time. Hear the pounding on the front door, as the enhancement inspectors demand entry. See yourself blush when they make you urinate in front of them. Cower at the possibility that a lab might make an error and report a false positive test result, or that you might accidentally swallow something that would trigger an investigation. Then remember that all this is taking place because some puissant, "gifted" individuals have inflicted their personal conception of the good life on everyone else and, incidentally, preserved their own sway.

Less-Radical Methods

If the costs, both tangible and intangible, of a full-fledged, government-run war against biomedical enhancements are not acceptable, perhaps there would be less extreme ways to try to prevent people from using them. One alternative is a voluntary moratorium on enhancement research and development.

In 1972, Stanford biochemist Paul Berg, who would later win a Nobel Prize for his work on nucleic acids, published the results of experiments in which he combined DNA from two different organisms. The trick, he had discovered, was to use enzymes to cleave the DNA molecules apart at specific sites, called "sticky ends," where they could be made to join together through the use of other enzymes. Berg based his experiments on a virus called simian virus 40 (SV40), which in 1960 had been found in the same kind of monkey kidney cells that had been used to produce the Salk and Sabin polio vaccines in the 1950s, cells that were relatively easy to work with. In 1961, however, researchers discovered that SV40 produced cancers in hamsters. This led the U.S. government to screen stocks of polio vaccine to make sure they had not been contaminated with SV40.[52] Nevertheless, Berg decided to try to splice SV40 DNA into the DNA of *E. coli*, a bacterium that lives in the human intestinal tract, where it aids in digestion. A cancer researcher got wind of Berg's plan and warned him that he might inadvertently create a new cancer-causing organism that would flourish in humans. Abashed, Berg halted his experiment and brought the matter to the attention of a group of colleagues in 1973 at the annual meeting of the Gordon Research Conference on Nucleic Acids. The scientists were eager to proceed with their research, which was pioneering what would become known as recombinant DNA engineering. But they also agreed that there were dangers. Led by Berg, they published a letter in the prestigious journal *Science* calling for a voluntary, worldwide moratorium on further recombinant DNA experiments "until the potential hazards of such recombinant DNA molecules have been better evaluated or until adequate methods are developed for preventing their spread."[53] The moratorium appears to have been successful; recombinant DNA experimentation only resumed in February 1975, when an international interdisciplinary group assembled at the Asilomar conference center in California and recommended that the NIH establish guidelines to govern recombinant DNA research.[54]

Conceivably, researchers and physicians could adopt a similar moratorium against biomedical enhancement. In 1999, HUGO, the international genetic research organization, called for a worldwide ban on human cloning for reproductive purposes.[55] Two years earlier, the World Medical Association (WMA) issued a resolution calling "on doctors engaged in research and other researchers to abstain voluntarily from participating in the cloning of human beings until the scientific, ethical and legal issues have been fully considered by doctors and scientists, and any necessary controls put in place."[56] (The WMA position is striking in that it makes "doctors and scientists" the sole arbiters of whether cloning should take place. This appears to confirm the criticism of bioethicist George Annas and his colleagues that the WMA, which was formed in 1946 after the Nuremberg trials, is merely a self-appointed trade association dedicated to protecting physician prerogatives. Annas and others also have lambasted the organization for appointing a former SS physician as its president in 1992 and for refusing to bar South African medical associations from membership despite their government's practice of apartheid.)[57]

Even if major scientific and professional groups were to agree on a moratorium, a voluntary stance is unlikely to be able to withstand the enormous demand for effective enhancements, the innate curiosity of the research community, and rogue scientists determined to seize the limelight. As science writer Alan Lightman points out, the effectiveness of Berg's moratorium on recombinant DNA experiments was in marked contrast to the disregard of an earlier one in which Robert Oppenheimer and other nuclear researchers in 1949 urged that work on the hydrogen bomb be stopped.[58]

One step beyond a purely voluntary ban would be professional self-regulation. In 1994, for example, the American Medical Association's Council on Ethical and Judicial Affairs issued a policy statement on the genetic enhancement of children that said that "genetic interventions to enhance traits should be considered permissible only in severely restricted situations. . . . [There must be] clear and meaningful benefit to the fetus or child; no trade-off with other characteristics or traits, [and] equal access . . . irrespective of income or other socioeconomic characteristics."[59] That same year, the Council also came out specifically against germline genetic engineering and the use of gene transfer technology for enhancement purposes.[60] Because these policies were adopted by the Council on Ethical and Judicial Affairs, they are more than merely hortatory. According to the organization's bylaws, AMA members can be censured, suspended, or expelled from the association for violations of the AMA principles.[61] This is not just the loss of a plaque or of an opportunity to attend annual meetings in plush resorts; it can threaten physicians' status as specialists and as esteemed members of hospital medical staffs. Yet self-regulation has its limitations. Sociologists have emphasized that self-regulation is one of the defining characteristics of a profession, such as law or medicine, but physicians subject to domestic self-regulatory constraints are unlikely to be the only source of access to biomedical enhancements; instead, enhancements are liable to be available on the black market and in foreign countries.[62] Even ethical physicians seeking to abide by the rules may find it hard to resist the economic attraction of being part of the enhancement industry.

Another approach would be to try to cut off research funding for the discovery and development of enhancements. In 2001, for example, President Bush barred the use of federal funds for human embryonic stem cell research other than on stem cell lines derived from embryos that had been destroyed before the announcement of the president's policy.[63] But this did not limit the use of private or state financing of research. In 2004, voters in California passed Proposition 71, a ballot initiative that provided $3 billion in funding for stem cell research at California universities and research institutions; a new state agency was created to administer the program, the California Institute for Regenerative Medicine, which makes grants and loans for stem cell research and research facility construction.[64] Stem cell research programs also have been established at Harvard, Johns Hopkins, the University of Minnesota, and the University of Texas.[65]

Even if it appears impossible to implement a truly effective ban on biomedical enhancements, some enhancement opponents might still seek to enact prohibitory laws on account of their symbolic value. Making enhancements illegal sends a statement about how much their use disturbs us. This approach finds support in a popular movement within the legal academy that emphasizes what it calls an "expressive function" for law, the idea that laws can play an important social role by signaling what is and is not socially acceptable. For example, in explaining why some criminal laws remain on the books despite being almost impossible to enforce, such as laws that punish certain forms of consensual sex between adults (for example, sodomy), one law professor observes that "the criminal law is less an instrument of social control than an announcement of moral values. That is why foreseeably unenforceable laws are enacted and why laws demonstrated to be unenforceable are not repealed."[66] But symbolic laws may exact a net social cost. A realization that legislatures intentionally enact provisions that they know cannot be enforced could corrode respect for the law in general. This is especially likely if it is hard to tell which commands are symbolic, because this would make it hard to know which ones actually need to be obeyed. When Nevada kept its sodomy law in effect despite being unable to enforce it, advocates for repeal argued that this undermined the power and authority of law in general.[67] Other critics point out that unenforceable laws can get in the way of laws that should be enforced. Efforts to lock up sexual perverts, for example, can bag so many petty offenders that serious pedophiles and sexual sadists remain at large.[68] Finally, any positive impact from symbolically making biomedical enhancements illegal is likely to be outweighed by the negative effect of transforming the user, who merely wanted to look better, do better at work, or excel at school, into a criminal.

Loss of Benefit

So far I have identified a number of reasons why we should think twice about extending the ban on biomedical enhancements in sports to other realms of activity. But there is an even more compelling reason why a ban on enhancements must not be allowed to spread beyond sports. Although enhancements in sports may confer benefits on individual athletes and teams, they don't do much for society. About the only way they might be said to produce public good is by promoting national prestige in international competitions such as the Olympics, which could aid in winning confrontations such as the Cold War, and perhaps by making some sporting events more exciting for fans, which could boost revenues for sponsors and investors. Of course, not everyone would agree that sports should become a battleground for nations and ideologies, or that sports ought to cater to fans' more atavistic tastes.

Outside of sports, on the other hand, biomedical enhancements could produce a vast amount of societal benefit. Presumably, the enhancements would be relatively safe, because otherwise they might produce a net loss for society. But assuming that any health risks that they present stay within our collective comfort zones, effective biomedical enhancements could make a huge positive difference, not only in individuals' lives but also for the collective good. Muscle-building drugs that evoke howls of outrage from sports officials could enable rescuers to save lives by lifting heavier objects. Alertness drugs prohibited by the Olympics could prevent automobile accidents. Beta blockers that cost athletes their medals could help steady surgeons' hands. Cognition-enhancing chemicals banned in games like chess or bridge could help people to be more productive at work. Soldiers could be more combat-effective. People could lead better sex lives.

Even enhancements that at first might not seem capable of producing net social benefit may on closer reflection be seen to do so. Cosmetic surgery, which may look like little more than a method of catering to a person's vanity, might give people the self-esteem that allows them to become more engaged and productive members of society. Some have said that truly effective antiaging interventions might threaten many aspects of our social system, from the solvency of Social Security and Medicare, to expected career arcs, to the structure of the nuclear family. But antiaging technologies also might improve productivity and give people time in which to perfect socially valued skills and increase their wisdom. Even the use of cognition-enhancing agents to improve test scores, likely to be condemned as a form of cheating, might have a positive effect if it gets the test-takers into the habit of using enhancements whenever the quality of their performance is critical. This also would help negate the concern that enhancements would ruin the predictive value of tests such as college entrance examinations, because the tests would predict the level of future performance of test-takers—who are then expected to continue to use enhancements at critical times in the future.

The social benefits obtainable from biomedical enhancements could be especially important in an era of global shortages and increasing global competition. As noted earlier, enhancement enthusiasts such as James Canton of the Institute for Global Futures think that biomedical enhancement is the key to our economic survival. From their perspective, advanced economies must maintain their technological edge if they hope to vie with emerging industrial giants and cheap labor markets. Given that biomedical enhancement is one of the new technological frontiers, woe to the developed country that does not maintain a lead in enhancement research, development, and use.

Chapter 9

The War on Enhancements

Despite the tremendous tangible and intangible costs of trying to prevent people from using biomedical enhancements outside of sports, including the loss of substantial societal benefits to the extent that these efforts would have been successful had they proceeded unhindered, a campaign against enhancement use in general is in fact under way.

A major enemy in this campaign is genetic enhancement. The NIH officially refuses to fund research on genetic engineering for enhancement purposes.[1] Although this stance might be chalked up to a conviction that preventing, curing, or mitigating disease is a more worthy way of expending scarce research resources, the NIH position is undoubtedly also an attempt to mollify critics of genetic enhancement. The American Medical Association regards genetic enhancement as unethical. An opinion of its Council on Ethical and Judicial Affairs proclaims that "efforts to enhance 'desirable' characteristics through the insertion of a modified or additional gene, or efforts to 'improve' complex human traits—the eugenic development of offspring—are contrary not only to the ethical tradition of medicine, but also to the egalitarian values of our society."[2] As noted earlier, the AMA also opposes using gene transfer technology to enhance children unless certain conditions can be met: There must be "clear and meaningful benefit to the fetus or child; no trade-off with other characteristics or traits, [and] equal access . . . irrespective of income or other socioeconomic characteristics."[3] (The second of these conditions is indefensible. Exactly how can a body of physicians rule out the possibility that a significant gain in one ability—say, high-level cognitive functioning—can ever be justified if it is accompanied by a minor degradation of some other, arguably less important, trait, like a loss of half an inch in height?)

Nevertheless, the reasons that genetic enhancement is singled out as a major foe are understandable. As described in chapter 1, the science of human genetics is full of surprises, like the much smaller number of genes than had been expected and the stretches of DNA that previously were thought to be superfluous but turn out to have important regulatory functions. The techniques for genetic manipulation are new and poorly understood. Just when scientists think they've licked a major technical problem, like how to deliver modified genes to the right place in the body, their methods turns out to have hidden dangers. A good example, mentioned earlier, is the French effort to use gene therapy to cure a disease in infants called X-linked severe combined immunodeficiency syndrome (X-SCID). With the aim of producing white blood cells with a proper immune response, the French researchers took stem cells from the children's bone marrow, used a standard retrovirus to insert corrected DNA into the cells, and returned the modified cells to the children's bone marrow. At first, the procedure seemed to have succeeded: ten boys developed functioning immune systems. But it turned out that the retrovirus that the researchers had used to insert the corrected DNA into the stem cells had lodged in a position in the children's DNA that was too near a gene that, if stimulated, can cause leukemia, a form of cancer. Three of the boys contracted the cancer.

Caution when dealing with genetic enhancement thus stems from a legitimate fear of making mistakes. That a mistake involves genes also gives rise to the concern that it could spread out of control. Remember that it was this risk from Paul Berg's recombinant DNA *E. coli* experiment that led to the voluntary moratorium on recombinant DNA research. In the case of genetic engineering, the apprehension is that the mistakes could become so widespread that they corrupt the human gene pool itself, in the same way that it is feared that a failed experiment with genetically modified plants or animals could infect and destroy entire ecosystems. At the extreme, humanity might become infertile or incapable of surviving some new environmental insult, such as a previously unknown disease.

But Courtney Campbell, director of the Program for Ethics, Science, and the Environment at Oregon State University, points out that failure itself is not the problem: "Failure, after all, is an integral learning occasion in the trial-and-error methodology of science."[4] The real fear is that scientists will succeed—but not in the way they anticipated. As Campbell explains, Willard Gaylin, a psychiatrist who cofounded a bioethics think tank called the Hastings Center, gave a name to this fear in the title of an article he wrote in 1977 describing public concern over recombinant DNA technology. He called it "the Frankenstein factor."[5] According to Gaylin, the Frankenstein factor colors high-tech research "that is seen as changing or controlling the 'nature' of the species or controlling behavior." In Gaylin's view, the Frankenstein factor operates to distort the public perception of this kind of research by investing it with "an extra dimension of anxiety and concern" that is unwarranted. If scientific progress is to proceed unimpeded, it "must be shielded from the prejudice of ignorance."

The Frankenstein factor is attacked in a 1999 article on genetic enhancement in the magazine *Science*.[6] The author, physician and genetics researcher Jon W. Gordon warns not only that a ban on gene transfer for enhancement purposes would be "cumbersome" but also, more important, that "fear of genetic manipulation may encourage proposals to limit basic investigations that might ultimately lead to effective human gene transfer." Because he believes the fear to be unwarranted, its adverse impact on scientific progress, in his opinion, would be indefensible: "Gene transfer studies may never lead to successful genetic enhancement, but they are certain to provide new treatment and prevention strategies for a variety of devastating diseases. No less significant is the potential for this research to improve our understanding of the most complex and compelling phenomenon ever observed—the life process. We cannot be expected to deny ourselves this knowledge."

Gordon specifically seeks to allay the fear that germline genetic enhancement could have a deleterious effect on the human gene pool. In Gordon's opinion, "this solemn pronouncement is totally without scientific foundation." The reason, he maintains, is simple arithmetic: Worldwide, there are 11 million babies born each month. If one of them were enhanced, by the time he or she had a child, 2.64 billion unenhanced children would have been born. Even if a thousand genetically engineered children were born each year, they would comprise only 1 out of every 320,000 live births. Any alterations that they introduced into the gene pool "would be swamped by the random attempts of Mother Nature."

Gordon may be incorrect, however, when he assumes that germline genetic enhancement is unlikely to take place on a large scale. "Passive" forms of germline engineering, such as selecting embryos for implantation during IVF on the basis of genetic tests, are becoming increasingly widespread. In 2005, more than 52,000 children were born with the aid of assisted reproductive methods, which could have enabled their parents to employ preimplantation genetic testing.[7] At present the only "enhancement" test being used is gender selection, but this is bound to change as tests become available for more nonmedical traits. On a worldwide basis, the impact from preimplantation testing alone would be much greater than Gordon suggests.

Yet preimplantation testing is a fairly primitive form of genetic engineering, because it enables parents to select only from among a naturally occurring set of traits—indeed, only those traits that showed up in the dozen or so embryos fertilized in the laboratory. Even a large number of these births probably would not affect the gene pool as dramatically as active genetic manipulation, which could involve characteristics not found in nature. Gordon is correct that this active type of genetic engineering is much farther off. But it is impossible to predict the pace of science. Even if we are talking decades, or a century, the long-term integrity of the gene pool may be much less assured than Gordon believes.

This is why Campbell is unwilling to dismiss the Frankenstein factor as the misconceptions of, in Gaylin's words, the "scientifically illiterate." Unlike mistakes, which teach scientists to go back and change the methodology of their experiments to produce a better result, the horror of the Frankenstein factor is success and the fact that it is irreversible: "There is no going back; the monstrosity must be lived with." To Campbell's way of thinking, the problem is scientific hubris, and the way to avoid it is to adhere to nine principles he describes as "the elements of a caring and careful science and biotechnology," which revolve around "humility," "pausing," and "restraint." It therefore might follow that a war against genetic enhancement is justified in order to slow science down so that we are not blindsided by it. Even if the war ultimately is doomed to failure, it can buy us time to permit, in Campbell's words, "an exercise of imagination and responsibility to consider unanticipated and unwanted outcomes to counter the boundless progressive rhetoric of a 'brighter future.'"

The question is whether buying that time is worth the cost, in terms of the expense of enforcement and the damage that its intrusiveness would do to the fabric of civil society. "History has shown," Gordon asserts, "that effort is far better spent in preparing society to cope with scientific advances than in attempting to restrict basic research." Moreover, slowing things down is no guarantee that we can dodge catastrophe. Incremental rather than dramatic scientific developments may lull us into incorrectly assuming that progress is not taking place, with us "waking up" only after it is too late to react effectively. Remember the proverbial frog in the slowly heated pot, who, in contrast to the frog who jumps out when thrust into hot water, fails to notice the change in temperature and gets cooked.

So far we have been considering whether a war specifically targeting genetic enhancement can be justified. But genetic enhancement is not the sole enemy in the war against biomedical enhancements. Not surprisingly, the campaign against steroids in sports has spilled over into society in general. For example, steroids taken under proper medical supervision could give police and firefighters extra strength that could come in handy in their jobs, but the Drug Enforcement Administration actively goes after police and firefighters and turns the results of its investigations over to local law enforcement authorities for punishment.[8] In Ohio, for example, three police officers were charged with illegal steroid use in 2003. One of the leaders of this crusade against steroid use by law enforcement personnel is the former executive director of the Kentucky Chiefs of Police Association, who coauthored an article on steroid use by police in 1991.[9] He doesn't buy the argument that steroids could help cops stand up to physically threatening thugs, and he is convinced that officers take steroids merely to improve their appearance. Why would police officers need to take steroids to protect themselves, he argues, when "they give you a damn gun."[10]

Human growth hormone, another substance taken by athletes to enhance performance, also is the target of antienhancement crusaders outside of sports. As noted in chapter 7, in 1990 Congress placed HGH in a unique regulatory status by making it the only drug that it is a federal felony to distribute for off-label uses—for purposes other than those expressly approved by the FDA. Not only does this prohibition include physicians who give HGH to athletes, it also extends to doctors who prescribe injections of the hormones to as many as thirty thousand patients who believe that HGH may retard the aging process.[11] The FDA has sent warning letters—a notice that the agency believes that the addressee is in violation of the law—to several companies accusing them of marketing HGH for antiaging.[12]

It is true that, unlike steroids, which clearly help to build muscles, there is little evidence that HGH is effective against aging. A 2007 review of the available clinical studies found that healthy older individuals who were given HGH had less fat mass and more lean body mass than those not receiving HGH but that HGH did not improve maximal oxygen consumption, bone mineral density, lipid levels, or fasting glucose and insulin levels, all of which are considered important indicators of aging. The authors also reported significant amounts of joint pain and fluid retention among HGH users.[13]

One of the leading voices against the antiaging use of HGH is Dr. Tom Perls, an associate professor of medicine at Boston University. In 2004, Perls fired off a letter to the FDA after he saw an article in the Miami Herald in which an FDA official was quoted as stating that off-label prescribing of HGH was legal. The FDA wrote back and explained that Perls had misread the quotation.[14] Perls also operates a website dedicated to "antiaging quackery."[15] According to Perls's website, he decided to take on the antiaging industry "when he noted the pernicious and deceitful picture of older people painted by many antiaging clinics, websites and hucksters. Such marketing promotes terrible and completely unwarranted biases. Learning more about the most popularized treatment, Dr. Perls realized that the promotion of HGH is unquestionably dangerous and illegal quackery."[16] However, an article in the Boston University newspaper suggests that Perls incidentally may be furthering his own research interests: "Perls, a MED [Boston University School of Medicine] associate professor, whose own longevity research examines nutrition, lifestyles, and genes—not magic hormone energy potions—hopes that the JAMA study will ring the "death knell" for the use of HGH as an anti-aging agent."[17]

Antienhancement forces also are skirmishing against the use of beta blockers, such as propranolol. As mentioned in chapter 1, these drugs, which slow the heart rate, have been used by athletes who need to alternate suddenly between intense physical exertion and utter calm, for example, competitors in a biathlon. Such drugs also have become popular outside of sports for those who need steady hands, such as surgeons and musicians, especially among string players, who tend to skitter their bows across the strings when they become nervous. There does not seem to be any effort to stop the use by surgeons, but there is considerable controversy within the music world over the drug, and a music teacher at Rhodes College in Tennessee was fired after she recommended to her students that they take propranolol to combat performance anxiety.[18] It is conceivable that in the future, foes of enhancement may require musicians vying for prizes in competitions to give urine samples to show that they were not using the drug.

The War on Drugs essentially began as a war against mood alteration, and it continues to be aimed at these substances, although of course alcohol, the most widely used mood-enhancer of them all, usually gets a pass. In 1969 Richard Nixon sent Congress legislation placing marijuana and LSD in the top category of dangerous substances, along with heroin.[19] Public attention next focused on tranquilizers, which the Rolling Stones popularized as "mother's little helpers." According to one group of commentators, "doctors and patients alike enthusiastically welcomed the advent of the benzodiazapines. . . . Their safety and efficacy led to a general belief, again among much of the medical profession as well as the public, that benzodiazepines were the simple answer to overcoming the emotional strains of everyday living."[20] Doctors were criticized for prescribing them to patients who had not been diagnosed with well-defined anxiety disorders, even though mental illnesses, including anxiety disorders, are often poorly defined and difficult to diagnose.[21] In a paper in the journal *Neuroscience,* a professor of psychiatry from Great Britain, borrowing from Marx, called tranquilizers "the opium of the masses."[22] Barbara Gordon, in *I'm Dancing as Fast as I Can,* described the severe side effects she suffered. In 1979, the U.S. Senate held hearings on benzodiazepine "use and abuse."

After tranquilizers, criticism turned to antidepressants, especially the new class of selective serotonin reuptake inhibitors (SSRIs), and the flagship drug, Prozac, introduced in 1988. There had always been unease about Prozac. Peter Kramer, an early champion of the drug in his 1993 book *Listening to Prozac,* questioned whether those who were transformed by it had become their "real" selves, as some of them maintained. Lauren Slater's 1998 memoir *Prozac Diary* described how the drug changed her life, but in ways that were complicated and not always welcome. One of the most vigorous attacks against Prozac was waged by the Church of Scientology, which opposes psychiatry and psychotropic drugs in general. In 1989, it launched a campaign against the drug after a coroner's report found some in the blood of an employee who had killed nine people, including himself, at a Louisville, Kentucky, printing company. In 1991, the church's Citizens Commission for Human Rights unsuccessfully petitioned the FDA to ban Prozac. Heber Jentzsch, the church's president, decried Eli Lilly, the manufacturer of Prozac, for having "a multi-billion killer drug on the market, and they want to keep it no matter how many people die on it."[23] Lilly responded by reprinting and distributing to physicians 250,000 copies of a cover story in *Time* magazine entitled "Scientology: The Cult of Greed." Scientology in turn spent $3 million on a series of full-page attack ads in *USA Today,* including four specifically lambasting Prozac. Lilly's director of corporate communications countered that the church was motivated by its financial self-interest in selling its members its own costly, nondrug treatment programs.[24]

Concern then shifted to whether people who were taking SSRIs were truly depressed, just as tranquilizer critics had questioned whether their users were really anxious. Carl Elliott speculated in his 2003 book *Better Than Well: American Medicine Meets the American Dream* that Prozac was being used to enhance mood rather than to treat clinical depression. At the same time, sadness was becoming fashionable. In an essay entitled "In Praise of Melancholy," for example, English professor Eric Wilson states: "Melancholia, far from a disease or weakness of will, is an almost miraculous invitation to transcend the banal status quo and imagine the untapped possibilities for existence. Without melancholia, the earth would likely freeze over into a fixed state, as predictable as metal. Only with the help of constant sorrow can this dying world be changed, enlivened, pushed to the new."[25] The SSRIs thus impair the joy of being sad.

Antienhancement forces are going after more than just prescription drugs used as enhancements. They also are attacking one of the oldest and safest substances, caffeine. As noted earlier, the Olympics banned caffeine until recently, and now places it on a "monitoring list," which means that athletes will continue to be tested for the substance but will not be punished if the tests come back positive.[26] If caffeine use increases beyond levels considered acceptable, however, WADA could restore it to the list of prohibited substances. Caffeine is still banned in college sports. The National Collegiate Athletic Association has established a maximum level of 15 micrograms of caffeine per milliliter of blood.[27] Athletes can exceed this level if they drink more than about 500 milligrams of caffeine in an hour, the equivalent of approximately two large Starbucks coffees.[28]

The campaign against caffeine is being waged outside of sports as well. Major targets are caffeine supplements and especially energy drinks, such as Red Bull. In 2006, sales of energy drinks in the United States rose to about $3.7 billion, an increase of 51 percent over the preceding year.[29] Antienhancement critics purport to be concerned primarily about safety issues, citing research at Northwestern University that showed that, over three years, the Illinois Poison Control Center received 250 reports of caffeine overdoses, with the average age of the victims 21, as well as worries that the drinks could cause dehydration in high school athletes and that, according to a report from Brazil, drinkers who mixed alcoholic and energy drinks were less able to recognize when they were inebriated.[30] Many of these concerns relate to use by minors, because energy drinks contain about twice the amount of caffeine as the average caffeinated soft drink.[31] Yet Red Bull has been banned in both France and Denmark for adults as well as children. EU officials challenged the French ban in the European Court of Justice, claiming that it impermissibly restrained trade, but in 2004, the court ruled that the ban could stand so long as the French government could prove that the drink posed health risks to users.[32] Ironically, Red Bull claims to be the first supplement to be certified as being free of banned substances under the new standards established by Major League Baseball.[33]

Attacks on caffeine are not limited to caffeine supplements and energy drinks. The soft drink industry has bowed to pressure and is disclosing caffeine content on soft drink labels.[34] In its 2007 annual innovations issue, the *New York Times* magazine describes a new urinalysis technique that tests sewer water, enabling police and doctors to detect "what illicit drugs the population of an entire city is ingesting." According to the article, the single most popular of these "illicit" drugs is caffeine. In February 2006, the mayor of Shaker Heights, Ohio, issued a proclamation stating that caffeine is linked to heart disease, hypoglycemia, central nervous system disorders, and some cancers, and declaring March 2006 to be "National Caffeine Awareness Month" in the upscale Ohio city. She was not alone; many mayors have taken similar action. It turns out that the request for the proclamations, as well as the wording of the warnings, came from an outfit called the Caffeine Awareness

Alliance, headed by Marina Kushner. Kushner also is president of a company called Soy Coffee LLC, which markets a caffeine-free coffee substitute.[35] The embarrassed Shaker Heights mayor, claiming that she wasn't aware of the alliance's conflict of interest, withdrew the proclamation and handed out to city employees bags of coffee she bought from a local coffee shop.[36]

So far, the war on enhancements outside of sports is fitful. While this might be because it does not attract enough support, the more likely reason is that it is just getting started. New, safe, and effective performance-enhancement drugs and techniques are only now beginning to be discovered. Genetic research still has a long way to go before genetic enhancement engineering becomes a reality. The military is just starting to incorporate biomedical enhancements into warfighting. There is no question that opposition to expanded uses of biomedical enhancement outside of sports is waiting in the wings.

As this chapter has shown, prohibition, the approach taken by most sports, clearly is not the right approach for society in general. It would create a nightmare police state which in the end would be unable to stop widespread use. In the meantime, society would lose enormous social benefits.

Yet as pointed out in chapter 2, enhancement opponents have several valid concerns. Some enhancements are dangerous and others are hoaxes. If society is going to be able to capture the benefits of legitimate uses of enhancements, it needs access to enhancements that are safe and effective. Another concern is whether enhancements will be available to everyone or only to the well-off, in which case they would widen the gap between haves and have-nots, with perhaps disastrous societal consequences. Finally, some individuals may need protection against making unwise decisions about whether or not to use enhancements or to participate in risky enhancement research, including children and persons who face undue pressures to excel.

Clearly, then, there is a need for some controls on biomedical enhancements to promote the public good. If the model of sports is not the solution, we must look elsewhere.

Chapter 10

Promoting Safety, Efficacy, and Informed Decisionmaking

ALTHOUGH THE repressive stance of sports clearly is insupportable outside of sports, this does not mean that society should take a laissez-faire approach toward biomedical enhancement that permits people to manufacture and market enhancements without any government intervention and that leaves individuals entirely free to decide for themselves whether or not to use them. While this approach might appeal to a desire for personal liberty, it creates a number of problems, many of which ultimately may have the effect of impairing personal liberty.

A chief concern is protecting people from unsafe or ineffective enhancement products and services. The health risks of anabolic steroids and the lack of evidence that human growth hormone retards aging, for example, have already been described. Without government oversight, people attempting to enhance themselves might suffer serious injury or waste large sums of money on dangerous or useless interventions.

History bears out this concern. In the early nineteenth century, many people followed Samuel Thomson, who believed that all illness was caused by cold and could be treated by heat. Then there were the homeopaths, who, explains medical sociologist Paul Starr in his landmark book *The Social Transformation of American Medicine,* "saw disease primarily as a matter of spirit" and believed that an illness could be cured with small doses of drugs that, in healthy persons, produced the same symptoms as the disease produced in patients. Immunizations aside, this sounds bizarre today, but the Hahnemann Medical School in Philadelphia, the Boston University School of Medicine, and the medical school at the University of Michigan all began as homeopathic institutions.

Other schools of medical thought arose in the late nineteenth century. They included osteopathy and chiropractic, both of which focused on the misalignment of body parts as the source of all ailments. There also were religious-based schools of thought, such as mesmerism, the idea that healing could be accomplished by putting people into trances, which was popular with a number of New England Universalist ministers, and Christian Science, which believes in healing through prayer.[1] The nineteenth century also saw the growth of patent medicines, products such as Hamlins Wizard Oil, Dr. James' Soothing Syrup (which contained heroin), Lungardia (containing, among other things, turpentine and kerosene), Tuberculene (which contained creosote), and "Widow Read's Ointment for the Itch," produced by Benjamin Franklin's mother-in-law.[2]

To protect the public from these nineteenth-century practices, the nation turned to a combination of government programs and professional self-regulation. Followers of the so-called allopathic school in the nineteenth century, which we now know as modern scientific medicine, gained control of medical education and state medical boards and excluded rival practitioners or, as in the case of chiropractors, drastically curtailed their authority to practice the healing arts. In 1906, Congress passed the Pure Food and Drug Act, the forerunner to today's food and drug laws. The first successful prosecution under the 1906 act was against the maker of a patent medicine called "Cuforhedake Brane-Fude."[3] The Food and Drug Administration now enforces a system in which manufacturers who wish to market new drugs or medical devices must submit to the agency the results of large-scale trials showing that their products are safe and efficacious for the intended uses. FDA diligence, for example, spared the United States the worst effects of the thalidomide tragedy in the late 1950s and early 1960s by blocking the drug from being sold here.

The question is whether government regulators and medical professionals can protect us from unsafe or ineffective biomedical enhancements. The need for this protection is exacerbated by unscrupulous entrepreneurs, the modern equivalent of "snake oil salesmen," who sell dubious enhancement products to unsuspecting consumers. For example, there is a flourishing antiaging industry that makes a fortune selling HGH and other unproven regimens for antiaging purposes. A group of colleagues and I described these marketing efforts as follows in a 2004 article in the journal of the Gerontological Society of America:

> As the Internet has become a widely used medium of communication, antiaging Web sites, such as "Youngevity: The Anti-Aging Company," have proliferated. According to the American Medical Association, 2,500 physicians have established specialty practices devoted to "longevity medicine." An American Academy of Anti-Aging Medicine (A4M), created in 1993, has grown to 12,000 members and receives 1.8 million hits per month on its Web site; its net assets increased from $650,000 in 1997 to $5.3 million in 2000. The goal of the clinical anti-aging community is to extend the time its patients can live without the morbidities of the aging process: "memory loss, muscle loss, visual impairment, slowed gait and speech, wrinkling of the skin, hardening of the arteries, and all the other maladies we call aging." Some of its members go even further. The president of A4M has authored books with titles such as *Grow Young with HGH: The Amazing Medically Proven Plan to Reverse Aging.*[4]

The Role of the FDA

Unfortunately, the FDA's ability to ensure that biomedical enhancements are safe and effective is limited. To begin to understand the FDA's limits, bear in mind that there is no such thing as a completely safe medical intervention. Every drug or medical procedure is accompanied by risks. A substance as safe as pure water can be deadly, as a Sacramento radio station learned when a participant died after drinking too much of it during a contest called "Hold your pee for a Wii," in which a Nintendo console was awarded to the person who could consume the most water without going to the bathroom.[5] Even a test can be dangerous, for example, by yielding a false result. The real question is not how safe an intervention is but whether its risks are outweighed by its benefits. When the FDA approves a new drug or device as "safe," what the agency really is saying is that it considers the health hazards of the product to be acceptable in view of the potential health benefits. Under this approach, even steroids might be considered safe enough for some enhancement uses, such as by rescue workers.

The goal of "effectiveness" also is elusive. Current FDA practice is that a drug or device will be considered efficacious if it performs better in clinical trials than a placebo.[6] In many cases, even if there already is a drug or device that is considered standard treatment for the target condition, it may be withheld from patients serving as subjects, and the experimental intervention compared instead with a placebo.[7] Consequently, determining that a product is efficacious usually means merely showing that it is better than nothing, rather than that it is superior to existing options. Accordingly, an FDA finding that, based on clinical trials, a cognition-enhancing drug had been found to be efficacious might not actually mean that it was better at enhancing cognition than other drugs or techniques.

In addition, there often is disagreement about how well a drug or device has to work for it to be deemed efficacious. In medical terms, this is the issue of whether the product is "clinically" efficacious—that is, whether the difference it makes to an individual's health or well-being is significant enough to be considered worthwhile. Clinical efficacy in part is a question of how much of an effect the product produces. In one case that made it to the courts, a drug company challenged the FDA's refusal to deem its oral proteolytic enzyme product effective to reduce swelling after hand surgery despite studies showing that it did so. A federal court of appeals upheld the agency's argument that, although the product indeed reduced swelling better than a placebo, the amount of reduction, a mere quarter of an inch, was not clinically meaningful.[8] Clinical efficacy also is a matter of what type of effect is produced. In his classic analysis of so-called clot busters, drugs such as streptokinase and tissue plasminogen activator that are administered to heart attack patients to reopen blocked blood vessels, bioethicist Baruch Brody relates the FDA's deliberations over whether it should be enough for studies to show that a drug breaks up clots, or whether the manufacturer should have to go further and demonstrate that the removal of the blockage relieves the symptoms of the heart attack or improves the patient's chances for long-term survival.[9] In the case of biomedical enhancements, the question might be whether studies that showed, say, that a drug produced a 2 percent improvement in the ability to memorize a series of letters or single-digit numbers without corresponding impact on any other cognitive abilities should be deemed sufficient evidence of effective cognitive enhancement.

Even if studies showed that a drug worked, the findings may be contradicted by later research. One commentator identified the 45 most widely cited reports of efficacy from clinical trials published in three major medical journals between 1990 and 2003. When he examined subsequent research on the interventions, he found that it contradicted the efficacy findings in seven cases and that the newer data showed a much weaker effect in seven others.[10]

Furthermore, the bulk of the FDA approval process is focused not on whether a product is effective but on whether it is "efficacious." This refers to the fact that clinical trials take place under highly artificial conditions, where subjects are screened to make sure they fit certain narrow criteria, and where the experimenters are specially trained to employ the investigational drug or device correctly. Neither of these conditions obtain in the real world, where virtually any practitioner can provide a new technology to practically anyone they wish. As a result, a product that works well within the confines of an experiment may not work well once it becomes widely marketed. The FDA is expanding its efforts to monitor how well drugs and devices work after they are approved, but the agency primarily is focused on detecting adverse health effects rather than lack of effectiveness.

Finally, in establishing that a drug or device is efficacious, the FDA does not consider its cost. This means that the fact of a drug or device receiving FDA approval says nothing about whether the drug provides a decent bang for the buck or whether it is a better deal than existing alternatives. The agency concerns itself with cost issues only when a manufacturer explicitly claims that its product is more cost-effective than a competitor's.[11] In the case of medical interventions to treat injury or disease, the primary source of concern about cost-effectiveness comes from third-party payers, such as employers, government health care programs, and private insurance companies, who attempt to hold down spending by steering patients away from ineffective products and services and toward cheaper treatment alternatives. But it is important to realize that third-party payers do not pay for biomedical enhancements. When a person gets a facelift or takes a beta blocker to prevent stage fright, they pay for these things out of their own pockets. Consumers therefore cannot rely on their health plans to help them figure out whether or not an enhancement works or is worth the cost.

These limitations also would reduce the value of the FDA's review of the safety of enhancement products. The agency approved Botox injections to remove frown lines on the basis of the results of two studies with a total of 537 subjects, 450 of whom received Botox, and the rest injections of a placebo.[12] Did the studies show that Botox was safe? That depends. Almost half of the subjects who received the active drug (44 percent) reported adverse effects, including headache, respiratory infection, nausea, flulike symptoms, and drooping of the eyelid (blepharoptosis). Roughly the same incidence of side effects occurred in the subjects receiving the placebo injections, indicating that the problems were caused by the injection itself rather than by the ingredients in Botox. The one exception was the eyelid drooping, which occurred only in the group receiving Botox. So is Botox "safe"? The FDA thought so, yet the drug clearly caused problems. Moreover, these problems appeared within the confines of the clinical trial. It is safe to expect even more adverse effects to occur when the drug is administered in a less carefully controlled environment by less well-trained practitioners.

What about Botox's effectiveness? Data from the two clinical trials clearly showed that Botox was better than placebo injections at reducing frown lines. But again this was only under the unusual conditions of the studies. Furthermore, the studies only assessed glabellar frown lines—the lines that appear between the eyebrows. The FDA accordingly approved the drug only for reducing that one type of frown line, but the product is often administered to reduce wrinkles in other areas of the face and neck.[13] With regard to these off-label uses, there is no evidence of effectiveness from adequate and well-controlled experiments. In addition, the studies only compared Botox to a placebo. There are no data comparing Botox to other techniques for reducing wrinkles, such as conventional cosmetics. Finally, the studies relied on by the FDA tell us nothing about whether Botox is good value for the money. Even if Botox works better than regular cosmetics, its cost (about $400 a treatment) may make it non-cost-effective, meaning that a person could pay less for some other treatment and still obtain a satisfactory result.

But Botox is an anomaly, in that it is one of the few products that the FDA has reviewed and approved as an enhancement. (Others are breast implants, liposuction machines, and certain types of contact lenses.) This means that, by and large, enhancement drugs and devices that are currently available have not been subject to the rigorous type of clinical investigation required by the FDA for their enhancement uses and instead are prescribed for enhancement use on an off-label basis. Some information about the safety of these products would exist, because the basic compounds or instruments would have been studied in animals and humans as a prerequisite to being approved for their medical uses. But this safety information would suffer from the same limitations discussed earlier that characterize evidence of efficacy from clinical trials—the highly regimented and artificial conditions of the study, which may bear little resemblance to real-world use. More important, there is no telling whether even this limited safety profile would apply to a product's enhancement use, which may entail different types of people, different dosage strengths and frequencies, and even introduction into different parts of the body. FDA regulations require manufacturers to notify the agency when they learn of adverse events that occur in connection with any uses of their drug or device, including off-label uses, but it is well known that there is significant underreporting of adverse events in general and no reason to believe that the picture would be any rosier in connection with biomedical enhancements in particular.[14]

In addition to the phenomenon of off-label use, biomedical enhancements may fall through a number of other gaps in the government's regulatory framework. Some enhancements are marketed as dietary supplements. According to the Dietary Supplement Health and Education Act (DSHEA), enacted in 1994, a product can qualify as a dietary supplement if it does not make a claim to treat a specific disease, bears a disclaimer on the label that the product is not approved by the FDA, and is taken by mouth.[15] Before the passage of DSHEA, for example, the FDA would have regulated as a drug a product that made any of the following claims: "Increase Energy Level; Lose Fat & Gain Muscle; Improves Sleep; Improves Cholesterol Levels; Improves Kidney Function; Improves Immune Function; Increase Memory; Increases Muscle Mass & Tone; Increase Strength, Energy and Endurance; Increases Exercise Performance; Mental Clarity; Lowers Body Fat %'s; Skin & Hair Improved; Strengthens Immune System; Help Create Stronger Bones; Lowers Blood Pressure; Reduces Wrinkles and Create Tighter, Smoother Skin; Improves Sex Drive and Performance; Improves Immune and Heart Function; Bone Density; Healing Time; Improves Brain Function, Memory and Mental Focus."[16] Since none of the attributes mentioned is a disease, the product in question, an "HGH Complex Spray," can be sold as a dietary supplement: it "lowers blood pressure" rather than treating high blood pressure; "improves cholesterol levels" instead of slowing the progression of atherosclerosis; and so on.

The DSHEA law was deliberately designed by the dietary supplement industry to make the FDA regime governing dietary supplements much looser than the one that regulates drugs and medical devices. A drug or device manufacturer must persuade the agency that its product is safe and effective before it can be marketed. In the case of a dietary supplement, however, the burden shifts to the FDA to show that a product is unsafe before the agency can restrict its sale or remove it from the market. (The only exception is for an ingredient that was not marketed in the United States as a dietary supplement or an ingredient in food before the passage of DSHEA; in that case, before marketing a product containing the ingredient, the manufacturer must supply the FDA with "information, including published articles, that supports a reasonable expectation of safety." However, this is less of a showing than required of a manufacturer of a new drug or device, which must submit reports of "adequate tests by all methods reasonably applicable to show whether or not the drug is safe for use under the conditions prescribed, recommended, or suggested in the proposed labeling thereof.")[17] The agency has removed only one dietary supplement ingredient from the market because of its health risks, ephedra. Moreover, until recently, manufacturers of dietary supplements were not required to notify the FDA when they found out that their products caused injury, and there was little voluntary reporting.[18] In 2007, Congress passed a new law requiring dietary supplement makers to report "serious adverse events" to the FDA, but this is still weaker than the reporting requirements for drugs, whose manufacturers must notify the agency of all adverse events, rather than just ones that are "serious."[19]

Dietary supplements are a concern for organized sports. As baseball commissioner Bud Selig and baseball executive Robert D. Manfred Jr. explain, both the Olympics and the National Collegiate Athletic Association have established broad bans against the use of many nutritional supplements. But the unions that represent professional athletes are resistant to prohibiting products that may be purchased lawfully over the counter.[20]

Another category of biomedical enhancements that, with few exceptions, is exempt from FDA review is cosmetic surgery. This follows from the fact that the FDA does not have the statutory authority to regulate "the practice of medicine," which includes surgery. This can get confusing, however, because the FDA does have the authority to regulate medical devices, including devices that are employed during cosmetic surgery. It is based on this authority, for example, that the agency has reviewed the safety and efficacy of liposuction machines and breast implants. But a surgeon can devise a new way to perform a facelift or nose job without obtaining FDA approval, so long as the technique does not depend on the use of new types of equipment and can spread to other surgeons without anyone performing formal clinical studies to determine whether it is safe and efficacious. The FDA also does not regulate endogenous enhancements, that is, enhancements that employ substances found in the person's own body. For example, although the FDA regulates blood products used in transfusions, such as plasma and platelets, the agency has no authority over a person's own blood when it is withdrawn, stored, and later reinfused, a technique called "blood doping" that some athletes use to increase the supply of oxygen to their tissues.

The FDA's lack of jurisdiction over the practice of medicine also complicates its oversight of genetic technologies, including genetic interventions used for enhancement purposes. The FDA does regulate gene therapy, the introduction into the body of modified genes to prevent, cure, or mitigate disease, which the agency regards as falling within the definitions of both drugs and "biologics" in the Federal Food, Drug, and Cosmetic Act.[21] The insertion of modified genes for enhancement purposes, such as to promote muscle growth, clearly would fall within the statutory definition of a drug in the act, because that definition includes "articles (other than food) intended to affect the structure or any function of the body of man or other animals."[22] But the introduction of modified genes for enhancement rather than therapeutic purposes would not fit the definition of a biologic under the act, which is a "virus, therapeutic serum, toxin, antitoxin, or analogous product *applicable to the prevention, treatment or cure of diseases or injuries of man*."[23] This raises the question of whether it is too much of a stretch to consider genetic enhancement to be a "drug," which would place it within the agency's jurisdiction, rather than the practice of medicine, which lies beyond the agency's purview.

This question has come up in connection with human reproductive cloning. This technique would involve taking a person's cell and using chemicals or electricity to stimulate it to begin dividing so that it would become an embryo that could be implanted in the uterus and brought to term. The result, if successful, would be a child who was a virtual genetic replica of the person from whom the cell had been obtained. So far as is known, this has never been accomplished in humans, but people began to worry that it might be possible after British researcher Ian Wilmut announced in 1997 that he had successfully cloned Dolly the sheep from one of its mother's mammary cells. In 1998, while Congress was deliberating whether or not to enact a law prohibiting attempts to clone a living human being, the acting commissioner of the FDA, Michael Friedman, announced on the Diane Rehm talk show on National Public Radio that the FDA already had jurisdiction over human reproductive cloning. As improbable as it might seem, it sounded from his comments like the agency would regard cloning as a "drug."[24] A few months later, in a letter to the research community, Stuart Nightingale, the FDA's associate commissioner for medical affairs, asserted that the agency indeed intended to regulate reproductive cloning under its authority to regulate drugs, adding that the FDA would not permit any reproductive cloning experiments to take place.[25] Two years later, after American fertility doctor Panayiotis Zavos and Italian collaborator Severino Antinori announced that they would attempt to clone a human being outside the United States, Congress held a hearing on cloning at which Kathryn Zoon, then the director of the FDA's Center for Biologics Evaluation and Research, maintained that the agency had the authority to regulate human reproductive cloning not only as a drug but also as a medical device and a biologic.[26] But she didn't explain the rationale for the agency's position, prompting Richard Merrill, a law professor who was a former FDA chief counsel, to describe Zoon's testimony as "surprisingly delphic" and to complain that "repetition" of the assertion of the basis for jurisdiction served "as a substitute for explanation."[27]

The FDA also has asserted jurisdiction over an assisted reproductive technique called ooplasmic transfer, which is used to treat a certain type of infertility in which fertilized eggs do not implant themselves in the uterus due to the lack of proper enzymes in the ooplasm of the egg, the fluid that surrounds the nucleus. The technique, which was developed by a fertility clinic in New Jersey, entails taking a normal donor egg, removing ooplasmic fluid that contains working enzymes, and injecting that normal ooplasm into the infertile egg. The egg then can implant itself in the womb and develop into a fetus that can be brought to term. The problem is that, while this technique does not alter the DNA from the mother and father that is contained in the nucleus of the implanted egg, it does add a small amount of additional DNA from the donor of the normal egg that is found in structures in the ooplasm called mitochondria. Therefore, the cells of the resulting child, including its own eggs or sperm, contain DNA from more than just its parents. While this is not an intentional outcome but rather an incidental effect of the infertility technique, it technically makes ooplasmic transfer a form of germline genetic engineering, as both the clinicians themselves acknowledged and bioethicists Eric Juengst and Erik Parens reiterated in an editorial in *Science*.[28] As we will see in chapter 13, germline genetic engineering is widely regarded as forbidden, and in 2001, the FDA sent a letter to the research community asserting that ooplasmic transfer was an investigational use of a new drug that did not have FDA approval.[29]

The question is whether the FDA will continue to expand its authority over reproductive activities to the point that it tries to regulate the use of assisted reproductive techniques to enhance offspring. As discussed earlier in chapter 1, these techniques currently include the use of surrogate eggs and sperm chosen because of the superior attributes of their donors and the use of in vitro fertilization and genetic testing to identify embryos of the desired gender for implantation in the uterus. Ultimately, it might be possible to modify a child's genes actively in the course of the reproductive process. If the FDA did try to extend its authority this far, it is conceivable that organized medicine, including the powerful American Medical Association, would oppose it as an invasion of the practice of medicine.

One specific type of genetic enhancement that is relatively devoid of FDA oversight is genetic testing. As mentioned in chapter 1, parents could use genetic testing to obtain desirable donor sperm or eggs or, in conjunction with IVF, to implant the embryos with the best genetic traits. They could test fetuses for nondisease as well as disease characteristics and abort those that did not pass muster. They could test their children for specific genetic abilities. Genetic testing of adults could be a component of educational or occupational counseling, military training, or dating.

Genetic testing is a complex industry. Clinicians or researchers get test samples from the individuals being tested. These are usually blood samples, but increasingly DNA is being obtained by swabbing the inside of the cheek. The test samples are sent to laboratories for processing. These may be free-standing commercial laboratories or laboratories operated by hospitals or research facilities. The laboratories use machinery to process and analyze the samples as well as chemicals, called reagents, that they may make themselves or purchase, either as plain chemicals or as "test kits." Some genetic tests are patented, and the companies that own the patents either operate commercial laboratory services to process the samples exclusively or license the tests to independent laboratories, which in turn must pay royalties.

Each of these different technologies is regulated by different government entities. The Centers for Medicare and Medicaid Services (CMS) oversees the inspection and certification of laboratories. The Centers for Disease Control and Prevention (CDC) assures the accuracy and reliability of testing services provided by in-house hospital or research facility laboratories. The FDA is responsible for regulating the accuracy and reliability of commercial test products, including testing equipment, reagents, test kits, and the tests themselves. There also is some state regulation and some standards established by professional and industry organizations.

The result is a web of oversight that is both overlapping and incomplete. One of the most glaring gaps is that the FDA has reviewed only a small proportion of genetic tests in widespread use, and many of the devices relating to genetic testing have been marketed with reference to the "substantial equivalence" provisions of the Federal Food, Drug, and Cosmetic Act, which essentially allows a manufacturer to market a product without going through the full approval process for a new device. In 1998, the FDA announced that reagents used in genetic testing were "class I" devices, the class with the least FDA oversight, and added that the agency would not even require manufacturers to adhere to "good manufacturing practices," the minimum quality controls ever imposed on medical manufacturers. Furthermore, the agency has taken the position that it will not regulate reagents developed and used within a laboratory, as opposed to reagents sold to other laboratories. In response to the FDA's stance, commentators have urged that the agency expand its oversight of genetic testing laboratories but have no easy answer to the objection that genetic testing is the practice of medicine, placing it beyond the agency's purview.

One area of particular concern is home genetic testing. Currently there are approximately 24 companies selling DNA tests that are performed on samples that people send in themselves, without going through a physician or other health care professional. Medical professionals complain that, without their involvement, consumers can use the tests inappropriately, misinterpret the results, and be denied the necessary follow-up.[30] One company offers DNA testing to establish paternity and maternity, as well as ancestry tracing.[31] The Australian company that developed the ACTN3 genetic test for athletic ability sells it directly to consumers. At-home tests also are offered to tell people which drugs they should take and to give them dietary advice, the latter often accompanied by sales pitches for expensive supplements.[32] As additional genetic mutations for nondisease characteristics are identified, more of these tests can be expected on the market. There is virtually no regulation of at-home tests by the FDA or other branches of the government.

The Role of Health Care Professionals

Another main source of protection from unsafe and ineffective biomedical enhancements is physicians and other health care professionals. Their role is especially critical in connection with enhancement services, such as cosmetic surgery, that are not subject to prior FDA approval.

But the expertise provided by health care professionals is only as good as the information on which it is based. And often this information is faulty or inadequate. This problem was pointed out dramatically by Dartmouth health services researcher John Wennberg and his colleagues in a series of studies in the 1980s on the frequencies at which patients received a number of high-tech medical procedures, such as heart bypass surgery, in different geographic locations.[33] Although the researchers found dramatic differences in the rates, they could not discern any valid explanations for the variations. It appeared that, to a considerable extent, doctors in different places did not agree on whether a patient with the same malady really needed the surgery or not. The resulting lack of confidence in physician expertise was one of the major factors that led health insurers to try to save money by implementing managed care, under which the insurers scrutinize the recommendations of the patients' physicians before agreeing to pay for expensive care.

As bioethicist Haavi Morreim points out, "Standard medicine is not nearly so scientific as is usually assumed. Among other factors, there are far too many phenomena to study; limited research resources are often directed as much by political and commercial interests as by medical needs; actual practices do not reflect well the science that has been gathered; the most pristine science is often the least useful in the real world care of ordinary patients."[34] Morreim mentions a number of modern practices that were thought to be effective but turned out not to be when subjected to rigorous investigation, including pulmonary artery catheterization, angioplasty, bypass surgery, hormone replacement therapy, high-dose chemotherapy with autologous bone marrow transplantation for breast cancer, and the overuse and underuse of antibiotics. Physician and legal scholar David Hyman and his colleague Charles Silver call attention to arthroscopic knee surgery for osteoarthritis, a procedure that is performed on about three hundred thousand Americans every year, at an estimated cost of $1.5 billion, despite a 2002 study in the *New England Journal of Medicine* that found that patients who received the surgery were less mobile than patients with the same condition who did not.[35] Dr. Stephen C. Schoenbaum, executive vice president of the Commonwealth Fund and former president of the Harvard Pilgrim Health Care company, admits: "We don't have the evidence [that treatments work], and we are not investing very much in getting the evidence." In fact, it is estimated that only about 25 percent of mainstream medical practices have been proven to be effective. David Eddy, one of the leading experts on improving the quality of health care put it succinctly: "The problem is that we don't know what we're doing."[36]

Physicians are surprisingly likely to be unfamiliar with new technologies. A 1991 report by an NIH task force on genetic testing, for example, noted that, on average, practitioners who did not specialize in medical genetics missed almost 30 percent of the answers to questions about genetics that a panel of fellow nongeneticist physicians deemed important. Five years later, a survey of primary care physicians found that more than 20 percent of them had not heard of genetic testing for susceptibility to breast cancer.[37]

Even if adequate scientific information existed about the safety and efficacy of biomedical enhancements and even if health care professionals were up to speed on the data, it is not clear that they would give good advice to their patients or (through regulatory agencies) the public. Numerous commentators have pointed out the degree to which medical practitioners face a conflict between their own self-interest and the interests of their patients. This certainly is not new: laws have long been on the books precluding doctors from receiving payments from colleagues for referring patients to them and barring doctors from referring patients to clinical laboratories and other facilities in which the doctors have a financial stake. More recently, some have voiced concerns about connections between physicians and drug companies that could lead to inappropriate prescribing practices and to financial relationships between industry and medical researchers that could jeopardize the well-being of research subjects.[38] A survey published in 2007 found that 94 percent of physicians had a relationship with the pharmaceutical industry. Drug manufacturers had paid for meals for 83 percent of them and had given drug samples to 78 percent. More than a third of the physicians reported being reimbursed by drug companies for attending professional meetings or continuing medical education classes, and 28 percent said they were paid for consulting, speaking, or enrolling their patients as subjects in clinical trials.[39] Drug companies employ approximately one sales representative for every three physicians in the country.[40]

These types of incentive could lead physicians and other health care professionals to skew their advice about biomedical enhancements and cause the people who rely on that advice to take excessive risks or waste money on ineffective products and services. For instance, some physicians sell dietary supplements directly to their patients for weight loss or antiaging effects. One Long Island obstetrician claimed that he made $83,000 in one month selling one company's products out of his office.[41] Some of the dietary supplements contained ephedra until the FDA banned the ingredient from the market for safety reasons.

As mentioned, there are laws that punish physicians who take "kickbacks" for referrals and engage in other types of financial folderol. But the primary check on conflicts of interest is the physician's professional integrity, reinforced by a set of special legal principles that regards all professionals—lawyers, academics, and accountants, as well as doctors—as "fiduciaries" and that penalizes them for taking advantage of patients for the physician's own self-interest.

The problem is that, in recent years, the principle that health care professionals owe patients a fiduciary duty to act in the patients' best interest has been under intensive attack. A number of conservative legal scholars want to scrap it in favor of allowing patients to negotiate with physicians to establish the terms of their relationship, in short, to make the relationship an ordinary business arrangement where the parties are at arm's length and patients must protect themselves against being taken advantage of, just as if they were buying a used car. Haavi Morreim argues that physicians who enroll their patients in clinical research are not fiduciaries for the patients because they owe their primary allegiance to the study rather than to the subjects.[42] The Supreme Court, worried that vigorous application of the fiduciary standard would conflict with managed care, which rewards practitioners for supplying fewer services to patients, has suggested that patients harmed by physician disloyalty may not sue them for breach of a fiduciary duty, only for ordinary malpractice. This would weaken patients' cases and deprive them of key remedies.[43]

Aside from individual health care professionals, professional organizations might be a source of guidance on biomedical enhancements. The American College of Medical Genetics urges people not to use home genetic test kits because of the potential risks.[44] As noted earlier, the American Medical Association in 1994 declared that it was unethical for physicians to enhance children genetically if it would involve a "trade-off with other characteristics or traits" or if they could not assure "equal access . . . irrespective of income or other socioeconomic characteristics," and the organization also forbids germline genetic engineering and the use of gene transfer technology for enhancement purposes.[45] The American Association for the Advancement of Science has come out against germline genetic enhancement.[46] The American Academy of Pediatrics "strongly condemns the use of performance-enhancing substances and vigorously endorses efforts to eliminate their use among children and adolescents."[47] These organizations might be better informed than individual practitioners about the scientific evidence concerning enhancements. On the other hand, it may be difficult to tell whether a professional organization is acting to protect the public or to further its members' financial self-interest. How much of the opposition by the American College of Medical Genetics to home genetic tests sold directly by manufacturers, for example, is attributable to its desire to preserve a larger piece of the lucrative genetic testing business for its members?

In short, physicians and other health care professionals may not have the information they need to advise people about using biomedical enhancements, and even if they did, it is not clear that they can be trusted to dispense this advice solely for the benefit of others.

Other Sources of Protection

Individuals considering using biomedical enhancements have a few other sources of protection from unscrupulous entrepreneurs. The

Federal Trade Commission is charged with promoting truth-in-marketing. Armed with jurisdiction from a variety of legislative sources, the commission has focused some attention on enhancements. It has gone after companies that make bogus claims for human growth hormone antiaging products, as well as products advertising female breast and male sexual enhancement.[48] The commission has attacked enhancement product claims both for lack of efficacy and for safety problems. It took action against the manufacturer of a male sexual enhancement product, for example, because the product contained yohimbine, an ingredient known to increase blood pressure and to interact with other medications.[49] But the FTC resources for carrying out its consumer protection responsibilities are limited and must be spread over many types of products and services. Moreover, the FTC's job in ensuring truthful marketing is complicated by the ease with which manufacturers and distributors can reach potential customers. There are not only ubiquitous print ads, television commercials, and infomercials but also numerous websites hawking enhancement products. Occasionally the commission goes after Internet firms. In 1997–1998, it conducted "Operation Cure. All," which netted more than 1,600 sites making false claims worldwide, 800 in the United States alone. But the commission itself admitted that this was only "the tip of the iceberg."[50]

In some cases, enhancement entrepreneurs are vulnerable to other sorts of legal attacks. The owner of a company called Berkeley Premium Nutraceuticals was indicted along with his mother and other company executives on federal charges of conspiracy, fraud, and money laundering. In addition to allegedly charging customers' credit cards without authorization, the company's former vice president for operations testified that evidence of effectiveness, positive testimonials and survey responses from users, and physician endorsements featured in ads for the company's male enhancement product, Enzyte, were all a hoax: the physicians and testimonials were fictitious; the surveys had been doctored; and the evidence that the pills increased penis size by an average up to 24 percent had been fabricated.[51] Physicians who provide injurious enhancement products to patients might be liable for medical malpractice, but organized medicine is persuading legislatures to make it harder and harder for patients to bring malpractice suits against doctors. People who are injured by enhancement products might bring suits against the manufacturers, but here too, the legal remedies are being cut back. At the end of 2007, for example, the Supreme Court of

Ohio upheld a meager $350,000 state limit on damages in products liability cases.[52]

Enhancement consumers also lack the oversight that health insurers and other third-party payers provide in regard to the safety and efficacy of medical interventions. The ECRI Institute, for instance, reviews medical products and services for employer health benefit plans; it is very desirable for the manufacturers of medical equipment and the providers of medical services to be accepted by it. One example of its role was a legal dispute over whether insurers should pay for a type of therapy for female urinary incontinence in which a woman is seated on a special chair and subjected to magnetic pulses, ostensibly to strengthen the pelvic floor muscles. Citing an ECRI assessment, among other sources of expertise, a federal court ruled in favor of the insurers and against the manufacturer.[53]

Health insurers also can help protect consumers from unsafe or ineffective products and services, although in doing so they open themselves up to charges of denying patients medically necessary care to increase their profits. One of most celebrated controversies pitting health insurers against physicians and patients was the battle over high-dose chemotherapy with autologous bone marrow transplantation, a treatment for advanced breast cancer in which some of the patient's bone marrow is removed and treated, the remaining bone marrow killed by large doses of radiation, and the treated marrow reinfused. Although the insurance industry vigorously opposed the procedure as experimental, it generally was forced to pay for it. As summarized by Peter Jacobsen and Stefanie A. Doebler, "The procedure cost upwards of $100,000 and was also expensive in terms of risks and side effects. When their health insurers refused to cover the treatment, many women sought payment through the judicial system. The result was a series of nearly a hundred courtroom battles, not to mention thousands of settlement negotiations, in which judges and juries were forced to determine whether women would have access to a new procedure that offered their only hope for survival. Without it they would almost certainly die. By the time studies were published conclusively showing that the procedure was ineffective, more than 30,000 women had already received the treatment, which often shortened their lives and added to their suffering, at a total cost of approximately $3 billion."[54]

When it comes to biomedical enhancements, consumers lose whatever benefit they might obtain from insurer expertise because insurance does not pay for enhancement, so insurers have no reason to expend resources to determine whether they are safe or effective. The legislation governing the Medicare program, for example, prohibits paying for "items or services . . . which are not reasonable and necessary for the treatment of illness, or to improve the functioning of a malformed body part," and includes a specific exclusion for "cosmetic surgery."[55] States have adopted the same coverage exceptions under their Medicaid programs. Private health insurance plans follow suit, including in their policies language such as the following: "Coverage is not provided for services and supplies . . . for surgery and other services primarily to improve appearance or to treat a mental or emotional condition through a change in body form."[56]

Improving the Situation

Despite the foregoing difficulties, increasing the safety and effectiveness of products and services remains the best way to respond to the potential health concerns of biomedical enhancements without sacrificing the social benefits. A number of steps might be taken to achieve this objective. An obvious suggestion is to plug some of the gaps in the scope of FDA regulatory authority. As mentioned earlier, one of the most serious gaps is the lack of data on the safety and efficacy of off-label uses of approved products. Clearly it would be foolhardy to try to block physicians from using drugs, devices, and biologics for unapproved uses. Doing so would deprive many patients of drugs on which they depend. One study found that more than 20 percent of all prescriptions written by doctors in their offices were for unapproved uses, with the percentage of off-label prescribing for cardiovascular ailments as high as 46 percent.[57] The study also found that 50 to 80 percent of cancer patients receive chemotherapy on an off-label basis. Some estimates of overall off-label use are as high as 60 percent, and as high as 80 to 90 percent in pediatrics.[58] Although off-label prescribing is in reality a form of unregulated, largely informal human experimentation, it is widely viewed as a vital means of caring for patients and discovering potential new uses for existing medicines.

Many enhancement products are unapproved or "off-label" uses of products approved for medical purposes. Botox, which the FDA had approved to treat certain facial disorders, had been employed cosmetically to reduce frown lines for years before the manufacturer obtained FDA approval for this use. According to the manufacturer's own data, almost

350,000 prescriptions for the alertness drug modafinil were being written annually in the United States when the only condition for which it was approved to treat was narcolepsy, which only affects about 135,000 people in the United States.[59] As for the legal restriction on promoting a product for an unapproved use, the 2004 recent case against Warner-Lambert for promoting Neurontin illegally for off-label uses, which the company settled by paying a $430 million penalty, shows that the practice nevertheless takes place.[60] Prohibiting off-label prescribing for enhancement purposes also would be a bad idea. There is no reason to think that the unapproved use of enhancements poses a greater risk of harm than the unapproved use of drugs for medical purposes. Given the extent of off-label prescribing for medical purposes, the reverse is much more likely to be the case. Moreover, much of the potential benefit from enhancements, described in chapter 8, would be lost.

One response to the phenomenon of unapproved use that does make sense, however, is to require manufacturers who derive substantial revenues from off-label sales of their products to make some concerted effort to determine the risks entailed by those uses. For example, the FDA could require manufacturers that enjoy off-label sales of a product beyond a certain dollar amount or more than a certain percentage of the overall sales of the product to conduct studies to ascertain whether persons who use the product on an unapproved basis suffered different or more serious adverse effects than the side effects that showed up in the studies conducted for FDA approval. The resulting safety information then could be made available to prescribing physicians and the general public. Because these studies would not need to establish efficacy, they would be less expensive and time-consuming than the full-scale clinical trials that must be submitted to obtain an FDA-approved use.

In addition, the FDA could make a much more intensive effort to monitor what actually happens to people who use products for enhancement purposes. This not only would help remedy the lack of information about off-label uses, it would also provide real-world information to augment the limited information derived from highly stylized clinical trials. Current FDA regulations require manufacturers in some cases to conduct studies on new drugs after they are approved. These so-called postmarketing studies are routinely required for drugs that have gone through an accelerated ("fast-track") approval process and for drugs that are labeled for use by children. The FDA also sometimes asks manufacturers to perform these studies on other drugs.[61] However, manufacturers have not always complied with these requirements and undertakings.[62]

As noted earlier, manufacturers of drugs and devices are required to report to the agency all adverse events they find out about, including those that occur in the course of unapproved use, but this system does not function well. Manufacturers have little incentive to disclose adverse events because it would reduce sales, and because they might be sued by patients alleging that the companies knew about the problems and still failed to take the drugs off the market or to issue special warnings.[63] One option would be to provide some sort of protection for manufacturers who reported, such as immunity from product liability suits or a reduction in the damages available to injured patients, but this would be unfair to patients who suffer serious injury. Another alternative would be to impose more severe penalties on companies for failing to disclose problems that they became aware of, but this might merely encourage them to become cleverer at concealment. The best solution would seem to be to augment the FDA's passive role, in which it merely receives information, with an active role in which the agency goes out and collects safety data. FDA personnel carry out all sorts of facility inspections in the discharge of their duties, so they could be given the authority to inspect a sample of hospital or physician medical records and collect mentions of adverse drug events.[64] The agency would need additional resources to carry out this task. It also might be necessary to insulate the inspection system from undue institutional influence so that it is not weakened by a reluctance to embarrass the agency personnel who had reviewed and approved the products in the first place.[65] Of course, there is little chance that such a system would be adopted to protect people only from dangerous biomedical enhancements, but then there is no reason why it should be limited to enhancement products.

Increasing the FDA's authority to regulate dietary supplements would help fill another chink in the agency's ability to protect enhancement users. Dietary supplement manufacturers could be required to sponsor full-scale clinical investigations and obtain FDA approval before marketing, but this would be extremely expensive. Furthermore, there is a limited supply of experimental resources, whether it be clinicians competent to design and conduct studies to institutional oversight to people willing to serve as guinea pigs, and it would be a mistake to devote them to dietary supplements at the expense of more important subjects, such as assessing the safety and efficacy of potentially life-saving drugs and devices. As an intermediate step, the FDA could be empowered to conduct a review of dietary supplements in the same way it evaluates over-the-counter medications. Instead of requiring proof of efficacy for each OTC product, expert committees established by the agency review the available data on classes of products and decide whether and under what conditions they should be sold. Only products containing active ingredients not previously on the market must go through the regular drug approval process.

It would help if there was more work being done on cost-effectiveness, that is, whether it is worth, say, spending thousands of dollars to shed weight through liposuction or stomach clamping surgery instead of using drugs or more traditional dieting. Once again, this is a much bigger issue for drugs and other medical interventions than for enhancements, given the far greater amount of spending on them. A thorough discussion of the pros and cons of cost-effectiveness analysis is beyond the scope of this book, but the approach is controversial because there is no universally accepted methodology. One question is whether cost-effectiveness considerations should enter into the FDA approval process or instead be brought to bear only after products already are on the market, such as by health plans deciding whether or not to include a new product in their pharmacy benefits formulary (the list of drugs that the plan pays for). Another dispute centers on how the effectiveness of different interventions should be measured and compared. Relatively simple comparisons between medical interventions can be made on the basis of how much competing interventions cost to produce the same desirable outcome, such as an additional year of life or a pain-free day. Similar measures could be applied to enhancements, comparing, say, the cost of cognition-enhancing drugs to produce the same amount of improvement in a particular cognitive function. But cost-effectiveness comparisons are rarely that simple, because different alternatives produce different mixes of risks and benefits. For instance, how should we compare a pill that costs $10 and produces a certain amount of improvement in short-term memory with a pill that costs $100 and increases overall IQ permanently? Some method is needed to compare the relative value of short-term memory and IQ and then to factor in the different amounts of improvement in each faculty. One way to do this is to survey the population, for example, asking people to mark on a scale from 1 to 10 how important short-term memory is and then how important IQ is, and doing the same for different amounts of each benefit. But this quickly runs into problems. A person with good short-term memory may place less of a value on it than a person with poor short-term memory. Which one is correct?

A fascinating illustration of these difficulties occurred when the state of Oregon decided in the early 1990s to ration services under its Medicaid program on the basis of which ones were most cost-effective. A commission was appointed that constructed a priority list based in part on survey responses and discussions at public meetings about which states of health were more important than others. Predictably, a treatment that reduced pain but left someone bedridden was deemed less important than treatments that both reduced pain and restored mobility. But this meant that treatments for people with physical disabilities were deemed less cost-effective than treatments for people who were not disabled, and this ran afoul of antidiscrimination laws like the Americans with Disabilities Act. As a result, the Bush and later the Clinton administration refused to allow Oregon to proceed with its plan. Oregon went back to the drawing board, and after a couple of additional unsuccessful attempts, ended up with a "priority system" based more on alphabetical order than cost-effectiveness.[66]

An even tougher problem is what to do about biomedical enhancements like cosmetic surgery that are medical services rather than products and therefore largely exempt from FDA oversight. One alternative is to make them more like products by making them more proprietary. For example, if a surgeon who invented a new cosmetic surgery technique could patent it and other surgeons could adopt it only if they obtained a license, the inventor might have a greater incentive to invest in safety and efficacy studies, especially if such studies were a requirement for patenting the technique. It actually is possible to obtain a so-called medical procedure patent, but because of concern that these patents could retard the spread of new medical knowledge and expertise, Congress has barred the patent-holders from bringing patent-infringement actions against other medical practitioners who employ the technique.[67] Obviously, this has the effect of substantially eroding the value of patenting. A similar policy objection would hold against enhancement procedure patents, although perhaps there would be less concern about slowing the spread of new enhancement techniques than surgeries for medical conditions.

A better option would be for the government to pay for studies of the safety and efficacy of key enhancement procedures. There is an analogy for this in the NIH's National Center for Complementary and Alternative Medicine (NCCAM), which provides funds to conduct clinical investigations of nonmainstream medical technologies. In fact, NCCAM already has sponsored research on enhancement: one study found that people who meditated may process information in the brain more efficiently than people who do not.[68] It might be objected that the NIH should devote its scarce research grants to projects aimed at diseases rather than enhancement. But publicly funded enhancement studies to investigate the safety of widely used enhancement techniques could spare the nation a substantial amount of medical expenditures if people stop using popular enhancements because of their health risks, while efficacy studies could identify enhancement interventions with the potential for large-scale social benefit.

In addition to publicly funded safety and efficacy studies, additional government resources could be devoted to policing the enhancement marketplace and taking action against unscrupulous entrepreneurs. The enforcement budget for the Federal Trade Commission and state consumer protection agencies could be increased for this purpose. Again, there is the question of priorities. Would quackery and fraud in the enhancement industry be considered a more serious public concern than, say, consumer advertising in general? But once more, enforcement resources could be focused on selected sectors of the enhancement market, such as those that adversely affect large numbers of purchasers or that target customers who are especially vulnerable to marketing pressures.

More effort also could be made to educate physicians and other health care professionals about enhancements so that they can serve as better sources of information for their patients. Professional societies could take a greater interest in enhancements and in updating their membership on new developments. In an article on protecting consumers of antiaging interventions that colleagues and I published in the journal of the American Gerontological Society, we called for professional groups to create task forces on antiaging practices.[69] Professionals could get together and take action against perceived problems. In 2002, for example, an international group of 51 gerontologists published an exposé of the antiaging industry in *Scientific American*.[70] (As mentioned in chapter 1, their leader was sued for defamation and slander for $120 million by the founders of an antiaging industry group, but the suit eventually was dropped.)

There is a limit, however, to what public measures can accomplish in seeking to make health care practitioners less susceptible to financial and other conflicts of interest with their patients. It would be a terrible mistake to dismantle the fiduciary obligations that the law imposes on the patient-physician relationship. The last thing either patients or their caregivers need is less trust between them. Not only would this lead to increased malpractice litigation, it could also compromise the effectiveness of medical treatment itself; as Mark Hall observes, trust is an aid in the healing process.[71] (Ironically, Hall is one of the leading scholars in favor of eliminating physicians' fiduciary duties toward patients.) However, the job of preserving fiduciary obligations is at least as much a matter for the professions themselves as for the courts. It is therefore imperative that professional organizations like the AMA and the American College of Physicians vigorously oppose any efforts to weaken their role as fiduciaries. As discussed earlier, the alternative to a fiduciary relationship is an ordinary business relationship, in which the parties deal with each other at arm's length. Why would a physician want to be seen as a common tradesperson?

Professional organizations also have a critical role to play in dealing with members' conflicts of interest. The rules of proper behavior are made clear in their codes of ethics. Opinion 8.06 of the American Medical Association's Council on Ethical and Judicial Affairs states for example that "physicians who choose to sell health-related products from their offices should not sell any health-related products whose claims of benefit lack scientific validity." Opinion 8.20 states that "treatments which have no medical indication and offer no possible benefit to patients should not be used."[72] These precepts must be enforced against all practitioners, including those who take advantage of their patients' ignorance and vulnerability to give them enhancements that the physicians should know are unsafe or ineffective.

The problem of enhancement tourism—people going abroad to secure enhancements that are illegal in the United States—is more intractable, chiefly because economies are becoming increasingly global. The best hope would be international cooperation to protect people against highly dangerous products and services, but as the War on Drugs demonstrates, this is costly, subject to national variance, and not very effective.

In the end, there is both a practical and an ethical limit to how much people can be protected from unsafe or ineffective biomedical enhancements. Products that have been approved by the FDA can be abused, and government regulators cannot completely prevent black markets from furnishing people with enhancements that are unapproved or illegal. Indeed, as we saw earlier in connection with the discussion of soft paternalism, there is a fundamental lack of agreement about just how much regulating the government ought to do. It would be folly for the hysteria over doping in sports to lead the government to over-regulate enhancements in a vain attempt to keep people from taking risks. But the government clearly has a crucial role to play in providing good information about safety and effectiveness for people who want to protect themselves, and investing in good information is a far more sensible approach than waging a hopeless war against enhancements.

But what about people who can't protect themselves? In discussing the need for a better understanding of enhancement safety and effectiveness, we have been assuming that decisions about whether or not to use enhancements would be made voluntarily by competent individuals. What protections are appropriate for people who are not competent, either by virtue of their age or mental status, or who are under so much pressure to use enhancements that their choices to do so may no longer be voluntary?

Chapter 11

Protecting the Vulnerable

SOME INDIVIDUALS MAY not be in a position to make voluntary, informed choices for themselves about whether or not to use biomedical enhancements. The term that most bioethicists use to describe them is *vulnerable*. The concept of vulnerability is a bit tricky. Some bioethicists, such as Daniel Callahan, regard everybody as "vulnerable."[1] Chilean professor Michael Kottow, for example, describes it as the universal human condition of being "intact but fragile."[2] According to this viewpoint, vulnerability is what triggers the duty to behave justly toward one another. Other scholars reserve the term for certain populations, for example to describe people who are "medically vulnerable" in that they are especially susceptible to being in poor health or suffering bad outcomes from medical treatment. The term is also commonly used to describe populations that are at a high risk of being misused as research subjects, a topic discussed in the next chapter. Here, vulnerability refers to impediments that get in the way of making rational choices about enhancements. For people with these impediments, the availability of good information about the safety and effectiveness of enhancements is not enough; they need additional help in making good decisions.

But who exactly are "they"? What are the kinds of impediments to good decisionmaking that determine different forms of vulnerability?

Age is one: the law regards most minors as incapable of making proper choices about weighty matters. As a result, minors generally cannot enter into binding contracts, including contracts entitling them to obtain health care from physicians. In addition to age, federal regulations designed to protect vulnerable persons in human experiments cite economic and educational disadvantage.[3] Some commentators point to membership in socially marginalized groups.[4] The federal research regulations list children, prisoners, pregnant women, mentally disabled persons, fetuses, and newborns as vulnerable. Broader interpretations of vulnerability focus on relationships in which there are inequalities of power, knowledge, or resources, and on individuals who are cognitively impaired or subject to intimidation.[5]

Vulnerability usually is considered an all-or-nothing proposition: either someone is vulnerable or they are not. But vulnerability is more properly thought of as a matter of degree. The question is not so much whether a person is vulnerable but *how* vulnerable they are. One way to think of this is to imagine a continuum that represents the ethical goals of decisionmaking, with "autonomy" at one end and "protection from harm" at the other. The opposite ends of the continuum also correspond to how much capacity a person has to make informed, voluntary choices, with more capable and secure persons accorded maximum decisionmaking freedom at one end of the spectrum, while toward the other end, more impaired or exposed persons are given less freedom, and at some point, no longer allowed to make decisions for themselves at all. Vulnerability then can be thought of as a condition that moves an individual away from the autonomy end of the continuum and toward the protection end. The more vulnerable a person is, the less freedom they should have to make their own decisions.

As we saw in chapter 6, there are a number of types of individuals who qualify as vulnerable when it comes to making decisions about whether or not to use biomedical enhancements. Some of these groups, as noted earlier, are mentioned in the federal research regulations: the economically and educationally disadvantaged, children, prisoners, pregnant women, mentally disabled persons, fetuses, and newborns. Other vulnerable groups that were identified in chapter 6 are employees, athletes, soldiers, and students. The members of these groups are subject to external and internal pressures that could expose them to enhancements in ways that would strike most people as unreasonable.

Some of these groups obtain a modicum of protection from the harms that could be caused by dangerous enhancements. Athletic organizations ban the use of virtually all enhancement drugs, including those that are harmful. Additional measures have been taken to prevent children from using enhancements in sports. Florida and New Jersey have initiated small-scale steroid testing programs for high school athletes. In May 2007, the Texas legislature mandated random steroid testing of all public high school athletes, and in January 2008, a Kansas City company called the National Center for Drug-Free Sport signed a $6 million contract to run the program for two years.[6] The company will select Texas high schools at random and then pick student-athletes randomly from a list furnished by the school. Students who test positive will be suspended from competition for 30 days and must pass another test before being allowed to resume playing. A second failed test will bring a one-year suspension. After a third positive test, the suspension will be permanent. Each test costs about $140.

Outside of sports, the government has the right to intervene when parents abuse their children, which would include situations in which parents gave their children enhancements that pose a significant risk of substantial harm to the children's health. State legislatures have begun cracking down on teenage use of tanning booths; more than half of the states require parental permission, and some prohibit teen use altogether. According to Joe Nation, the California assemblyman who authored a bill to ban teen access, "There is a big difference between going to the beach and a tanning salon. When kids go to the beach they put on sunscreen."[7]

With regard to workers, federal law requires employers to provide places of employment that are free from recognized hazards that are causing or are likely to cause death or serious physical harm to employees; this might be interpreted to prohibit employers from requiring workers to use dangerous enhancements. Government regulations permit employers to offer their employees wellness programs, which are somewhat analogous to enhancements in that the employers' goal is to reduce costs and maintain productivity. But the regulations forbid employers from forcing employees to participate.

Finally, surrogate decisionmakers, such as family members or legal guardians, are appointed for persons with mental disabilities that render them incapable of making rational choices.

Yet some of the groups that are vulnerable to outside pressure receive little protection. Members of the military who are ordered to use dangerous enhancements have no legal recourse against the government. Although the Federal Tort Claims Act allows people injured by government actions to sue the government to obtain compensation, the Supreme Court has ruled that this does not extend to injuries suffered by members of the military that "arise out of or are in the course of activity incident to service."[8] This rule, known as the Feres doctrine after the 1950 case in which it was established, is interpreted extremely broadly. In one instance, for example, a federal court refused to permit an underaged woman in the Air Force who was raped after she passed out at a party to sue the military for allowing the party to take place and for not protecting her from her assailant, an airman who had a prior criminal record for violent crime.[9] The airman was court-martialed for the attack, but this would not be likely to happen to superiors who ordered soldiers to use hazardous enhancements in the course of carrying out legitimate military duties.

There also might be little protection for students facing pressure from schools eager to improve performance in academic competitions, standardized test scores, or college placements. For example, public schools in 29 states are still permitted to use corporal punishment. An Ohio law passed in 1994 purported to ban it, but it allowed local school districts to set up their own paddling policies, subject to certain procedures. Although a far cry from the 68,000 paddlings in 1984, 270 occurrences were reported in the 2005–2006 academic year.[10] In 1977, the Supreme Court refused to hold that corporal punishment was "cruel and unusual" under the Eighth Amendment on the basis that public schools are "open to public scrutiny." "The schoolchild has little need for the protection of the Eighth Amendment," said the justices. "Though attendance may not always be voluntary, the public school remains an open institution. . . . At the end of the school day, the child is invariably free to return home. Even while at school, the child brings with him the support of family and friends and is rarely apart from teachers and other pupils who may witness and protest any instances of mistreatment."[11] The Court noted that teachers and school officials might be liable if the punishment exceeded what was "reasonably necessary for the proper education and discipline of the child," but if the use of enhancements were deemed reasonably necessary for legitimate educational objectives, schools could have a significant amount of freedom to pressure pupils to use enhancements despite parental objections.

Even where vulnerable groups did receive special protection, the protections might be inadequate. The surrogates who are supposed to make decisions for people who lack the mental competence to do so on their own, for example, are often in a position to take advantage of the situation, and about 30 percent of all crimes against the elderly involve financial abuses, affecting between three and five million seniors a year.[12] This is more of an issue in connection with allowing mentally incompetent people to serve as subjects in risky enhancement experiments, discussed in the next chapter, but surrogates might be induced by financial rewards from manufacturers or service providers to purchase unsafe or ineffective enhancements for their charges.

At the other end of the age spectrum, parents have a great deal of discretion about how to raise their children. Although critics bewail parents who give kids stimulants to help them do better in school or who provide adolescents with cosmetic surgical procedures such as nose jobs or breast augmentation, there is no public effort to stop these practices. Indeed, there is a tug of war between proponents of more protection for children and advocates for greater parental autonomy. One group thinks that the legal standard of "abuse and neglect" is too lax, giving parents too much freedom to harm their children, such as by "indoctrinating" them with parental beliefs.[13] The other group thinks that "abuse and neglect" is too draconian and that the state should interfere only, for example, if there is "clear and convincing evidence" that the parents' actions represent "likely and serious harm" to their children.[14] In a highly competitive society in which educational advantage is key to success, many parents may be willing to give their children enhancements just as they now buy them tutoring and "help them" with their homework.

In fact, rather than wanting to protect persons susceptible to external pressure, society in a number of instances might want to force them to use risky enhancements. This is likely not only within the military but also in the case of persons whose jobs would pose a serious risk to the public if they were not performed well, such as airline pilots, tanker captains, and power-plant operators, as well as those whose work impacts national security, such as higher-level government officials, intelligence operatives, and others in sensitive positions. If enhancement use is mandated by the government, then there is some protection for users in the form of constitutional constraints on government action, such as requirements that it meet standards of due process and equal protection. But the Constitution gives the government a large amount of discretion when national interests are at stake, especially when the interest is national security.

Finally, even if individuals could be protected from outside pressures to use dangerous enhancements, they still might succumb to internal compulsion. As noted earlier in chapter 6, for example, employers don't have to require employees to use enhancements; employees desiring to get ahead or just desperate to hold onto their jobs will use them on their own. The same is true of athletes, students, members of the military, and anyone who could expect to gain from enhancement use in competitive situations.

Could we reduce or eliminate this internal competitive drive? In Sweden, young children take part in school sports in an "egalitarian" fashion, with every child making the team and getting a chance to play.[15] For some workers, advancement is based mostly on seniority. But at some point, competition seems inevitable. Discerning audiences are not thrilled by mediocre performances. Beauty remains a key factor in forming sexual relationships. Seniority may be an acceptable basis for promotion in the postal service, but hardly for positions of critical public importance. Even in Sweden, when children reach a certain age, school sports cease to be egalitarian. So long as resources are scarce, they cannot be had by all, and traits such as ability and appearance inevitably will be among the metrics of social success.

But even if complete protection for vulnerable populations against external and internal pressures is impossible, some steps can be taken. By far the most critical is to make sure that safe and effective biomedical enhancements are readily available and that people have access to good information about the risks and benefits of enhancement alternatives. Those who are determined to force others to use enhancements and those who feel they have no alternative but to use them at least will have enhancements on hand that reflect a reasonable balance between benefit and harm.

If the pressure to excel is great enough, however, there will be a temptation to employ enhancement techniques that are potentially dangerous in the hope of obtaining a competitive advantage. Therefore, whenever possible, vulnerable persons should be given the opportunity to participate in enhancement-free competitions. For example, if a major sports organization decides to allow the use of enhancements, it also should hold enhancement-free events for athletes who are willing to be tested and have their results considered separately. In addition, those in a position to coerce others, including employers, athletic coaches and trainers, and schools, should be punished if they give their charges enhancements that are unreasonably hazardous.

The key term here is *unreasonably.* While it may seem impossibly vague and imprecise, it is a standard that has long been used by the law to evaluate behavior on the basis of the facts of particular cases and under circumstances where greater specificity and precision cannot be achieved in advance. The determination of whether or not a person has acted reasonably is typically made by a jury, ostensibly of one's peers. Thus, a jury decides if someone who caused an automobile accident was driving reasonably, and where the behavior in question involves special expertise, as in education or sports, the jury hears testimony from experts about what they think is reasonable. A reasonableness standard would require juries to consider whether employers, athletic personnel, or educators who mandated the use of specific enhancements acted as they should have under the circumstances.

Parental decisions deserve special deference, however, in recognition of the parents' right to raise their children as they deem appropriate and the assumption that they are likely to be better suited than anyone else to judge what is best for them. Accordingly, parental decisions should be presumed to be reasonable, and they should be publicly accountable only for actions that a jury finds "abusive." In addition, authority figures such as employers, educators, and athletic coaches and trainers should not be permitted to give biomedical enhancements to minors without parental permission. But parental permission shouldn't automatically absolve an authority figure from the obligation to act responsibly. Parents too are vulnerable to external pressure, such as pressure from school administrators to medicate energetic children inappropriately. Hence, even if a parent consents, authority figures should be held accountable if they gave children enhancements in a manner that is later deemed to have been unreasonable.

Chapter 12

Access and Inequality

As chapter 3 made clear, one of the most challenging problems created by biomedical enhancements is how they should be distributed. A main theme in my previous book, *Wondergenes,* was the unfairness that would result if access to highly effective biomedical enhancements were distributed as it is now, on the basis of ability to pay. Some enhancements, like caffeine and nicotine, are cheap enough to be available to virtually anyone. But more powerful and exotic enhancements are likely to be out of the reach of the average person, and some may be available only to the affluent. As I argued in *Wondergenes,* this could threaten the belief in equality of opportunity that sustains liberal democratic societies in the face of actual inequality, paving the way for social turmoil and the collapse of the liberal state.

In *Wondergenes,* as here, I rejected the idea that we could simply prevent anyone from obtaining enhancements. Instead I described a number of steps that society might take to level the playing field when people with greater resources interact with their less fortunate brethren and suggested using them to prevent the enhanced from taking unfair advantage of the unenhanced. I proposed, for example, that people seeking to purchase an enhancement be required to get a license, which the government would issue on condition that they used their enhanced abilities only in socially acceptable ways. I also suggested that enhanced individuals be handicapped when they compete with persons who are not enhanced. It is relatively easy to see how this might be accomplished in the sports context, with enhanced athletes required to run farther or finish in less time. Outside of sports, we might handicap enhanced people by requiring them to disclose the fact that they are enhanced, by expecting them to subordinate their interests to those of weaker parties, and by undoing the deals they make if they seem in retrospect to be unfair.

But there is a serious defect in all these approaches. For them to be effective, we will have to be able to identify persons who have been enhanced in order to know whom to handicap or whether enhanced individuals have misused their licenses or taken unfair advantage of other persons. In short, we would have to employ the same measures to detect the use of enhancement that would be needed to enforce an outright ban, measures that I concluded in chapter 8 were impractical as well as intolerably intrusive. The only difference between the remedial measures I proposed in *Wondergenes* and complete prohibition is that, under the former, society would be able to obtain some benefits from enhancement use, because people would be allowed to use them so long as they did so in the public interest. But the regime that we would have to create to produce this benefit would be so repressive that it would hardly be worth it. In *Wondergenes* I acknowledged that the surveillance and intrusion that would be needed to level the playing field would be harsh, but I defended it on the grounds that it would avoid a direr dystopia in which the enhanced and the unenhanced clashed for power in an increasingly unstable political environment. I pointed out that, when we deem it necessary, "we put up with the intrusion and the cost of leveling the playing field." The example I gave was sports: "Athletes are forced to submit to physical examinations and to provide samples of body fluids for testing, often under conditions that deny them minimal privacy. If they don't like it, we tell them, don't play sports." Similarly, I stated, "if you don't like being leveled to promote competitive fairness, don't become enhanced." But sports is not an apt analogy. While we may have a choice about whether or not to play competitive sports, none of us can avoid the competitive scramble for scarce societal resources, and as Chapter 8 makes clear, the arbitrary rules that govern sports are not suitable for application elsewhere.

If banning biomedical enhancements would be foolhardy and if restricting their use to socially desirable ends would require a repressive police state, the only alternative is to make sure that enhancements are available, not only to the well-off but to everyone. In other words, access to enhancements should be subsidized for those who cannot otherwise afford them. I rejected this approach in *Wondergenes* because I felt it would cost too much. Using a highly conservative estimate that everyone would need at least ten thousand dollars worth of enhancements, I calculated that this would amount to almost twice the entire federal budget. But I was not only forgetting that many people would be able to afford enhancements without government aid; I was also making the mistake of rejecting the possible because it is not the ideal. The key question is not whether we can afford to subsidize all enhancements for everyone, but whether we can provide enough access to avoid a future blighted by inequality, chaos, and oppression. The answer is that we should try.

One possibility would be to provide free or subsidized enhancements to those poorer persons who had the least amount of socially desirable traits and who were plagued by the worst luck. While this might seem the most just method for equalizing social opportunity, it would face serious difficulties in attempting to determine who qualified for the benefit. Bear in mind that we're talking about enhancement, not remediation. So the beneficiaries would not be persons who were abnormally ill-equipped for success; these presumably would be covered by programs for people with disabilities. Instead we would be subsidizing persons who, while "normal," are not as endowed than others. But who would this be? Would someone with an IQ, say, of 120 be entitled to publicly funded cognitive enhancement because there are other people with higher IQs? How about if we agreed on some arbitrary cutoff, say an IQ of 120, and said that everyone with normal intelligence who fell below that cutoff would be entitled to cognition-enhancing drugs to boost their IQs by 20 points? While persons who previously had IQs of 120 would be better off at 140, now there would be a huge gap between those with IQs of 140 and above and those with less than 120. What if the entitlement to enhancements were based, like some notions of normalcy, on what percentile of the population one falls into? That is, everyone below a certain percentile would receive subsidized enhancement. But then the population immediately below them would fall into that percentile and be entitled to the subsidy, and so on.

This problem arises with any benefit program that is not universal:

a tax cut for persons making $99,999 or less a year is not entirely fair to persons earning exactly $100,000. But when we express cutoffs in terms of income or wealth, we seem less concerned, perhaps because we recognize that there are many other valuable attributes besides money, including health, beauty, and brains. In terms of moral and social acceptability, then, we probably could get by with an enhancement subsidy based on income. It wouldn't be perfectly fair, but it might be fair enough.

Implementing the subsidy would be relatively straightforward. If the nation ever adopted a comprehensive scheme of subsidized national health insurance, enhancements could be included in the package of basic benefits that would be guaranteed for everyone. In the meantime, Congress could include enhancements among the products and services covered by Medicaid and other publicly funded health insurance programs or give out vouchers that could be used for enhancement purchases. Vouchers also could be given to low-income taxpayers who are not eligible for government health insurance programs.

This raises the question of whether individuals would be left free to decide which enhancements to purchase with their vouchers from among all those that are lawfully being sold, or if instead they would only be allowed to purchase certain enhancements that are approved by the government. Consider flexible spending accounts, before-tax money that employees can set aside to pay for medical care that is not covered by their health insurance plans. These accounts are governed by Internal Revenue Service regulations that exclude payment, among other things, for cosmetic surgery, weight loss programs (except for people who are diagnosed with a weight-related illness such as obesity or hypertension), and over-the-counter drugs not prescribed by a physician.[1] An enhancement voucher program presumably would provide much broader coverage, so that someone might be able to use an enhancement voucher for a facelift, rather than be restricted to enhancements that would be expected to produce greater societal benefit. But there still might be concern that unscrupulous entrepreneurs could induce people to purchase products or services of dubious value, such as unproven but lawfully marketed dietary supplements or antiaging substances, although this concern would be lessened if we adopted the more vigorous regulatory regime for assuring that enhancements were safe and efficacious that was described in chapter 10.

If publicly funded access to enhancements is not to employ a voucher system, the question is which enhancements should be covered, on the assumption that it would be too expensive to cover them all. The answer could be left up to elected representatives, expert commissions, or government bureaucrats. When the Clintons put forward their national health insurance program in the early 1990s, they proposed creating a national health board of presidential appointees who would decide what medical services would be covered. The government decision-maker might look to John Rawls's notion of "primary goods"—those that every rational person should want. By identifying the enhancements that would fit that definition, experts might be able to generate a list of the enhancements to which everyone should be given access. Fritz Allhoff argues, for example, that eyesight, speed, strength, mental acuity, mathematical and spatial reasoning, language faculties, creativity, and musical ability are primary goods, while height, skin color, eye color, and sex are not.[2] But this leaves the question of which primary goods should take priority, in the likely event that it is too expensive to cover enhancements for all of them.

One possibility would be to employ some means of achieving a public consensus on which enhancements to cover first. This could be a simple set of surveys or opinion polls or perhaps a more elaborate method such as public discussion forums. When the Oregon legislature in the early 1990s decided to expand its Medicaid program to make more people eligible for benefits, an effort described earlier, the state employed a combination of telephone surveys and public meetings to create a list of medical treatments in order of importance. Based on calculations of how much it would cost to cover the treatments for the expanded Medicaid population, the state legislature then decided how far down the list it could afford to go in covering treatments under the program, given the state budget. But care must be taken to make sure that the public input is accurate and unbiased. At the public meetings held in Oregon, for instance, the attendees did not consist of the people who would be directly affected by losing access to treatments that Medicaid previously had paid for, namely, those receiving Medicaid, but predominantly comprised female health care workers such as nurses, 67 percent of whom had college degrees and 30 percent of whom had incomes exceeding $50,000 a year. (At the time, the state deemed families of four that were earning more than about $7,000 a year to be ineligible for Medicaid because they had too much income.)[3] So these meetings did not provide a sense of what treatments were most important to those who would receive access to them or be denied it but rather to those who would be paying for the program, and that seems wrong.

If some method were used to limit or prioritize which biomedical enhancements were to be subsidized, it would seem advisable to offer people a choice among a set of alternatives rather than giving them access only to one particular type of enhancement. Instead of covering just enhancements that improved cognition, for example, subsidies could instead be available for enhancements that improved other high-priority mental or physical traits, such as strength, dexterity, artistic or musical ability, or drive, assuming relatively safe and effective enhancements of that sort existed. This would increase decisionmaking autonomy and to some degree allow for different opinions about what personal characteristics were most prized. It also would serve to reduce the concern that naturally talented elites would simply make use of the same enhancements as the less advantaged, thereby preserving their privileged social status. Subsidized access that allowed different people to enhance different talents would create a population with a greater diversity of enhanced talents, and this might help negate the advantages enjoyed by the naturally gifted. For example, although naturally bright persons who used a cognitive enhancement might still remain intellectually superior in comparison with less-bright people with access to the same enhancement, they might not have as much energy or be as musical as a less-bright person who chose to enhance those traits instead. Of course, the elite might be able to afford to enhance multiple traits—to become smarter *and* more energetic *and* more musical—but subsidized access to enhancements would keep the achievement gap from growing as wide as it would if high-tech enhancements were available to the well-off alone, and it would produce more social benefit by enabling more people to be better at what they chose to do.

If we can't afford to provide health care for all, it might be objected, why would we want to spend money on subsidizing access to biomedical enhancements? One response is that we are bound eventually to adopt some form of national health insurance and that we can wait until then to think about adding enhancements to the list of covered services for low-income individuals. But it also might be argued that this objection incorrectly assumes that any health-oriented intervention deserves a higher priority for government funding than any enhancement. At first, it might seem obvious that medical benefits are inherently more valuable than enhancement benefits. Health is often described as a "special," "basic," or "primary" good, without which it is impossible to attain "normal species functioning" or to enjoy a reasonable range of opportunities.[4] Enhancement, on the other hand, might seem less essential, because a person who is enhanced most likely starts out within the normal range for the enhanced trait. But some enhancement benefits may correctly be perceived as more valuable than medical benefits. An enhancement that potentially increases cognitive function, for example, might be deemed more valuable than a substance to treat a minor skin irritation. The same might be said for compensatory enhancements described above, supranormal abilities given to persons with disabilities to make up for deficiencies in other traits, or for enhancement for members of the military, which could make it easier to attain important national security objectives. In fact, if access to enhancements proved as important an ingredient of social success as seems likely, it could be viewed as analogous to access to basic education, which is widely regarded as a right and without which it is almost impossible to succeed.

So far there has been only one attempt to provide subsidized access to something that might be considered a biomedical enhancement. In 1998, the director of the federal agency that oversees the Medicaid program directed all states to cover Viagra for Medicaid beneficiaries; given the widespread use of the drug by men seeking to enhance their sexual performance, it is certain that at least some of the prescriptions under Medicaid ended up being used for this purpose. The federal directive explained that, with the exception of diet pills, smoking cessation products, and infertility treatments, the law required states to provide coverage of any prescription drug that had been approved by the FDA and that this included Viagra, which was approved for erectile dysfunction.[5] But in 2005, reports appeared that between January 2000 and March 2005, 198 sex offenders in New York had received Medicaid-reimbursed Viagra after their convictions, and in 2006, Congress voted to bar both Medicare and Medicaid from paying for impotence drugs altogether. Charles Grassley (R-Iowa), the chair of the Senate Finance Committee who introduced the bill, pointed to an estimate by the Congressional Budget Office that this would save the government $2 billion between 2006 and 2015. The Chairman of the House Energy and Commerce Committee, Joe Barton (R-Tex.), urged passage after scoffing that "blind adherence to the misguided rules within the federal bureaucracy regularly produces outcomes that are either hilarious or outrageous, but this is unique. Only a Medicaid bureaucrat could give Viagra to rapists and think it was okay."[6] The idea of paying for sex offenders to obtain Viagra does sound odd, but the government's action also arguably makes it more difficult for poor men on Medicaid to have children. Convicted sex offenders are readily identified as a result of state and federal enactment of "Megan's laws," which require them to be publicly registered. If the objective was to prevent them from getting Viagra, the government could have required physicians or pharmacists to check the registries before prescribing the drug.

Indeed, according to one commentator, the assumption that society can draw a clear line between therapies and "lifestyle" drugs when it comes to a product like Viagra is false. "On one end of the spectrum," states Alison Keith in an article in *Health Affairs,* "treatment for smoking cessation may be considered a lifestyle issue; in fact, quitting smoking is one of the most beneficial things that one can do to improve one's long-term health prospects. One could also argue that treatment for arthritis or migraines primarily affects lifestyle and not the ability to survive. In the extreme, one might argue that recent innovations in the treatment of stroke are principally lifestyle enhancements, aimed at preventing a lifestyle burdened by immobility or other lost functions. The point, of course, is that virtually all medical treatment affects patients' ability to live the lives they prefer. There is simply no bright line distinguishing lifestyle from medical necessity."[7] The motivation behind Keith's views might be suspect, however, because she wrote this in her position as the director of economic policy for Pfizer, the manufacturer of Viagra.

So far I have explained why I have rejected a major recommendation in my earlier book, *Wondergenes.* Another suggestion I made in that book, however, remains viable, and that is to implement a national enhancement lottery. This would be particularly important if subsidized access to enhancements were severely limited for budgetary reasons, because a lottery or something like it (game show prizes, for example) would be the only lawful way that poor people could gain access to a wider selection of enhancements. As I described it in *Wondergenes,* "Winners would be chosen at random, and would receive a voucher entitling them to whatever genetic enhancements were legally available. The lottery would be open to everyone, but it would be voluntary. Individuals who objected to genetic enhancement on the basis of morality or religion could decline their winnings. Everyone automatically would be given one chance to win, and no one could purchase tickets. The odds of winning could be adjusted upward or downward, and the drawings held at variable frequencies, so that a sense of equality of opportunity in obtaining access to genetic enhancements was created and maintained."[8] Interestingly, in 2007 a London company called Europa International, which sells cosmetic surgery services to Britons for a group of Prague cosmetic surgery clinics, established a lottery in which tickets can be purchased for £1.50 by text or phone message, and the winner receives £6,000 toward the cost of the cosmetic surgery of their choice at the Czech Republic clinics.[9] While this was a marketing gimmick, and it did evoke some criticism in Britain, it suggests that a lottery with a more public-spirited enhancement objective might be feasible.

Finally, if government funding of enhancements is going to be counted on to increase access and maintain the belief in equality of opportunity, it is important that the cost of enhancements to the government be as low as possible. At present, the government extracts steep price discounts for the drugs its purchases. For example, the Veterans Administration pays only about 42 percent of the average wholesale drug price.[10] This same discount scheme could be applied to enhancements purchased by government subsidy programs. In addition, the government could contract with certain groups of enhancement providers to furnish services to persons with enhancement entitlements; in return for the high volume of customers that they would get, the providers would be expected to charge lower prices. It also is conceivable that the government could simply dictate the prices of the enhancements that it purchases. This is especially likely if the enhancement were regarded as critical to national security or well-being, or if the seller were attempting to keep the price too high. For example, when the military decided it needed an anthrax vaccine, it negotiated a price with the vaccine's sole supplier, although it later increased the price to spur the expansion of production facilities to meet increased demand.[11] As a last resort, the government could set up its own enhancement manufacturing facility. This too was considered in response to the shortage of anthrax vaccine supplies, but was abandoned as not being cost-effective.[12]

Chapter 13

Abominations

As THE BEGINNING chapters showed, biomedical enhancements cover a broad spectrum. At one end are familiar ones like caffeine and nose jobs. At the opposite extreme lie enhancements that transform people in such bizarre ways that they would induce in others powerful feelings of awe or revulsion. The future might see DNA from different species combined to produce a chimera, a creature that is part animal and part human. One of the characters in Michael Crichton's book *Next*, for example, is a part-human, part-chimpanzee named Dave. But Dave is a souped-up ape, not an enhanced human. A better illustration is Julian Savulescu's conceptualization of people who are given genes for longevity from tortoises, memory from elephants, and night vision from owls and rabbits, or "Cheetah-man," Daniel Lee's drawing of a relay runner with unmistakable feline features, which appeared on the cover of Andy Miah's 2004 book about genetic modification of athletes.[1] The future also might see transhumans, beings whose human genes have been genetically advanced in such an extreme fashion that they no longer seem human.

These possibilities are so disturbing that many people might insist on banning them, even if we do not block less dramatic forms of biomedical enhancement. Biotech critic Jeremy Rifkin and biologist Stuart

Newman tried to obtain a patent on a "humanzee" to prevent others from actually creating one.[2] Bioethicist George Annas promotes a "Convention on the Preservation of the Human Species," an international treaty that would bar germline genetic manipulations.[3]

It certainly makes sense to discourage exotic enhancements until they are reasonably safe. Imagine the outrage if premature attempts were to lead to women dying in pregnancy or giving birth to monsters. Germline genetic enhancement currently is objectionable for this reason: it is relatively untried and risks causing severe and unpredictable physical harm both to recipients and future generations. Even if it avoided these problems, it could create a new genetic aristocracy, a "genobility," as I called it in *Wondergenes*, in which elite status would be even more a matter of inheritance than it is now and in which the gap between the gifted and the rest of society would grow to unbridgeable proportions. Some experts believe that germline gene therapy would be a safer and more effective way of preventing certain genetic diseases. Biophysicist Burke Zimmerman argues that it would avoid the need for repeatedly treating one generation after the next (assuming treatments were even available) and that correcting problems at the earliest stages of development could prevent early forms of damage.[4] But it may be more difficult to maintain that germline genetic *enhancement* would yield benefits substantial enough to offset the risks.

That said, attempts to ban extreme forms of enhancement would raise the same practical and constitutional problems mentioned in chapter 8. Because germline enhancement most likely would be performed in conjunction with in vitro fertilization, prohibitory laws could target the physicians and IVF clinics rather than the parents and children, which might alleviate some of these concerns. But huge enforcement problems would remain. Imagine what it would take to detect that someone's germ cells had been manipulated, especially if this had taken place abroad. We also might need to sanction germline enhanced persons whose forebears had slipped through the enforcement net, which might seem unfair because it would punish children for the sins of their ancestors. And some commentators, such as John Robertson, even would object to restrictions that applied only to IVF physicians and clinics as impermissible government interference with reproductive liberty.

Moreover, many of the more extreme forms of enhancement would be accompanied by inherent disincentives. Assuming that the changes were visible, as in the case of chimeras with obvious nonhuman features, the same revulsion that animates opponents of this type of enhancement might well cause those who had been enhanced in this way to be shunned by society. They might obtain some mileage from their celebrity as freaks, much in the same way shock artists like Ron Athey make money poking themselves with needles during performances.[5] But it would be difficult for them to lead anything like a normal life. Indeed, if their alterations were great enough, they might not be able to reproduce, at least not in the usual ways. Knowing this, it is unlikely that many people would avail themselves of the technology, even if it did exist.

But of course it wouldn't be the enhanced individuals themselves who made that choice. Transgenic or transhuman enhancement almost certainly would have to take place before people were born. If parents were to doubt or ignore the adverse impact on their children, the parents clearly would be responsible and, if they were found guilty of child abuse, would merit severe punishment. But the children would suffer as well, and society would face the tragic task of trying to ease the suffering of what they had spawned.

Chapter 14

Research on Enhancement

BECAUSE BY FAR the best way to ensure that biomedical enhancements promote the public good is to make them as safe and effective as possible, it is critical that good information be available about their risks and benefits. Good information includes knowledge about the chemical formulation of the drug or the electrical and mechanical design of the device, as well as data about the effects that the enhancement produces in laboratory and animal testing. But by far the most important information comes from human experiments.

The United States, along with other nations and international organizations, has developed an elaborate system of ethical norms and legal rules to govern biomedical research using human subjects. The principles they embody were developed to safeguard against abuses such as the Nazi medical experiments that came to light following World War II; indeed, the first set of rules to protect human subjects was adopted by military judges at Nuremberg as part of their verdict against the Nazi doctors. But the Nazis were not the only ones who conducted unethical medical experiments. In the early 1960s, mentally disabled children in a state school on Staten Island were deliberately infected with hepatitis, some of it extracted from feces, to test the efficacy of treatment with gamma globulin. Around the same time, patients at Jewish

Chronic Disease Hospital in New York were unknowingly injected with live cancer cells to learn about organ transplant rejection. But next to the abuses of the Germans and Japanese during World War II, the most infamous case is the U.S. Public Health Service syphilis experiment at Tuskegee. Begun in 1932, the study involved 410 African-American syphilitic men in rural Alabama. The purpose of the study was to follow the course of the untreated disease. Subjects were not informed what was wrong with them, and they were not treated, even in the 1950s after penicillin had been recognized as standard, effective therapy. In fact, U.S. public health officials actively discouraged treatment by local physicians, the state health department, and the army. Subjects were offered a $50 burial subsidy to stay in the study, and in 1958, each survivor was given $25 and a certificate of appreciation. The first paper describing the study appeared in the medical literature in 1936, and reports continued to be published through the 1960s. In 1969, a committee of the U.S. Centers for Disease Control and Prevention (CDC) reviewed the experiment and authorized it to continue. By the time the press exposed the study in 1972 and halted it, only 74 men remained alive.

Revulsion against the experiment at Tuskegee led Congress to enact the National Research Act of 1974. This created the President's Commission for the Study of Ethical Problems in Medicine and Biomedical and Behavioral Research, which in turn produced the Belmont Report, the primary source of ethical principles for human subjects research, which forms the basis for the so-called Common Rule, the federal regulations governing human experimentation. The Common Rule requires experiments to be approved by institutional review boards (IRBs), committees created by the institutions that conduct the research and comprised primarily of employees of those institutions who perform their duties as an uncompensated add-on to their regular jobs. (Experiments funded by the government or intended to be submitted to the FDA also must obtain government approval.) To approve the proposed experiment, the IRB reviewers must satisfy themselves that the benefits are maximized and the risks minimized and that the risks are reasonable in relation to the anticipated benefits, including benefits to subjects and the importance of the knowledge to be gained.[1] Furthermore, the reviewers must ensure that the investigators will obtain the informed consent of the subjects. This requires that the subjects be given a description of the proposed experiment, together with information about reasonably foreseeable risks and any benefits to the subject or to others that may reasonably be expected from the research.[2] Additional requirements kick in for obtaining informed consent for specific populations (e.g., pregnant women, fetuses and newborns; prisoners; and children).[3] Special safeguards may also be imposed to protect other populations deemed "vulnerable to coercion or undue influence, such as . . . mentally disabled persons, or economically or educationally disadvantaged person."[4]

It is open to question how well these protections work. In a 2004 critique in the journal *Nature Medicine,* Ezekiel Emanuel, the head of bioethics at the Clinical Center of the National Institutes of Health, and his colleagues wrote that "today, almost no one feels satisfied with protections for human participants in clinical research." The authors listed a host of criticisms:

> Clinical investigators are frustrated by a review process that seems bureaucratic and inefficient. Institutional review board (IRB) and ethics committee members and staff feel overworked, sometimes baffled by ambiguous regulations, and uncertain of calls for accreditation. Regulators, stymied by their limited authority, worry about criticism for inaction despite harm to research participants. Commercial sponsors of research see the system as inefficient and repetitive. Foreign researchers and governments often view the requirement to follow U.S. regulations as culturally insensitive and even imperialistic. The public finds each alleged case of unethical practice and the recent deaths of several research participants troubling and indicative that the system is broken.[5]

But the need for data about the safety and effectiveness of biomedical enhancements raises an even more fundamental issue. By and large, current protections for human subjects were designed for experiments aimed at diagnosing, preventing, curing, or treating illnesses and medical conditions. How would these rules be applied to enhancement research? And even if they could be made to work well, would they be able to protect human enhancement subjects adequately?

Assessing Risk and Benefit

One concern raised by enhancement research is how to decide if the risks from an experiment would be outweighed by the potential benefits. The degree of potential benefit depends on the nature of the benefit as well as its amount: The more important or valuable the potential benefit, the greater the risks that researchers ethically can impose on subjects. As the Declaration of Helsinki proclaims: "Medical research involving human subjects should only be conducted if the importance of the objective outweighs the inherent risks and burdens to the subject."[6] The Nuremberg Code agrees that "the degree of risk to be taken should never exceed that determined by the humanitarian importance of the problem to be solved by the experiment."

It might be wondered, therefore, whether it would be unethical to conduct an enhancement study unless it offered a much better ratio of benefits to risks than a health-oriented study. Suppose there were a drug that increased muscle mass in people with muscle-wasting diseases but also caused liver damage in a small number of patients. Should an IRB approve a study to see if the drug increased muscle mass in normal individuals? Similarly, should an IRB approve a study to measure patient satisfaction with a new surgical technique for facelifts, given that any surgical procedure carries with it a certain risk of scarring? Would a risk of scarring that was acceptable in a study in which the technique was used to correct a facial deformity also be acceptable in a study of cosmetic use?

On the one hand, it might seem obvious that medical benefits are inherently more valuable than enhancement benefits. It would be highly unlikely, for example, that the National Institutes of Health would invest a significant portion of scarce research funds in enhancement rather than health-oriented research. If enhancements have less inherent value than medical interventions, then it might seem unethical to expose enhancement subjects to the same amount of risk as subjects in health-oriented experiments. A study of a new plastic surgery technique with more than a minimum of risk might be justified in subjects who required nasal reconstruction but not in subjects who sought nose jobs. Moreover, some enhancement technologies, such as those involving genetic factors in illness, are new and their risks poorly understood. As one commentator states, "If the safety of a treatment is relatively unknown . . . a larger potential benefit might reasonably be required."[7] Finally, commentators argue that because subjects in enhancement studies are healthy, whereas subjects in medical experiments are ill to begin with, enhancement subjects have more to lose, and therefore researchers must offer them greater benefits for a given amount of risk. Nicholas Agar states, for example, that "the cost/benefit analysis is different for enhancement. While those who are experimenting with treatments for serious diseases may only succeed in substituting one kind of misery for another, those experimenting on human enhancement are likely to substitute a miserable life for a happy one."[8]

But the value of a benefit clearly depends on the nature of the benefit. It is reasonable to expect that some health-oriented benefits would be regarded as more valuable than some enhancement benefits. Most people probably would agree that an experiment to test a potentially life-saving drug or medical device posed an opportunity for greater benefit than an experiment to test a new nonprescription contact lens like Bausch and Lomb's MaxSight, which reduces glare for athletes and makes them appear more fearsome. On the other hand, as noted earlier, some enhancement benefits may be perceived to be more valuable than medical benefits, so that an enhancement that would potentially lead to a substantial increase in cognitive function, for example, might be deemed more valuable than a substance to treat a minor skin irritation. In short, in both health-oriented and enhancement research, the potential benefit necessary to justify a set of risks will depend on the specifics of the study in question.

A second question is how much to defer to the subjects in assessing potential enhancement benefits. The Common Rule takes a highly paternalistic approach, allowing investigators to approach potential subjects to seek their informed consent to participate only after experts, in the form of institutional review boards, government sponsors, government regulators, and the investigators themselves, are satisfied that the potential benefits outweigh the risks. This may be justified in the case of health-oriented research on the grounds that physicians and other medical experts are best suited to gauge medical benefits and risks. But it is not clear that these experts possess any particular advantage when it comes to making the value judgment about whether a given degree of risk outweighs a given probability of benefit. One neurologist observes: "As neurologists, we may have special understanding of the potential benefits and risks of quality of life therapies in so far as they work through the nervous system. But we have no special insight into the pursuit of happiness."[9] And as noted earlier, despite being opposed in general to biomedical enhancement, the President's Council on Bioethics also doubts that medical experts are particularly well suited to evaluate enhancement benefits: "There are difficulties when medical practice moves beyond therapy. Where the goal is restoring health, the doctor's discretion is guided by an agreed-upon and recognizable target. But a physician prescribing for goals beyond therapy is in uncharted waters.

Although fully armed with the means, he has no special expertise regarding the end—neither what it is nor whether it is desirable."[10] This could be taken to imply that subjects in enhancement studies should be given more leeway than subjects in health-oriented research in accepting risks in return for potential benefits.

But it is important to recognize that experts continue to play a crucial role in protecting subjects even in enhancement experiments. Only experts are likely to possess the ability to determine if a proposed study was properly designed, so that the risks to subjects can be justified in light of valid and reproducible results; or if the investigators had misrepresented the potential benefits, deemphasized risks, failed to disclose information necessary for informed consent, devalued subjects' welfare, or possessed certain types of unacceptable conflicts of interest. Experts also can prevent subjects from falling prey to the enhancement equivalent of the so-called therapeutic misconception, in which subjects mistakenly assume that they will derive some direct enhancement benefit from participating in the study, without realizing that they may be randomly assigned to a group of subjects that receives a placebo instead of the experimental enhancement or that the experimental intervention may turn out to provide no enhancement benefits to the subjects who actually receive it.

Another question is whether the mechanisms inherent in the Common Rule to prevent unethical experimentation are adequate to protect against the potential adverse social impacts of biomedical enhancements. Consider a proposal to study a biomedical enhancement that would be so expensive that few people would be able to afford it. Is it ethical to conduct a study that, if successful, might exacerbate social inequality? What if the subjects themselves could not afford the enhancement once the study ended? One solution might be to provide subjects with ongoing free or subsidized access to the enhancements. But even if the subjects themselves could obtain the enhancement, what if it was likely to be used much more extensively by a different population outside of the study? For example, the use of prescription stimulants is more prevalent in populations with higher socioeconomic status and better access to health care.[11] Would it be ethical to include subjects with lower socioeconomic status in a study to determine if a prescription stimulant improved cognitive performance?

This certainly is a legitimate ethical question, although it is not unique to enhancement research, because expensive, new medical treatments may be unaffordable for many, and health disparities based on race and income are well documented.[12] But it is not at all clear that IRBs have the authority to consider this objection, whether in enhancement or health-oriented research. On the one hand, the Common Rule says that an IRB may approve a study only if it concludes that the risks are reasonable in relation to the anticipated benefits, including benefits to subjects and the importance of the knowledge to be gained. Conceivably, the knowledge to be gained from a study of an enhancement that would increase inequality or that might not be available to people in the subjects' social class might not be deemed important enough to justify imposing any substantial risks on the subjects. But another section of the federal regulations specifically prohibits IRBs from considering "possible long-range effects of applying knowledge gained in the research (for example, the possible effects of the research on public policy)."[13] If social inequality is deemed to be a public policy concern, the rules may preclude IRBs from taking it into account in evaluating proposed human experiments.

Research on Vulnerable Populations

Earlier we saw that certain individuals might not be able to make voluntary choices about whether or not to use biomedical enhancements. The same factors that limit their ability to decide to use an enhancement also would compromise their ability to give informed consent to participate in enhancement experiments. The Common Rule establishes special protections for so-called vulnerable populations, specifically mentioning pregnant women, fetuses and newborns, prisoners, and children as well as other populations deemed "vulnerable to coercion or undue influence, such as . . . mentally disabled persons, or economically or educationally disadvantaged person."[14] One question is whether the protections are adequate. A second question is whether there are other distinct groups that merit special attention.

Embryonic and in Utero Research

Some enhancements might be administered to developing embryos or fetuses. This includes genetic testing following in vitro fertilization to identify the "best" embryos for implantation into the womb, manipulation of embryonic and fetal DNA to produce enhancement effects, and the administration of enhancement drugs in utero. Attempts to produce these technologies would require experiments to determine how to make them work, experiments that would be carried out on organisms that were incapable of giving their consent. This raises the question whether the research would be ethical.

Federal regulations currently permit research to take place on fetuses that holds out the prospect of "direct benefit" to subjects.[15] Because the regulations do not define the term "direct benefit," there is no obvious reason why this would not apply to enhancement as well as health-oriented research. The only special protection for fetuses is that the researchers must obtain the assent of the parents.[16] Fetal enhancement research might pose a significant health risk to pregnant women, but some parents would be willing to accept this risk in return for the possibility of enhancing their children. Again, the only current protection for the woman is the requirement that both she and the father consent to the experiment.

As we shall see, there is a far more elaborate set of rules governing research on children. It is interesting to speculate why the same protections do not apply to fetuses as well, particularly when such powerful political forces are dedicated to preserving fetal interests against the threat of abortion, forces that have held sway over the executive branch of the government, which regulates human subjects research, for the past several years. Given the acrimonious public debate over embryonic stem cell research, it is even more surprising that there are no regulations governing embryonic research, except for President Bush's limitation on the use of federal funds for new sources of stem cells. Embryos and fetuses clearly do not enjoy the same legal and ethical status as children, but it would seem appropriate to protect them against outlandish medical or enhancement experimentation.

Research on Prisoners

Except for children, prisoners are the group that receives the most research protections under existing federal regulations. They may not be offered significant inducements to agree to serve as experimental subjects, such as better living conditions, food, amenities, money, or favorable consideration regarding parole. They may not participate in research that poses greater risks than those that would be accepted by nonprisoners. A majority of the members of the IRB that approves the proposed study cannot be associated with the correctional institution housing the subjects, and at least one member of the IRB must be a prisoner or prisoner representative. Finally, the research proposal must be approved by the Department of Health and Human Services after public notice.[17]

These protections, like most of the rest of the Common Rule, were adopted in 1974, following the revelations about the Tuskegee study. At the same time that the public learned about Tuskegee, reports came out about experiments at places like Holmesburg, the Philadelphia prison in which inmates were enrolled in numerous trials that exposed them to everything from dandruff treatments to dioxin and other radioactive, hallucinogenic, and carcinogenic chemicals.[18] Beginning in 1951, experiments were conducted at Holmesburg on behalf of several government agencies and more than 30 drug companies, most under the direction of the University of Pennsylvania, which had a research facility in the prison. Subjects could earn as much as $1500 a month, compared with the 15 or 25 cents a day they could earn at other jobs. The government estimates that, before 1970, about 90 percent of all new drugs were tested on prisoners at places like Holmesburg.

In 2006, a committee of the prestigious Institute of Medicine of the National Academy of Sciences recommended that the restrictions on using prisoners in medical research be relaxed to ease the shortage of available subjects. The recommendations would permit research on risky drugs so long as the drugs had completed preliminary human testing (FDA phases I and II) and offered the possibility of direct benefit to the subjects themselves and so long as at least half of the subjects were nonprisoners.[19]

At first it might seem unlikely that anyone would want to try to enhance criminals. Give them steroids to see if it made them stronger? Cognitive enhancers so they were smarter and harder to catch? But as the IOM report indicates, prisoners constitute a readily available and relatively easily managed study population. Moreover, it is conceivable that someone might want to test whether certain enhancements could make them more tractable while in jail or less likely to commit additional crimes if released. For example, convicts with enhanced cognitive ability might be able to get good enough jobs that they no longer felt the need to make money illegally.

Research on Workers

Another setting where there may be special demand for enhancement research is in the workplace. Not only might researchers find it convenient to conduct studies under such relatively controllable conditions, but employers and employees would also have a strong interest in enhancements that could improve on-the-job performance, and workers may feel compelled to agree to serve as subjects to avoid adverse consequences from their bosses, or just to have the chance to perform better.

The NIH office responsible for protecting research subjects is cognizant of the risks that workers might face: "The issues with respect to employees as research subjects," it states, "are essentially identical to those involving students as research subjects: coercion or undue influence, and confidentiality."[20] Yet the Common Rule provides no special protections for workplace research, and there is no mention in labor laws of the perils that subjects might face. Although it may seem odd to say so, given the possibility of coercion or undue pressure to participate, workers seem somewhat similar to prisoners. Consideration should be given to prohibiting employers from penalizing employees who decline to serve as research subjects, to requiring the IRB that reviews the research proposal to be independent of the employer, and to including employee representation among its members.

An interesting question arises concerning how much risk employees should be allowed to accept. On the one hand, they should be protected from research that poses risks greater than those that would be accepted by subjects who are free of workplace pressure. On the other hand, enhancements that substantially improve performance at work could be of tremendous benefit to the workers themselves, such as by preserving their jobs. As a result, it might be ethical to allow them to accept greater risks than subjects outside the workplace. Indeed, it might be appropriate to permit enhancement studies to be conducted in the workplace, while health-oriented research that poses similar risks but does not specifically target workplace illnesses would be unethical.

Research on Students

Students who are children would be entitled to the same research protections as other children. But adult students would seem to fall into a category similar to workers. The NIH recognizes the special vulnerability of university students, commenting in a guidebook for IRBs:

> The problem with student participation in research conducted at the university is the possibility that their agreement to participate will not be freely given. Students may volunteer to participate out of a belief that

> doing so will place them in good favor with faculty (e.g., that participating will result in receiving better grades, recommendations, employment, or the like), or that failure to participate will negatively affect their relationship with the investigator or faculty generally (i.e., by seeming "uncooperative," not part of the scientific community). Prohibiting all student participation in research, however, may be an over-protective reaction. An alternative way to protect against coercion is to require that faculty-investigators advertise for subjects generally (e.g., through notices posted in the school or department) rather than recruit individual students directly. As with any research involving a potentially vulnerable subject population, IRBs should pay special attention to the potential for coercion or undue influence and consider ways in which the possibility of exploitation can be reduced or eliminated.[21]

These are good suggestions, but as in the case of workers, the regulations themselves furnish no protections aimed specifically at subjects in educational environments.

At a minimum, students should not be penalized for refusing to serve as subjects, the IRB that reviews the research proposal should be independent of the educational institution, and students should be included among its members. As with workers, though, risks that might be unacceptable in other contexts might appear to be justified in studies of experimental enhancements that offer potential academic benefits to the subjects.

Research on Athletes

Athletes might accept large experimental risks due to external pressure from their coaches, trainers, fans, family members, and teammates. There is also, of course, great internal pressure to win. Remember the survey of the 200 world-class athletes in which half stated that they would be willing to take a drug that enabled them to win every competition for five years, but then would kill them.[22] Conceivably, a significant percentage also would be willing to participate in an experiment to assess the safety and efficacy of a dangerous performance-enhancing drug, if they stood to benefit enough from it. In an investigation to gauge the safety and efficacy of a corticosteroid to treat Duchenne muscular dystrophy, 10 of the 30 patients in the experimental group developed cataracts.[23] If the steroid had the potential to enhance sports performance, athletic subjects might feel that the improvement in performance outweighed the risk to their eyesight. Furthermore, as Dena Davis has pointed out, athletes may represent a convenient supply of subjects, especially in college settings.[24] Yet there are no special protections for them. As in the case of students, regulations should prohibit athletes from being punished for refusing to serve as subjects, such as by being kept out of competition. Moreover, research with athletes should be reviewed by an IRB that has no connection with the team or sport, and athletes should be included among its members. There is precedent for this last suggestion in the World Anti-Doping Agency's (WADA's) Athletes Committee, composed of 13 Olympic and Paralympic competitors who act as advisors to the agency.[25]

One concern raised by the prospect of using athletes as subjects is that the experimental enhancements they are given may be prohibited in their sporting events. This helps explain why so little good safety data is available on the use of performance-enhancing drugs in sports. As the director of the biological psychiatry laboratory at Harvard Medical School's McLean Hospital commented, "You can't ethically do a study of 100 guys, feed 50 of them high doses of drugs, and then sit back and see who drops dead."[26] To avoid this complication, researchers could follow the lead of WADA, which excludes active competitors from serving as subjects in tests to validate its drug testing methodologies. But this could reduce the value of the test results, because the physiological characteristics of noncompeting athletes may differ significantly enough from those of athletes who are actively competing that the results of the experiments would not apply to the actual target population. Moreover, as noted earlier, it is not clear that IRBs currently have the authority to consider the policy issues raised by testing banned or potentially banned substances.

Another problem raised by research on athletes is that, even if the experimental enhancement were not banned, subjects who received it might gain an unfair competitive advantage over other athletes who do not have access to it. For example, the technology might be sufficiently new that it has not yet been addressed by the rules, as is the case with nitrogen tents, mentioned in chapter 1. It is not clear how serious this problem is. For one thing, the advantage derived from the experimental enhancement may not present any greater ethical challenge than if athletes were given access to an experimental dietary regimen, training technique, or piece of equipment. So long as the advantage persisted only for a reasonably short length of time—allowing other competitors to gain access to the regimen or device once they become aware of its usefulness—it may not be unethical to allow subjects to derive some benefit from the experimental enhancements in competition, perhaps as some compensation for agreeing to be exposed to the study risks.

But if access to the experimental enhancement were deemed to confer an unfair advantage on subjects, IRBs currently may not have the authority to take this into consideration in deciding whether or not to approve the study. It is true that that the Belmont Report names "justice" as one of the three cardinal principles of research ethics (the other two being respect for persons and beneficence). However, the emphasis, codified in the Common Rule's requirement that the selection of subjects be "equitable," is on the potential injustice of exposing subjects to the risks of the study, not providing them with the potential benefits.[27] The Belmont Report only hints at the potential injustice from gaining access to the benefits of a study, stating that "whenever research supported by public funds leads to the development of therapeutic devices and procedures, justice demands both that these not provide advantages only to those who can afford them and that such research should not unduly involve persons from groups unlikely to be among the beneficiaries of subsequent applications of the research."[28] This does not respond directly to the justice issue raised by enhancement research in sports, that by participating in research, the subjects might obtain an unfair advantage in athletic competitions.

Research on Members of the Military

As described in chapter 1, the military is engaged in a large-scale program of enhancement research. Much of it is being carried out using members of the civilian population as subjects under the standard rules for human subjects research, just as would be the case in a university or research institution setting. But a good deal of it is conducted on members of the military, and this raises the question of whether they are in a position to refuse to participate.

The military has a checkered past when it comes to human experiments on its members. Beginning in 1952, the Army tested incapacitating agents, including nerve agents, nerve agent antidotes, psychochemicals, and irritants, on 7,120 service personnel without adequate informed consent. The program was only halted in 1975.[29] In the 1950s and 1960s, the Defense Department, in cooperation with the CIA, gave LSD and the hallucinogen quinuclidinyl benzilate to servicemen without their consent; many of the experiments were conducted under a program known as MKULTRA, which was established to offset reported Soviet and Chinese progress in perfecting brainwashing techniques.[30] One of the oddest sets of experiments took place during the 1960s with soldiers who were Seventh-Day Adventists. Believing that they were forbidden by their religion from engaging in combat, certain SDA draftees agreed to participate in experiments to develop vaccines and treatments for germ-warfare agents, including Q fever, tularemia, Rift Valley fever, malaria, sandfly fever, anthrax, Queensland fever, Rocky Mountain spotted fever, encephalitis, and plague.[31] A number of successful vaccines resulted, including for yellow fever, hepatitis A, anthrax, and plague, as well as potentially effective immunizations for tularemia, Queensland fever, and Venezuelan equine encephalitis.[32] Many subjects volunteered for the project, called Operation Whitecoat, to avoid being sent to Vietnam. The Operation Whitecoat investigators apparently took pains to ensure that they obtained the informed consent of subjects, telling them, for example, that one possible outcome, albeit an unlikely one, could be death.[33] But afterward, questions were raised about whether the participants really had a choice, because the experiments were endorsed by SDA officials, and as one subject later pointed out, "We grew up to trust the church."[34]

In response to these incidents, the military took a number of steps to protect soldiers who were asked to serve as experimental subjects. The Department of Defense adopted its own regulations embodying the Common Rule.[35] It gave the individual services discretion to establish additional protections. The U.S. Army, for example, requires most human subjects research to go through two layers of IRB review, one by the IRB at the institution that actually conducts the experiments and the second by the Human Subjects Research Review Board, a unit under the command of the Army Surgeon General.

With two exceptions, military research cannot take place without the informed consent of the subjects. One exception is for "emergency research," studies of techniques to treat soldiers with medical emergencies who, because they are unconscious or otherwise non compos mentis, cannot make their own decisions.[36] (The FDA has established a similar exception for this type of research in nonmilitary patients.) One product that the military is interested in for this type of experimentation is PolyHeme, a type of blood substitute that is much easier to store than real blood.

The second exception permits soldiers to be given investigational drugs without their consent when the president certifies that this is "in connection with the member's participation in a particular military operation." This exception was created during the first Gulf War, when the military anticipated that the Iraqis might use chemical and biological agents and wanted to be able to give soldiers experimental botulism and nerve gas vaccines under combat conditions in which obtaining their informed consent would be impractical.[37] Originally, the exception permitted the commissioner of the FDA to waive the informed consent requirement upon request by the secretary of defense, but in 1998, after reports had surfaced about Gulf War Syndrome and other health problems alleged to have been caused by the vaccines, Congress insisted that in the future, the president must take action before the informed consent requirement could be waived.[38]

How adequate are these protections for military subjects in enhancement research? The Department of Defense and the service arms seem to have established comprehensive programs to ensure that their research is conducted in an ethical manner. But the realities of military life create doubts about their practicality, and the exigencies of combat make it unlikely that any system of protections for subjects would be entirely effective. The requirement of a presidential order to waive the requirement of informed consent is certainly important, but the existence of this exception signifies that the military may feel compelled to dispense with formal clinical trials altogether and simply dispense investigational enhancement drugs on the battlefield to meet operational needs. The military recognizes the importance of insulating soldiers who are solicited to participate in experiments from undue pressure from their superiors. For example, both service and Department of Defense regulations provide that "unit officers and non-commissioned officers (NCOs) are specifically restricted from influencing the decisions of their subordinates to participate or not to participate as research subjects" and add that "unit officers and senior NCOs in the chain of command are required to be absent during research subject solicitation and consenting activities."[39] Service regulations also require that informed consent forms include a statement that "participation is voluntary, that refusal to participate will involve no penalty or loss of benefits to which the subject is otherwise entitled, and that the subject may discontinue participation at any time without penalty or loss of benefits to which the subject is otherwise entitled."[40] But as one set of commentators points out, it may be almost impossible for soldiers to distinguish when they are being asked to serve as experimental subjects and when they are being told to do something by their commander: “Service members are obligated to obey all lawful orders from superiors, and may feel compelled to respect the orders from senior officials conducting research. . . . The contrast of a service member as both a vulnerable subject who must be protected from a commander’s coercion and, simultaneously, a warrior who may at any time be ordered into harm’s way is not well explored.”[41] Finally, the instinct for self-preservation is likely to lead soldiers to grasp at any means of improving their chances of surviving battle, including exposing themselves to risks in order to gain access to experimental enhancements. One solution might seem to be to restrict military enhancement research to subjects who are noncombatants, but this may encounter the same problem of lack of experimental verisimilitude as sports testing carried out in noncompetitors.

Research on Children

The Common Rule permits children to participate in research if the investigators have obtained the permission of the parents, as well as the “assent” of the children if that is possible. Some ethicists might think that it is unethical for parents to enroll their children in any enhancement trials, on the grounds that biomedical enhancement is contrary to a child’s best interest. Parents might be deemed to be sacrificing the children’s welfare in order to further the parents’ own ambitions or social status or to be valuing the children too much in terms of their capabilities, that is, “commodifying” them. But children already have served as subjects in some biomedical enhancement research. For example, there have been at least seven studies on the effects of caffeine in normal children, at least some of which were subject to some sort of ethical oversight.[42] Moreover, there is little objection to parents placing their children in experimental educational settings to try to make them better learners. Why then should parents be prohibited from enrolling their children in a study simply because it involves a biomedical enhancement?

Even as staunch an opponent of biomedical enhancement as Thomas Murray seems to agree. In his book *The Worth of a Child,* Murray takes issue with bioethicist Paul Ramsey, who maintains that “no parent is morally competent to consent that his child shall be submitted to hazardous or other experiments having no diagnostic or therapeutic significance for the child himself."[43] Murray argues that "protecting a child's physical safety may be very important but it is not the entirety of our moral obligations to our children; risks, especially very small ones, may be accepted in the service of other goods and values." Consequently, Murray thinks that parents ought to be permitted to enroll children of "normal-but-short" stature in experiments to see if human growth hormone would make them taller: "I do not believe we can say that parents who enroll their children in this experiment clearly violate their obligations to their children . . . . They hope that their children will benefit from participating, even if the benefit does not so clearly fall into the realm of 'Therapeutic.'" (Technically, the use of HGH that Murray is describing does not qualify as an enhancement, because the term *normal* to describe these children is misleading. The children's height is more than two standard deviations below the population mean, which by convention makes them abnormally short, but they are called "normal-but-short" because, unlike people who are dwarfs, their short stature is not attributable to a hormonal deficiency.)

Yet saying that children might be permitted to serve as subjects in some enhancement studies does not mean that there can be no limits on parental consent, because some parents might be willing to enroll their children in excessively risky trials in the hope that the children would receive experimental interventions that gave them a competitive advantage. As we saw earlier, the law does impose a limit on how much risk parents can impose on their children. So the question is how to protect children from participating in enhancement research that society would regard as too dangerous.

Children are one of the populations that the Common Rule lists as vulnerable, and the regulations contain four separate sets of provisions intended to protect them as subjects. One provision, section 404, applies to research with children that entails no greater than "minimal risk." The regulations define minimal risk to mean that "the probability and magnitude of harm or discomfort anticipated in the research are no greater in and of themselves then those ordinarily encountered in daily life or during the performance of routine physical or psychological examinations or tests."[44] A 1977 report of the President's Commission for the Protection of Human Subjects of Biomedical and Behavioral Research lists among minimal risk procedures: "routine immunization, modest changes in diet or schedule, physical examination, obtaining blood or urine specimens, developmental assessments. . . , questionnaires, observational techniques, noninvasive physiological monitoring, [and] psychological tests and puzzles," and a committee of the Institute of Medicine analogizes minimal risk to a well-child visit to the doctor.[45] This level of risk is so low that few if any experiments in which children were given biomedical enhancements would be likely to qualify.

Similarly, enhancement studies are unlikely to fall under section 406 of the regulations, which pertains to research that presents only a "minor increase over minimal risk." Although this term is not defined in the regulations, most biomedical enhancements probably would be deemed to create a greater risk than this, and besides, section 406 requires the study to yield "generalizeable knowledge about the subjects' disorder or condition which is of vital importance for the understanding or amelioration of the subjects' disorder or condition," and an enhancement by definition does not address a disorder or condition.

Interestingly, an NIH panel that reviewed a study in which normal-but-short children were to be given HGH concluded that the study could proceed under section 406. The implications of this decision for enhancement research troubled bioethicist Carol Tauer:

> Although the NIH panel states specifically that very short stature in non-GH-deficient children is a statistical rather than a medical abnormality, the panel applies a regulation explicitly designed for approving research on the medical treatment of sick children. Such an application of 46.406 creates a precedent for approving greater than minimal risk research with healthy children in order to study any condition researchers or clinicians would like to be able to modify. If there are people who regard the condition as disadvantaging and who seek "treatment" for it, then that condition would seem to qualify for studies under 46.406.
>
> An "enhancement" modification is designed to alter a condition that is considered undesirable, either absolutely or relatively. Given the precedent in the NIH committee report, 46.406 could be used to approve greater-than-minimal-risk research on children to test enhancement uses of genetic therapies. While the ethical literature and public policy statements on human gene therapy continue to assert that enhancement applications are not planned or intended, the conclusions of the NIH panel open the door for such research, even on children.[46]

Section 405 of the regulations allows an IRB to approve research with children that entails greater than minimal risk as long as there is a prospect of direct benefit to the individual subjects from the intervention in question; furthermore, the IRB must determine that the risks are balanced by the potential benefits to the subjects and that the ratio of risks to benefits is at least as favorable as that which would be provided by alternative treatments. The question is whether a direct enhancement benefit would count as a "direct benefit." The regulations fail to define the term, and a survey of the heads of IRBs showed that they were unclear about what it means.[47] The regulation does not speak in terms of a "direct *medical* benefit," but as noted at the beginning of this chapter, the entire focus of the Common Rule is on health-oriented research, and the regulation does require the potential benefit to be compared to the benefit from alternative "treatments." Still, because the regulation does not explicitly rule out enhancement research, it might allow enhancement research presenting more than minimal risk to be conducted on children if an IRB were convinced that the risks were outweighed by the potential benefits.

The final section of the regulations, section 407, is a catchall that applies to research on children that does not fall under one of the other three sections. It allows children to participate as subjects if a special review panel appointed by the NIH's Office of Human Research Protections finds that "the research presents a reasonable opportunity to further the understanding, prevention, or alleviation of a serious problem affecting the health or welfare of children."[48] Again, the question is whether an enhancement study would be deemed to address "a serious problem affecting the health or welfare of children." Ori Lev, Franklin G. Miller, and Ezekiel J. Emanuel in the department of bioethics at the Clinical Center of the National Institutes of Health take the position that enhancement research could be deemed to be health-oriented in that it can provide information that would enable enhancement users to avoid harmful enhancements.[49] In that case, a 407 panel might be willing to approve even relatively risky enhancement research on children.

While no 407 panels have been convened to review enhancement research as such, one study that did receive approval through the 407 process, although it was never carried out, involved administering to normal children methylphenidate and dextroamphetamine, which are controlled substances approved for treating ADHD but which, as noted in chapter 1, are also used off-label to enhance cognition. The purpose of the study was to see whether magnetic resonance imaging could be useful as a means of diagnosing children with ADHD. To find this out, the researchers needed to determine if children with ADHD who were taking the drugs exhibited different brain images than siblings who were given the drugs but did not have ADHD.

Because none of the special protections for research on children clearly apply to enhancement studies, one possible conclusion is that such research is forbidden. In a 2001 case, *Grimes v. Kennedy Krieger Institute*, a Maryland court seemed to reach a similar conclusion.[50] The case involved a study of different methods for abating lead levels in Baltimore. The goal was to see if there was an approach that might go some way toward reducing lead levels in children's blood but at the same time would be affordable for landlords providing housing to low-income families. The judge ruled that the IRB should not have approved the study because, while it was under way, some of the children were left in housing where they continued to be exposed to unhealthy levels of lead. In the judge's opinion, even though the results of the study might prove helpful to other children or to the community at large, the study impermissibly imposed health risks on the children without the prospect of a direct benefit to them. While the study in question was not enhancement research, the court rendered a sweeping decision that, at first blush, would appear to preclude any enhancement studies in which children serve as subjects: "We hold that in Maryland a parent, appropriate relative, or other applicable surrogate, cannot consent to the participation of a child or other person under legal disability in nontherapeutic research or studies in which there is any risk of injury or damage to the health of the subject." Only on closer analysis does it become clear that the court was not using the term "nontherapeutic" to refer to research with a nonmedical goal, such as enhancement research, but in the technical sense in which the term is used in the regulations governing research on children, that is, to quote a footnote in the opinion, to medical research that "is not designed to directly benefit the subjects utilized in the research, but, rather, is designed to achieve beneficial results for the public at large." In other words, the *Grimes* opinion would not necessarily preclude enhancement research on children—only enhancement research that did not offer the prospect of direct enhancement benefit to the subjects.

An alternate interpretation of the existing regulatory scheme is that because the regulations were only meant to govern health-oriented research, research on children that is not health-oriented, including enhancement research, can proceed if it fulfills the general requirements for protecting human subjects, namely, that an IRB judges that the risks are outweighed by the potential benefits and that adequate steps have been taken to obtain the informed consent of the subjects or, because children are not legally competent to give consent, the assent of their parents or legal representatives. But this leaves children without adequate protections. If the authors of the Common Rule correctly perceived that children deserve special protection from risky research designed to diagnose, cure, treat, or prevent disease, it would seem to follow that children also need special protection from risky research that does not have such health-oriented goals. In that case, what should those protections be?

First, the Common Rule should acknowledge that an enhancement benefit may comprise a direct benefit for pediatric subjects and that a potential for an enhancement benefit may outweigh a certain amount of risk. Second, IRBs should determine whether a study that would be acceptable for competent adult subjects would be too risky for children. In an obvious sense, the IRB would have to take into account relevant physiological differences between children and adults. For example, a long-term study of steroids that might be ethical in adults would be unethical for children because of the adverse effects of steroids on bone growth. Beyond that is the question of the extent to which an IRB or government regulator should be allowed to second-guess parents who are willing to give consent for their children to participate in enhancement trials. On the one hand, as we have seen, parents are entitled to broad discretion in deciding how to raise their children. On the other hand, some parents may be overzealous in attempting to give their children a competitive advantage, thereby exposing them to unreasonable risks. The general legal standard by which parental actions are judged is, as we said, "abuse and neglect," which is typically interpreted to permit a large measure of tolerance for parental decisionmaking. But this standard has to govern not only parental decisions made in the public realm, such as decisions about whether or not to consent to children participating in biomedical research, but also decisions within the confines of the family, such as how children are clothed, fed, and disciplined. Given the private nature of the realm in which such decisions are made, it is fitting that parents be given wide latitude and spared from excessively intrusive public scrutiny. Only when their private behavior toward their children is egregious should the state feel entitled to intervene. But enrolling children in studies is a more public act (even though the subjects' identities must be kept confidential). Accordingly, it seems appropriate to permit an IRB to scrutinize parental decisions about enrolling children in enhancement research more extensively than just to prevent abuse and neglect. For example, an IRB might be authorized to disapprove a proposed enhancement study on children if the IRB felt that no reasonable parents, being adequately informed about the risks and potential benefits and having paramount regard for their children's welfare, would give permission for their children to serve as subjects.

Research on the Educationally or Economically Disadvantaged

The Belmont Report lists people who are educationally or economically disadvantaged as among the classes of vulnerable subjects, but the primary concern seems to be that investigators could take advantage of the subjects for the investigators' own ends:

> One special instance of injustice results from the involvement of vulnerable subjects. Certain groups, such as racial minorities, the economically disadvantaged, the very sick, and the institutionalized may continually be sought as research subjects, owing to their ready availability in settings where research is conducted. Given their dependent status and their frequently compromised capacity for free consent, they should be protected against the danger of being involved in research solely for administrative convenience, or because they are easy to manipulate as a result of their illness or socioeconomic condition.[51]

Enhancement research, however, raises a different danger: that people who are disadvantaged will agree to accept study risks that seem unreasonable to people in less desperate situations in exchange for a chance to improve their lot with the aid of an experimental enhancement.

This triggers one of the great controversies in research ethics. On the one hand, it could be argued that people who are in desperate straits should be protected from accepting risks that ordinary persons would find unacceptable. On the other hand, the fact that these people are so desperate means that they stand to gain greater benefit than others, and ethically, the prospect of greater benefit can offset a larger amount of risk. For example, studies of drugs with serious side effects might be ethical if the subjects were seriously ill with conditions for which there were no satisfactory remedies, but not if the subjects were in less danger. But this does not mean that the disadvantaged should be given no special protections, any more than it means that patients with fatal, nontreatable illnesses should be allowed to enroll in any study that offers a potential benefit, no matter how small the benefit or how great the risk. As my colleague Sharona Hoffman points out, "Many scholars have noted that the decisionmaking capacity of individuals suffering from prolonged or serious illnesses is often impaired and have recommended that research protocols designed to involve such patients be subjected to heightened scrutiny by IRBs. Seriously ill patients may experience depression, extreme anxiety, rage, denial, or desperation to find a cure, all of which may cloud their judgment and their ability to evaluate the benefits and risks of a clinical trial."[52] There is still a need to make sure that people who are economically or educationally disadvantaged give valid informed consent to participate, namely, that they understand the nature of the study and that, in their desperation, they don't fall prey to the therapeutic misconception (thinking that all subjects will obtain some benefit) or fail to appreciate the magnitude of the risks that are involved.

Research on Genetic Enhancement

Given the amount of fear generated by the concept of genetic enhancement, it might be thought that any research on its safety or efficacy should trigger special scrutiny. But from an ethical standpoint, many forms of genetic enhancement differ little from their nongenetic counterparts. Research on enhancement drugs made using recombinant DNA technology, for example, would not seem to pose any greater ethical concerns than research on enhancement drugs made through conventional chemistry. Genetic testing for enhancement purposes would raise troubling privacy and confidentiality issues, but so would any experiment that employed human biologic samples containing DNA. Gene insertion and deletion techniques might seem more exotic than traditional biomedical interventions, and therefore require a more thorough safety evaluation before being used in humans, but they do not seem to raise particularly novel ethical issues. Only research on germline genetic manipulations would seem to raise special ethical objections, but many of these same concerns would be raised by other forms of embryonic enhancement research, discussed earlier.

In any event, a proposal to conduct an experiment using genetic technology already triggers special regulatory oversight. In 1976, the NIH created the Recombinant DNA Advisory Committee (RAC) and later gave it the authority to review protocols for conducting gene modification experiments in human subjects. In a 1985 policy statement, the RAC made it fairly clear that it would not consider protocols to enhance human traits.[53] In 1997, the NIH ceded the regulatory function of the RAC to the FDA. But the RAC still has an advisory role, and it reviews genetic research protocols that are referred to it by the FDA or by manufacturers or that are the subject of requests for NIH grants. If germline and other troubling forms of genetic enhancement research get closer to reality, it may make sense to restore the RAC's full-scale regulatory oversight over these types of proposed studies.

In summary, enhancement research on human subjects should be permitted in certain circumstances. But greater protections are needed for subjects who might be vulnerable to coercion or undue pressure.

Conclusion

AT THE END of the introduction to this book, I asked three questions: should we stop biomedical enhancement, can we, and were we meant to? The answers to the first two questions are now clear. We cannot stop it, nor should we. Substantial benefits can be had by using the right kinds of enhancement for the right reasons, and the costs of trying to avert the wrong kind of enhancement altogether are too high. Activities like sports and games may decide to continue to pay those costs in order to sustain certain arbitrary sets of rules, but elsewhere, enhancements should be regulated, not banned.

This does not mean that regulation will be easy or cheap. When it comes to biomedical enhancement, we need to identify an appropriate boundary between private spheres, in which competent individuals are allowed to make their own decisions about whether or not to use enhancements, and public realms, in which government regulation is necessary. New regulatory mechanisms must be created and adequately funded. The likelihood that enhancements will be used for societal benefit rather than purely for personal gain must be maximized. Enhancements that bear significantly on social success must be made widely available. Clearly, these are enormous challenges.

What about the final question? Is biomedical enhancement an insult to “creation”? Mormonism notwithstanding, even the most covetous deity is not likely to deny humans their morning dose of caffeine. But the technology of enhancement aims at more than modest increases in alertness, strength, or cognitive skill. Its trajectory extends to the ultimate rules and tools of evolution. The lesson of this book is that there is little that can be done to knock it off this course. We will find out if we were “meant” to do these things only once they have been done. We cannot run the ship of life aground, nor steer it much. About all we can do is trim the sails.

Notes

Chapter 1. The Technological Horizon

1. Julian Savulescu, Justice, fairness, and enhancement, *Annals of the New York Academy of Sciences* 1093 (2006): 324.

2. Tim Johnson, What is 20/20 vision? available at www.uihealthcare.com/topics/medicaldepartments/ophthalmology/2020vision/index.html, last visited June 7, 2007.

3. H. Gilbert Welch, Lisa Schwartz, and Steven Woloshin, What's making us sick is an epidemic of diagnoses, *New York Times,* Jan. 2, 2007, F1.

4. R. Petersen, G. Smith, S. Waring, R. Ivnik, E. Tangalos, and E. Kokmen, Mild cognitive impairment: Clinical characterization and outcome, *Archives of Neurology* 56 (1999): 303–8.

5. L. Hayflick, Anti-aging medicine: Hype, hope, and reality, *Generations* 25, no. 4 (2001): 20–26.

6. President's Council on Bioethics, Beyond therapy: Biotechnology and the pursuit of happiness (Washington, D.C.: President's Council on Bioethics, 2003), p. 192.

7. J. S. Olshansky, L. Hayflick, and B. A. Carnes, Position statement on human aging, *Journals of Gerontology Series A: Biological Sciences and Medical Sciences* 57 (2002):B292–97.

8. John M. Hoberman, Sport and the technological image of man, in William J. Morgan and Klaus V. Meier, eds., Philosophic inquiry in sport, 2nd ed. (Champaign, IL: Human Kinetics, 1995), p. 203.

9. House of Commons, Science and Technology Committee, Human enhancement technologies in sport, advance copy, Feb. 22, 2007, p. 29.

10. Greg Bishop, Getting a boost, boom and bust, *Seattle Times,* Oct. 11, 2005, p. D6.

11. Ibid.

12. Blair Tindall, Better playing through chemistry, *New York Times,* Oct. 17, 2004, section 2, p. 1.

13. Joel Garreau, A dose of genius: "Smart pills" are on the rise. But is taking them wise? *Washington Post,* June 11, 2006, p. D1.

14. Tindall, Better playing through chemistry, section 2, p. 1.

15. Ibid.

16. FDA not wild about Pfizer ad. CNN.MONEY, Nov. 15, 2004, available at http://money.cnn.com/2004/11/15/news/fortune500/pfizer_ad.reut/index.htm?cnn=yes, last visited May 30, 2007.

17. American Society of Plastic Surgeons, available at www.plasticsurgery.org/media/statistics/loader.cfm?url=/commonspot/security/getfile.cfm&PageID=23625, last visited June 11, 2007.

18. CBS News, Schoolgirls use steroids, too, available at www.cbsnews.com/stories/2005/04/25/health/main690876.shtml, last visited June 11, 2007.

19. Jodi Mailander Farrell, More teens see implants as a right, 2004, available at www.breastimplantinfo.org/news/mhearldimplnt1204.html, last visited May 30, 2007.

20. Chuck Yarborough, People watch, *Cleveland Plain Dealer,* Apr. 20, 2005, p. E2.

21. Natasha Singer, More doctors turning to the business of beauty, *New York Times,* Nov. 30, 2006, p. A1.

22. Carl Elliott, Better than well (New York: W.W. Norton, 2003), p. 247.

23. Claudia Dreifus, An economist examines the business of fertility, *New York Times,* Feb. 28, 2006, p. F5.

24. Rita Rubin, Giving growth a synthetic hand use of hormone sparks debate, *Dallas Morning News,* July 7, 1986, p. A1.

25. Nicholas Bakalar, Ugly children may get parental short shrift, *New York Times,* May 3, 2005, p. D7.

26. Bruce Gottlieb, What can't a beauty queen do? *Slate,* May 27, 1999, available at http://slate.msn.com/id/1002887, last visited June 14, 2007.

27. Arthur W. Frank, Emily's scars, surgical shapings, technoluxe, and bioethics, *Hastings Center Report* (March-April 2004): 20.

28. Jessica C. Dixon, Note: The perils of body art: FDA regulation of tattoo and micropigmentation pigments, *Administrative Law Review* 58 (2006): 679.

29. Frank, Emily's scars, 20.

30. BBC News, Apr. 8, 2004, available at http://news.bbc.co.uk/go/pr/fr/-/1/hi/health/3610379.stm, last visited June 11, 2007.

31. Center for Science in the Public Interest, Health action newsletter: The caffeine corner: Products ranked by content, available at www.cspinet.org/nah/caffeine/caffeine_corner.htm, last visited Nov. 17, 2003.

32. David A. Norris, How a coffee played a role in Civil War, CNN/living, available at www.cnn.com/2007/LIVING/wayoflife/10/29/mf.coffee.confederacy/index.html, last visited Nov. 5, 2007.

33. A. H. Rezvani and E. D. Levin, Cognitive effects of nicotine, *Biological Psychiatry* 49 (2001): 258–67.

34. G. Romain, Nicotine patches memory problems, available at www.betterhumans.com/News/news.aspx?articleID=2003-12-05-4, last visited Feb. 4, 2004.

35. Freud's cocaine capers, *Time*, Jan. 6, 1975, available at www.time.com/time/magazine/article/0,9171,912660-1,00.html, last visited June 14, 2007.

36. Garreau, Dose of genius, D1.

37. Andrew Pollack, A biotech outcast awakes, *New York Times*, Oct. 20, 2002, section 3, p. 1.

38. Earnings Call Transcript, Remarks of Frank Baldino, CEO, Cephalon, available at http://seekingalpha.com/article/19829, last visited June 13, 2007.

39. Jerome P. Kassirer, These two make quite a team, *Washington Post*, Oct. 10, 2004, p. B01.

40. Garreau, Dose of genius, D1.

41. Jonathan Moreno, Mind wars: Brain research and national defense (Washington, D.C.: Dana Press, 2006), p. 118.

42. Pallab Ghosh, Drugs may boost your brain power. BBC News, Apr. 16, 2007, available at http://news.bbc.co.uk/2/hi/health/6558871.stm, last visited Apr. 17, 2007.

43. J. A. Yesavage, M. S. Mumenthaler, J. L. Taylor, L. Friedman, R. O'Hara, J. Sheikh, J. Tinlenberg, and P. J. Whitehouse, Donepezil and flight simulator performance: Effects on retention of complex skills, *Neurology* 59 (2002): 123–25.

44. Ulric Neisser, *Cognitive Psychology* (New York: Appleton-Century-Crofts, 1967).

45. Ghosh, Drugs may boost your brain power.

46. Available at www.pfizer.com/product_overview.asp?drug=AR&country=US&lang=EN&spec, last visited Oct. 30, 2006.

47. Alex Baenninger, Jorge Alberto Coasta e Silva, Ian Hindmarch, Hans-Juergen Moeller, and Karl Rickels, Good chemistry: The life and legacy of Valium inventor Leo Sternbach (New York: McGraw-Hill, 2004).

48. Carl C. Elliott, A philosophical disease: Bioethics, culture, and identity (New York: Routledge, 1999).

49. Caleb Hellerman, Are antidepressants good for a boost if you're already healthy? available at www.cnn.com/2006/HEALTH/conditions/11/13/unnatural.highs/index.html, last visited Nov. 28, 2006.

50. Paul J. Ford, From treatment to enhancement in deep brain stimulation: A question of research ethics, *Pluralist* 1 (2006): 35–44.

51. Donald W. Goodwin, Alcohol and the writer (Riverside, NJ: Andrews and McMeel, 1988), quoted in Christopher Lehmann-Haupt, Books of the Times; Odd angles on alcoholism and American writers, Nov. 7, 1988, avail-

able at http://query.nytimes.com/gst/fullpage.html?res=940DE3D61431F934A35752C1A96E948260&sec=&spon=&pagewanted=1, last visited Feb. 21, 2008.

52. Jan Carl Grossman, Ronald Goldstein, and Russell Eisenman, Undergraduate marijuana use as related to openness to experience, *Psychiatric Quarterly* 48 (1974): 93–108; and Russell Eisenman, Jan Carl Grossman, and Ronald Goldstein, Undergraduate marijuana use as related to internal sensation novelty seeking and openness to experience, *Journal of Clinical Psychology* 36 (2006): 1013–19.

53. Salim Muwakkil, Truth is, some drug users are creative and productive, *Baltimore Sun,* Sept. 1, 1999, p. 17A.

54. Meg Nugent, Pursuit of happiness may lead to the fridge: Food and mood linked, experts say, *Times-Picayune* (New Orleans), Jan. 14, 2007, p. 22.

55. Scottish ice-cream maker develops mood-enhancing ice-cream. Feb. 26, 2002, available at www.foodnavigator.com/news/printNewsBis.asp?id=43248, last visited Feb. 25, 2008.

56. Noah Shachtman, Be all that you can be, *Wired* 15 (2007): 3, available at www.wired.com/wired/archive/15.03/bemore.html?pg=1&topic=bemore&topic_set=, last visited Feb. 23, 2008.

57. Moreno, Mind wars.

58. Shachtman, Be all that you can be.

59. Ibid.

60. British House of Commons, Science and Technology Committee report: Human enhancement technologies in sport.

61. M. Stoil, Amphetamine epidemics: Nothing new, *Addiction and Recovery* 10 (1990): 9.

62. Rhonda Cornum, John Caldwell, and Kory Cornum, Stimulant use in extended flight operations, *Airpower Journal,* Spring 1997, available at www.airpower.maxwell.af.mil/airchronicles/apj/apj97/spr97/cornum.html, last visited Nov. 12, 2008.

63. Robert Schlesinger, Defense cites stimulants in "Friendly fire" case, *Boston Globe,* Jan. 4, 2003, p. A3.

64. Thom Shanker and Mary Duenwald, Threats and responses: Bombing error puts a spotlight on pilots' pills, *New York Times,* Jan. 19, 2003, p. 1.

65. Lianne Hart, Use of "go pills" a matter of "life and death," Air Force avows, *Los Angeles Times,* Jan. 17, 2003.

66. Ibid.

67. The court-martial, *St. Louis Post-Dispatch,* editorial, July 3, 2003, p. C12.

68. Schlesinger, Defense cites stimulants, A3.

69. Doug Simpson, U.S. pilot defends attack in secret, *Toronto Star,* July 2, 2004, p. A01.

70. Ian Sample, Wired awake, *The Guardian,* July 29, 2004, Science section, p. 4.

71. J. A. Caldwell Jr., J. L. Caldwell, N. K. Smythe, and K. K. Hall, A double-blind, placebo-controlled investigation of the efficacy of modafinil for sustaining the alertness and performance of aviators: a helicopter simulator study, *Psychopharmacology* 150 (2000): 272–82.

72. Sample, Wired awake, Science section, p. 4.

73. Ibid.

74. Mark Dodd, Navy to check on breast surgery, *The Australian,* Sept. 17, 2007, p. 7.

75. Hayflick, Anti-aging medicine, 20–26.

76. E. T. Juengst, R. H. Binstock, M. Mehlman, S. G. Post, and P. Whitehouse, Biogerontology, "anti-aging medicine," and the challenges of human enhancement, *Hastings Center Report* (July-August 2003): 21–30; and F. Fukuyama, Our posthuman future (New York: Picador, 2002).

77. J. Fries, Aging, natural death, and the compression of morbidity, *New England Journal of Medicine* 303 (1980): 130–35.

78. Olshansky, Hayflick, and Carnes, Position statement on human aging, B292–97.

79. Hayflick, Anti-aging medicine, 20–26.

80. Duff Wilson, Aging: Disease or business opportunity? *New York Times,* Apr. 15, 2007, section 3, p. 1.

81. Hayflick, Anti-aging medicine, 20–26.

82. National Institute of Aging, 2001–2005 strategic plan, available at www.nia.nih.gov/AboutNIA/StrategicPlan/ResearchGoalB/Subgoal1.htm, last visited June 14, 2007.

83. D. Sinclair and A. L. Komaroff, Can we slow aging? *Newsweek* 148 (2006): 80–84.

84. The creation of Yao Ming, *Time Asia,* adapted from Brook Lamar, *Operation Yao Ming* (New York: Penguin Books, 2005), available at www.time.com/time/asia/covers/501051114/story.html, last visited May 29, 2007.

85. Available at www.eharmony.com/singles/servlet/about/dimensions, last visited Feb. 27, 2007.

86. Gina Kolata, Psst! Ask for donor 1913, *New York Times,* Feb. 18, 2007, p. 5.

87. Genetics and IVF Institute, available at www.givf.com/donoregg/aboutourdonors.cfm, last visited Feb. 27, 2007.

88. California Cryobank, Inc., available at www.cryobank.com/pdf/profile.pdf, last visited Feb. 27, 2007.

89. Fertility Alternatives, available at www.fertilityalternatives.com/eggdonors.html#16, last visited Feb. 27, 2007.

90. Paul Olding, The genius sperm bank, BBC News, available at http://

news.bbc.co.uk/go/pr/fr/-/2/hi/uk_news/magazine/5078800.stm, last visited June 18, 2007.

91. *Cleveland Plain Dealer,* Jan. 6, 2007, p. A6.

92. Denise Grady, Girl or boy? As fertility technology advances, so does an ethical debate, *New York Times,* Feb. 6, 2007, p. D5.

93. K. Hudson. Preimplantation genetic diagnosis: Public policy and public attitudes, *Fertility and Sterility* 85 (2006): 1638–45.

94. Available at www.drugfreesport.org.nz/c/News/Former+Track+Coach +Convicted+of+Doping.html, last visited May 25, 2007.

95. Department of Health and Human Services, National Institutes of Health, Recombinant DNA Research; Request for Public Comment on "Points to Consider in the Design and Submission of Human Somatic Cell Gene Therapy Protocols," Appendix M. 50 *Federal Register* 2940 (1985).

96. NHGRI researchers explore genetics of canine speed, available at www.genome.gov/25521028, last visited May 8, 2007.

97. L. A. Whittemore et al., Inhibition of myostatin in adult mice increases skeletal muscle mass and strength, *Biochem Biophys Res Commun* 300 (2003): 965–71.

98. Steven Dickman, Gene mutation provides more meat on the hoof, *Science* 277 (1997): 1922–23.

99. Andrew Gumbel, Mutant gene led to athlete's son being born musclebound, *The Independent,* June 24, 2005, p. 28.

100. Markus Schuelke, Kathryn R. Wagner, Leslie E. Stolz, Christoph Hübner, Thomas Riebel, Wolfgang Kömen, Thomas Braun, James F. Tobin, and Se-Jin Lee, Myostatin mutation associated with gross muscle hypertrophy in a child, *New England Journal of Medicine* 350 (2004): 2682–88.

101. Michael Dobie, Of mighty mice and super men, *Newsday,* Mar. 20, 2005, p. B10.

102. Jeff Alexander, Rare condition gives boy incredible strength, *Chicago Tribune,* May 29, 2007, available at www.chicagotribune.com/news/local/michigan/chi-ap-mi-exchange-musclebo,1,508637.story?coll=chi-newsap_mi-hed, last visited May 30, 2007.

103. J. Savulescu and B. Foddy, Comment: Genetic test available for sports performance, *British Journal of Sports Medicine* 39 (2005): 472.

104. Nan Yang, Daniel G. MacArthur, Jason P. Gulbin, Allan G. Hahn, Alan H. Beggs, Simon Easteal, and Kathryn North, ACTN3 genotype is associated with human elite athletic performance, *American Journal of Human Genetics* 73 (2003): 627–31.

105. Andy Coghlan, Elite athletes are born to run, *New Scientist,* Aug. 30, 2003, p. 4–5.

106. Tuomo Rankinen, Molly S. Bray, James M. Hagberg, Louis Perusse, Stephen M. Roth, Bernd Wolfarth, and Claude Bouchard, The human gene

map for performance and health-related fitness phenotypes: The 2005 update, *Medicine and Science in Sports and Exercise* 38 (2006): 1863–88.

107. Mauro Costa-Mattioli, Delphine Gobert, Elad Stern, Karine Gamache, Rodney Colina, Claudio Cuello, Wayne Sossin, Randal Kaufman, Jerry Pelletier, Kobi Rosenblum, Krešimir Krnjević, Jean-Claude Lacaille, Karim Nader, and Nahum Sonenberg, Phosphorylation bidirectionally regulates the switch from short- to long-term synaptic plasticity and memory, *Cell* 129 (2007): 195–206.

108. Ian Sample, Gene discovery raises hope of treatment for memory loss, *The Guard*ian, Apr. 6, 2007, available at www.guardian.co.uk/medicine/story/0,,2051447,00.html, last visited Apr. 7, 2007.

109. José A. Apud, Venkata Mattay, Jingshan Chen, Bhaskar S. Kolachana, Joseph H. Callico, Roberta Rasett, Guilna Alce, Jennifer E. Iudicello, Natkai Akbar, Michael F. Egan, Terry E. Goldberg, and Daniel R. Weinberger, Tolcapone improves cognition and cortical information processing in normal human subjects, *Neuropsychopharmacology* 32 (2007): 1011–20.

110. BBC News, Aug. 24, 2004, available at http://news.bbc.co.uk/2/hi/science/nature/3592976.stm, last visited May 14, 2007.

111. Y. Tang, E. Shimizu, G. Dube, C. Rampon, G. Kerchner, M. Zhuo, G. Liu, and J. Tsien, Genetic enhancement of learning and memory in mice, *Nature* 401 (1999): 63–69; and Xiaohua Cao, Zhenzhong Cui, Ruiben Feng, Ya-Ping Tang, Zhenxia Qin, Bing Mei, and Joe Z. Tsien, Maintenance of superior learning and memory function in NR2B transgenic mice during ageing, *European Journal of Neuroscience* 25 (2007): 1815–22.

112. Y. Tang, E. Shimizu, and J. Tsien, Do "smart" mice feel more pain or are they just better learners? *Nature Neuroscience* 4 (2001): 453–54.

Chapter 2. Self-Satisfaction

1. President's Council on Bioethics, Beyond therapy: Biotechnology and the pursuit of happiness (Washington, D.C.: President's Council on Bioethics, 2003), pp. 28, 147.

2. Ibid., p. 147.

3. Bill McKibben, Enough (New York: Owl Books, 2004), p. 47.

4. Carl Elliott, The mixed promise of genetic medicine, *New England Journal of Medicine* 356 (2007): 2024–25.

5. President's Council on Bioethics, Beyond therapy, p. 144, emphasis in original.

6. Ibid., pp. 140, 155.

7. Ibid., p. 144, emphasis in original.

8. McKibben, Enough, p. 49.

9. Ibid., p. 47.

10. Carl Elliott, The tyranny of happiness, in Eric Parens, ed., Enhancing

human traits (Washington, D.C.: Georgetown University Press, 1998), p. 182, emphasis in original.

11. Peter Breggin and Ginger Ross Breggin, Talking back to Prozac (New York: St. Martin's Press, 2003), pp. 206–7.

12. Gerald McKenny, Enhancements and the ethical significance of vulnerability, in Parens, ed., Enhancing human traits, p. 235.

13. J. Mark Olsen, Depression, SSRIs, and the supposed obligation to suffer mentally, *Kennedy Institute of Ethics Journal* 16 (2006): 283–303.

14. President's Council on Bioethics, Beyond therapy, 150.

15. Ibid.

16. Ibid., p. 147.

17. Ibid., p. 147, 149.

18. McKibben, Enough, p. 209, emphasis in original.

19. Michael Sandel, The case against perfection, *Atlantic Monthly,* April 2004, p. 54.

20. Erik Parens, Authenticity and ambivalence: Toward understanding the enhancement debate, *Hastings Center Report* 35 (2005): 34, 37–38.

21. President's Council on Bioethics, Beyond therapy, p. 140.

22. Ibid., p. 145, emphasis in original.

23. Eric Parens, Is better always good? The enhancement project, in Parens, ed., Enhancing human traits, p. 12.

24. Ronald Cole Turner, Do means matter? In Parens, ed., Enhancing human traits, p. 156.

25. Your Guide to the Most Popular Nutritional Supplements and Dietary Supplements, available at www.nutritional-supplement-info.com, last visited Feb. 23, 2005.

26. Juan A. Carrillo and Julio Benitez, Clinically significant pharmacokinetic interactions between dietary caffeine and medications, *Clinical Pharmacokinetics* 39 (2000): 133.

27. Guangping Gao, Corinna Lebherz, Daniel J. Weiner, Rebecca Grant, Roberto Calcedo, Beth McCullough, Adam Bagg, Yi Zhang, and James M. Wilson, Erythropoietin gene therapy leads to autoimmune anemia in macaques, *Blood* 103 (2004): 3300–3302.

28. Pearl Y. Martin, Jenny Laing, Robin Martin, and Melanie Mitchell, Caffeine, cognition, and persuasion: Evidence for caffeine increasing the systematic processing of persuasive messages, *Journal of Applied Social Psychology* 35 (2005): 160–82.

29. Thomas Croghan and Patricia Pittman, "Lifestyle" and live-saving [*sic*] drugs, *Pittsburgh Post-Gazette,* Nov. 28, 2004, p. B1.

30. Arthur W. Frank, Emily's scars, surgical shapings, technoluxe, and bioethics, *Hastings Center Report* (March-April 2004): 22.

31. Greg Bishop, Getting a boost: changing your genes, *Seattle Times,* Oct. 9, 2005, pp. C1, C12.

32. *Poe v. Ullman,* 367 U.S. 497, 542 (1961).

33. *Schloendorff v. Society of New York Hospital,* 105 N.E. 92, 93 (New York, 1914).

34. Thomas Emerson, Toward a general theory of the first amendment, *Yale Law Review* (1963): 877–956.

35. Joel Feinberg, Harm to self (New York: Oxford University Press, 1986).

36. President's Council on Bioethics, Beyond therapy, p. 306.

37. F. H. Buckley, Perfectionism, *S. Ct. Econ. Review* 13 (2005): 133–63, 134.

38. Aristotle, *The Politics,* trans. E. Barker (1958), 317.

39. *Planned Parenthood v. Casey,* 505 U.S. 833, 851 (1992).

40. Patrick Devlin, The enforcement of morals (New York: Oxford University Press, 1965), p. 111.

41. Ibid., p. 111.

42. Ibid., p. 14.

43. Peter Cane, Taking law seriously: Starting points of the Hart/Devlin debate, *Journal of Ethics* 10 (2006): 21–51.

44. H. L. A. Hart, Law, liberty, and morality (Palo Alto: Stanford University Press, 1963), p. 50.

45. Buckley, Perfectionism, 157, 144.

46. Charles Taylor, Atomism, in Charles Taylor, Philosophy and the human sciences: Philosophical papers (Cambridge, 1985).

47. Robert P. George, Making men moral (New York: Oxford University Press, 1993), p. 20.

48. Leon Kass, The wisdom of repugnance, *New Republic,* June 2, 1997, p. 17.

49. Ibid.

50. James Fitzjames Stephen, Liberty, equality, fraternity (Indianapolis: Liberty Fund, 1993), p. 13.

51. Devlin, Enforcement of morals, p. 17.

Chapter 3. Social Reward

1. Eryn Brown, Sometimes, nips and tucks can be career moves, *New York Times,* Feb. 12, 2006, section 3, p. 6.

2. Ibid.

3. D. S. Hamermesh and J. E. Biddle, Beauty and the labor market, *American Economic Review* 84 (1994): 1174–94.

4. Markus M. Mobius and Tanya S. Rosenblat, Why beauty matters, *American Economic Review* 96 (2006): 222–35.

5. Matthew Bailey, Kids who play with caffeine, *Sunday Telegraph* (Sydney, Australia), June 3, 2001, p. 13.

6. Joan Ryan, It isn't a scandal in kid sports: Supplements help boost performance, *San Francisco Chronicle,* Mar. 16, 2004, p. B1.

7. Rob Walker, Muscular metaphor: How one company found the right words to tap the baby-boomer penchant for personal development, *New York Times Sunday Magazine,* May 6, 2007, p. 38.

8. There's hell toupee for bad cows, *Pittsburgh Post-Gazette,* Feb. 11, 2004, p. D2.

9. John Horton, Geauga champion steer tests positive for steroid, *Cleveland Plain Dealer,* Dec. 2, 2007, p. B1.

10. International Olympic Committee, Factsheet: The IOC Commission and the fight against doping, available at http://multimedia.olympic.org/pdf/en_report_838.pdf, last visited June 23, 2005.

11. National Institute on Drug Abuse, NIDA InfoFacts: Steroids (Anabolic-Androgenic), available at www.drugabuse.gov/Infofacts/Steroids.html, last visited June 8, 2005.

12. Restoring Faith in America's Pastime: Evaluating Major League Baseball's Efforts to Eradicate Steroid Use: Hearing before the House Committee on Government Reform, 109th Congress, 2005, (statement of Sen. Jim Bunning), available at http://reform.house.gov/.

13. Donald M. Hooton, testimony, Restoring Faith in America's Pastime: Evaluating Major League Baseball's Efforts to Eradicate Steroid Use: Hearing before the House Committee on Government Reform, 109th Congress, 2005, available at http://reform.house.gov/.

14. Carl Lewis, testimony, Restoring Faith in America's Pastime: Evaluating Major League Baseball's Efforts to Eradicate Steroid Use: Hearing before the House Committee on Government Reform, 109th Congress, 2005, available at http://reform.house.gov/.

15. Anahad O'Connor, Wrestler found to have taken testosterone, *New York Times,* July 18, 2007, p. A15.

16. Fred Hartgens and Harm Kuipers, Effects of androgenic-anabolic steroids in athletes, *Sports Medicine* 34 (2004): 513, 516.

17. William N. Taylor, Anabolic steroids and the athlete (Jefferson, NC: McFarland, 2002).

18. Eric Kutscher, Brian Lund, and Paul Perry, Anabolic steroids: A review for the clinician, *Sports Medicine* 32 (2002): 285–96.

19. Hartgens and Kuipers, Effects of androgenic-anabolic steroids in athletes, 513–54.

20. Kutscher, Lund, and Perry, Anabolic steroids, 285–96.

21. Manuel Estrada, Anurag Varshney, and Barbara E. Ehrlich, Elevated

testosterone induces apoptosis in neuronal cells, *Journal of Biological Chemistry* 281 (2006): 25492–501.

22. F. H. Bronson and C. M. Matherne, Exposure to androgenic-anabolic steroids shortens life span of male mice, *Medicine and Science in Sports and Exercise* 29 (1997): 615–19.

23. M. Parssinen et al., Increased premature mortality of competitive powerlifters suspected to have used anabolic agents, *International Journal of Sports Medicine* 21 (2000): 225–27.

24. Shalender Bhasin et al., The effects of supraphysiologic doses of testosterone on muscle size and strength in normal men, *New England Journal of Medicine* 335 (1996): 1–7.

25. Thomas W. Storer, Lynne Magliano, Linda Woodhouse, Martin L. Lee, Connie Dzekov, Jeanne Dzekov, Richard Casaburi, and Shalender Bhasin, Testosterone dose-dependently increases maximal voluntary strength and leg power, but does not affect fatigability or specific tension, *Journal of Clinical Endocrinology and Metabolism* 88 (2003): 1478–85.

26. Shalender Bhasin, Linda Woodhouse, Richard Casaburi, Atam B. Singh, Ricky Phong Mac, Martin Lee, Kevin E. Yarasheski, Indrani Sinha-Hikim, Connie Dzekov, Jeanne Dzekov, Lynne Magliano, and Thomas W. Storer, Older men are as responsive as young men to the anabolic effects of graded doses of testosterone on the skeletal muscle, *Journal of Clinical Endocrinology and Metabolism* 90 (2005): 678–88.

27. Hartgens and Kuipers, Effects of androgenic-anabolic steroids in athletes, 513–54.

28. Harrison Pope, Elena Kouri, and James Hudson, Effects of supraphysical doses of testosterone on mood and aggression in normal men, *Archives of General Psychiatry* 57 (2000): 133–40; Ann Clark and Leslie Henderson, Behavioral and physiological responses to anabolic-androgenic steroids, *Neuroscience and Biobehavioral Reviews* 27 (2003): 413–36; Shalender Bhasin et al., The effects of supraphysiologic doses of testosterone on muscle size and strength in normal men, *New England Journal of Medicine* 335 (1996): 1–7; Kutscher, Lund, and Perry, Anabolic steroids, 285–96; and Hartgens and Kuipers, Effects of androgenic-anabolic steroids in athletes, 513–54.

29. Anahad O'Connor, Wrestler found to have taken testosterone, p. A15; and Hartgens and Kuipers, Effects of androgenic-anabolic steroids in athletes, 513, 516.

30. John M. Tokish, Mininder S. Kocher, and Richard J. Hawkins, Ergogenic aids: A review of basic science, performance, side effects, and status in sports, *American Journal of Sports Medicine* 32 (2004): 1543–53; and Linn Goldberg, M.D., testimony, Steroid Use in Sports, Part II: Examining the National Football League's Policy on Anabolic Steroids and Related Substances:

Hearing before the House Comm. on Government Reform, 109th Congress, 2005, available at http://reform.house.gov/.

31. Nick Evans, Current concepts in anabolic-androgenic steroids, *American Journal of Sports Medicine* 32 (2004): 534–42.

32. Ingemar Thiblin and Anna Petersson, Pharmacoepidemiology of anabolic androgenic steroids: A review, *Fundamental and Clinical Pharmacology* 19 (2005): 27–44.

33. Carl Lewis, testimony, Restoring Faith in America's Pastime: Evaluating Major League Baseball's Efforts to Eradicate Steroid Use: Hearing before the House Committee on Government Reform, 109th Congress, 2005, available at http://reform.house.gov/.

34. American Association of Neurological Surgeons, available at www.neurosurgerytoday.org/what/patient_e/concussion.asp, last visited July 12, 2007.

35. Study finds common sports injuries could be lethal, *Parks and Recreation* 42 (2007): 19(1).

36. Centers for Disease Control and Prevention, Nonfatal sports and recreation related injuries treated in emergency departments, United States, July 2000–June 2001, *Morbidity and Mortality Weekly Report* 51 (2002): 736.

37. Mark Juhn, Popular sports supplements and ergogenic aids, *Sports Medicine* 33 (2003): 921–39.

38. W. Jelkmann, Use of recombinant human erythropoietin as an antianemic and performance enhancing drug, *Current Pharmaceutical Biotechnology* 1 (2000): 11–31.

39. John M. Tokish, Minider S. Kocher, and Richard J. Hawkins, Ergogenic aids: A review of basic science, performance, side effects, and status in sports, *American Journal of Sports Medicine* 32 (2004): 1543–53.

40. Associated Press, Muscle-pain reliever is blamed for Staten Island runner's death, *New York Times*, June 10, 2007, section 1, p. 38.

41. Hartgens and Kuipers, Effects of androgenic-anabolic steroids in athletes, 513–54.

42. National Institute on Drug Abuse, NIDA InfoFacts: Steroids (Anabolic-Androgenic).

43. Rep. John Sweeney, statement, Anabolic Steroid Control Act of 2004: Hearing on H.R. 3866 before Subcommittee on Crime, Terrorism, and Homeland Security of the House Comm. on the Judiciary, 108th Congress 6, 2004.

44. Chairman Tom Davis, statement, Restoring Faith in America's Pastime: Evaluating Major League Baseball's Efforts to Eradicate Steroid Use: Hearings before the House Committee on Government Reform, 2005, available at http://reform.house.gov/.

45. Joseph Biden, statement, Steroids in Amateur and Professional

Sports—The Medical and Social Costs of Steroid Abuse: Hearings on the Steroid Abuse Problem in America, Focusing on the Use of Steroids in College and Professional Football Today before the S. Comm. on the Judiciary, 101st Congress 2, 1989.

46. Robert L. Simon, Good competition and drug-enhanced performance, in William J. Morgan and Klaus V. Meier, eds., Philosophic inquiry in sport, 2nd ed. (Champaign, IL: Human Kinetics, 1995), p. 209.

47. Bill McKibben, Enough (New York: Owl Books, 2004), p. 190.

48. Robert L. Simon, Good competition and drug-enhanced performance, p. 209.

49. Available at www.fundinguniverse.com/company-histories/Prince-Sports-Group-Inc-Company-History.html, last visited July 15, 2007.

50. International Tennis Federation, available at www.itftennis.com/technical/rules/history/racket.asp, last visited July 15, 2007.

51. Ronald Blum, Selig calls for tougher steroid policy, *USA Today,* June 1, 2005, available at www.usatoday.com/sports/baseball/2005-04-30-selig-steroids_x.htm, last visited July 9, 2007.

52. Jack Curry, Four indicted in a steroid scheme that involved top pro athletes, *New York Times,* Feb. 13, 2004, p. A1.

53. Tony Chamberlain, Rahlves walks away wistfully, *Boston Globe,* Feb. 21, 2006, p. D4.

54. Joanne Gerstner, Naoko Takahashi, 28, of Japan, celebrates victory in the women's marathon with Olympic-record time of 2:23.14, *Detroit News,* Sept. 24, 2000, p. 10D.

55. Todd Jones, Relax, Canada, you did it, *Columbus Post Dispatch,* Feb. 25, 2002, p. 1D.

56. Hubert Mizell, A reason to celebrate for Russia, *St. Petersburg (Florida) Times,* Feb. 12, 1992, p. 1C.

57. Jennifer Alsever, A new competitive sport: grooming the child athlete, *New York Times,* June 25, 2006, p. BU5.

58. Hermine H. M. Maes et al., Inheritance of physical fitness in 10-yr-old twins and their parents, *Medicine and Science in Sports and Exercise* 28 (1996): 1479–91.

59. Stefan Lovgren, The science of Lance Armstrong: Born, and built, to win, *National Geographic News,* July 22, 2005, available at http://news.nationalgeographic.com/news/2005/07/0722_050722_armstrong.html, last visited Nov. 5, 2007.

60. Times Online, Scientists create "mighty mice," Nov. 2, 2007, available at www.timesonline.co.uk/tol/news/uk/science/article2788843.ece, last visited Nov. 5, 2007.

61. Douglas Robson, Players experiment until their strings sing, *USA Today,* July 1, 2005, p. 15C.

62. Little League Online, www.littleleague.org/MEDIA/bats.asp, last visited July 16, 2007.

63. Brendan I. Koerner, Ready for hardball softball, *New York Times,* May 30, 2004, section 3, p. 2.

64. Nate Schweber, Ball field injury spurs push to limit metal bats in New Jersey, *New York Times,* Oct. 22, 2006, p. 29.

65. Brendan I. Koerner, For skiers, fashion follows function, *New York Times,* Feb. 5, 2005, section 3, p. 2.

66. William Saletan, The beam in your eye: if steroids are cheating, why isn't Lasik? *Slate,* Apr. 18, 2005, available at www.slate.com/id/2116858, last visited July 16, 2007.

67. Personal communication from Gary Green, M.D., May 16, 2007.

68. Clifton Brown, For Woods, winning the Majors is the only thing, *New York Times,* Apr. 3, 2000, p. D1.

69. Charles Krauthammer, Beer? Hot dogs? Steroids? *Washington Post,* June 2, 2006, p. A19.

70. Bausch and Lomb, available at www.bausch.com/en_US/consumer/visioncare/product/softcontacts/nikemaxsight.aspx, last visited July 16, 2007.

71. Ray Fittipaldo, Norwood a scary lion: 169-pound receiver with the red eyes is coming up big, *Pittsburgh Post-Gazette,* Sept. 15, 2006, p. D8.

72. Associated Press, New lenses give athletes edge, *Houston Chronicle,* June 8, 2006, sports section, p. 2.

73. Bernard Wysocki Jr., For a pro sports psychologist, lifer is a nonstop consultation, *Wall Street Journal,* Sept. 20, 2005, p. B1.

74. House of Commons Science and Technology Committee. Report: Human Enhancement Technologies in Sport, advance copy, Feb. 22, 2007, available at www.publications.parliament.uk/pa/cm200607/cmselect/cmsctech/67/67.pdf, last visited October 1, 2008.

75. U.S. Olympic Committee, available at www.usoc.org/12181_19094.htm, last visited July 16, 2007.

76. Daniel Coyle, How to grow a super athlete, *Play: New York Times Sports Magazine,* Mar. 2007, pp. 36, 39.

77. Personal communication from Peter Fricker, director of the Australian Institute of Sport, Dec. 7, 2006.

78. Andy Miah and Emma Rich, Genetic tests for ability? Talent identification and the value of an open future, *Sport, Education, and Society* 11 (2006): 259–73.

79. Gretchen Reynolds, Give us this day our daily supplements, *Play: New York Times Sports Magazine,* March 2007, p. 24.

80. W. M. Brown, Paternalism, drugs, and the nature of sports, in Morgan and Meier, eds., Philosophic inquiry in sport, p. 220.

81. Bruce Weber, Cheating matters (sometimes), *New York Times,* Dec. 16, 2007, p. WK3.

82. President's Council on Bioethics, Beyond therapy: Biotechnology and the pursuit of happiness (Washington, D.C.: President's Council on Bioethics, 2003).

83. Michael Sandel, The case against perfection, *Atlantic Monthly* 293 (2004): 50–54, 56–60, 62.

84. AAP News Release: AAP condemns use of performance-enhancing substances, Apr. 4, 2005, available at www.aap.org/advocacy/releases/apr substances.htm, last visited May 30, 2007.

85. Fred Hartgens and Harm Kuipers, Effects of androgenic-anabolic steroids in athletes, *Sports Medicine* 34 (2004): 513–54; J. Sturmi and D. Diorio, Anabolic agents, *Clinics in Sports Medicine* 17 (April 1998): 2; F. Kadi and A. Eriksson, Effects of anabolic steroids on the muscle cells of strength-trained athletes, *Medicine and Science in Sports and Exercise* 31 (1999): 1528–34; S. Basaria, CR 138: Anabolic-androgenic steroid therapy in the treatment of chronic diseases, *Journal of Clinical Endocrinology and Metabolism* 86 (2001): 5108–17; J. A. Lombardo and R. Y. Sickles, Medical and performance-enhancing effects of anabolic steroids, *Psychiatric Annals* 22 (1992): 19–23; A. D. Rogol and C. E. Yesalis, Anabolic-androgenic steroids and athletes: What are the issues? *Journal of Clinical Endocrinology and Metabolism* 74 (1992): 465–69; and H. A. Haupt, Anabolic steroids and growth hormone, *American Journal of Sports Medicine* 21 (1993): 468–73.

86. International Olympic Committee, Medical: The fight against doping and promotion of athletes' health, available at http://multimedia.olympic.org/pdf/en_report_838.pdf, last visited June 28, 2005.

87. AAP News Release, AAP condemns use of performance-enhancing substances, Apr. 4, 2005, available at www.aap.org/advocacy/releases/aprsubstances.htm, last visited May 30, 2007.

88. Greg Bishop, Getting a boost: changing your genes, *Seattle Times,* Oct. 9, 2005, p. C11.

89. Blog of Clarence Bass, available at http://cbass.com/Bowerman.htm, last visited July 16, 2007.

90. Barrie Houlihan, Dying to win (Strasbourg: Council of Europe Publishing, 1999), p. 112.

91. Bill McCollom. Speed jumps: Why fast skis matter and how the U.S. team got 'em, *Ski Racing,* Sept. 29, 2003, available at www.franconiaskiclub.com/PDFs/Speed%20jumps%20and%20fast%20skis.pdf, last visited June 18, 2005.

92. Roger Gardner, On performance-enhancing substances and the unfair advantage argument, in Morgan and Meier, eds., Philosophic inquiry in sport, p. 220.

93. Greg Bishop, Getting a boost: changing your genes, *Seattle Times,* Oct. 9, 2005, p. C11.

94. Roger Gardner, On performance-enhancing substances and the unfair advantage argument, p. 220.

95. Bishop, Getting a boost, p. C11.

96. Sandel, The case against perfection, p. 55.

97. *United States v. Holmes* 1842. 26 F. Cas. 360 (Cir. Ct. E.D. Pa.).

98. Ibid.

99. *Holmes v. New York City Housing Authority,* 1968. 398 F.2d 262 (2d Cir.); and *Hornsby v. Allen,* 1964. 330 F.2d 55 (5th Cir.).

100. Leonard Koppett, A thinking man's guide to baseball (New York: Dutton, 1967).

101. Sen. John McCain, statement, Steroid Use in Professional and Amateur Sports: Hearing before Senate Committee on Commerce, Science, and Transportation, 108th Congress, 2004, available at http://commerce.senate.gov/hearings/witnesslist.cfm?id=1100.

102. Nick Cafardo, This dose of news sounds an alarm, *Boston Globe,* Apr. 29, 2007, p. C10.

103. Mel Antonen, DH at 30: Hit, miss, *USA Today,* July 14, 2003, p. 1C; and Bill Dawson, DH at 30: Rule still enrages purists, but many hitters relish role, *San Diego Union-Tribune,* May 12, 2003, p. C2.

104. Available at http://ontrackandfield.com/main/catalog/2007/polevaulthistory.html, last visited July 14, 2007.

105. Forbes, available at www.hardballtimes.com/main/article/how-much-is-your-team-really-worth/, last visited July 19, 2007.

106. Julie Macur, The wheels come off a sport, *New York Times,* May 13, 2007, section 4, p. 1.

107. Michael McCarthy, Sports and entertainment are double-teaming fans, *USA Today,* June 16, 2005, p. 1C.

108. Harvey Araton, Football and taste, out of season, *New York Times,* Feb. 6, 2001, p. D1.

109. Randy Brown, XFL's failure a success for U.S., *Albany Times Union,* May 22, 2001, p. A9.

110. Stephen Romei, Outlaw football bombs in tasteless play, *Australian,* Apr. 27, 2001, p. 25.

111. Don Walker, He fold me: McMahon smacks down XFL due to tiny ratings, huge losses, *Milwaukee Journal Sentinel,* May 11, 2001, p. C1.

112. Jay Mariotti, Trashing the garbage of the XFL, *Sporting News* 225 (2001): 7.

113. Randy Brown, XFL's failure a success for U.S., *Albany Times Union,* May 22, 2001, p. A9; see also *Seattle Times,* May 15, 2001, p. B4.

114. Samuel Abt, Riders are still critical of the French police and courts for their role in drug affair, *New York Times,* Oct. 11, 1998, section 8, p. 9.

115. Catherine Carstairs, The wide world of doping: drug scandals, natural bodies, and the business of sports entertainment, *Addiction Research and Theory* 11 (2003): 263–81.

116. John Hoberman, A pharmacy on wheels (1998), available at www.mesomorphosis.com/articles/hoberman/tour-de-france-doping-scandal.htm, last visited July 19, 2007.

117. Dick Patrick, Drugs taint games, *USA Today,* Sept. 26, 2000, p. 1A.

118. Olympic Movement Anti-Doping Code Appendix A, §I(A)(a)(2003), available at www.sportgericht.de/Doping/Dopingliste/dopingliste2003.pdf, last visited June 10, 2005.

119. World Anti-Doping Agency 2004, Athletes Passport, April 2004, available at www.wada-ama.org/rtecontent/document/April_04.pdf, last visited June 10, 2005.

120. Robert L. Simon, Good competition and drug-enhanced performance, pp. 21–214.

121. Michael Lavin, Sports and drugs: Are the current bans justified? in Morgan and Meier, eds., Philosophic inquiry in sport, p. 236.

122. Thomas Murray, The ethics of drugs in sports, in Richard H. Strauss, ed., Drugs and performance in sports (Philadelphia: Saunders, 1987), p. 15.

123. Personal communications from Thomas H. Murray.

124. Simon Gardiner et al., Sports law, 2d ed. (London: Cavendish, 2001).

125. Sen. Jim Bunning, statement, Restoring Faith in America's Pastime: Evaluating Major League Baseball's Efforts to Eradicate Steroid Use: Hearing before the House Committee on Government Reform, 109th Congress, 2005, available at http://reform.house.gov/.

126. Glenn Dickey, Forget the purity notion when analyzing baseball, *San Francisco Chronicle,* Oct. 22, 1994, p. B2.

127. Will Manley, Will's world: Baseball, boomer, and censorship, *American Libraries* 34 (2003): 96.

128. Mike Huggins, The Victorians and sport (London: Hambleton and London, 2004), p. 57.

129. Barrie Houlihan, Dying to win (Strasbourg: Council of Europe Publishing, 1999), p. 34.

130. Amateur Athletic Foundation of Los Angeles, An Olympic games primer, available at www.aafla.org/6oic/primer_text2.htm, last visited May 25, 2007.

131. Selena Roberts, The road to success is paved with cheating, *New York Times,* Apr. 8, 2007, section 8, p. 3.

Chapter 4. The Hegemony of Meritocracy

1. Sharon Beder, Selling the work ethic: From puritan pulpit to corporate PR (New York: Zed Books, 2000).

2. Ibid.

3. University of Connecticut Press Release, available at http://news.uconn.edu/2007/July/rel07059.html, last visited July 20, 2007.

4. The pulse, *Cleveland Plain Dealer,* Jan. 6, 2007, p. B9.

5. Michael Sandel, The case against perfection, *Atlantic Monthly,* April 2004, p. 54.

6. Arthur Brooks, Who really cares: The surprising truth about compassionate conservatism (Cambridge, MA: Basic Books, 2006).

7. S. J. McNamee and R. K. Miller Jr., The meritocracy myth (Lanham, MD: Rowman and Littlefield, 2004).

8. M. Young, The rise of the meritocracy (London: Thames and Hudson, 1958).

9. McNamee and Miller, The meritocracy myth.

10. Ibid.

11. Ibid.

12. Ibid.

13. Dusty Horwitt, This hard-earned money comes stuffed in their genes, *Washington Post,* Apr. 18, 2004, p. B3.

14. Jerome Karabel, The legacy of legacies, *New York Times,* Sept. 13, 2004, p. A23.

15. Ibid.

16. Ibid.

17. Malcolm Gladwell, Examined life: What Stanley H. Kaplan taught us about the S.A.T., *The New Yorker,* Dec. 17, 2001, p. 86.

18. Nicholas Lemann, The big test: The secret history of the American meritocracy (New York: Farrar, Straus and Giroux, 1999).

19. Horwitt. This hard-earned money, p. B3.

20. G. W. Bush, State of the Union Address, 2004, available at www.whitehouse.gov/news/releases/2004/01/20040120-7.html, last visited Oct. 1, 2008.

21. Bruce Weber, Cheating matters (sometimes), *New York Times,* Dec. 16, 2007, p. WK3.

22. *PGA Tour, Inc. v. Casey Martin,* 2001. 532 U.S. 661.

23. BBC Sport 2008, "Blade runner" handed Olympic ban, http://news.bbc.co.uk/sport1/hi/olympics/athletics/7141302.stm, last visited Jan. 29, 2008.

24. Sandel, The case against perfection, p. 58.

Chapter 5. Access to Enhancements and the Challenge to Equality

1. American Society for Aesthetic Plastic Surgery, available at www.surgery.org/download/2006stats.pdf, last visited Sept. 13, 2007.

2. PharmacyChecker.com, available at www.pharmacychecker.com/Pricing.asp?DrugName=Provigil&DrugId=26022&DrugStrengthId=43729, last visited Sept. 11, 2007.

3. Matthew Harper, Genomics all mapped out, Forbes.com, available at www.forbes.com/sciencesandmedicine/2007/09/04/genomics-craig-venter-biz-sci-cx_mh_0904venter.html, last visited Sept. 13, 2007.

4. Newsfocus: The race for the $1000 genome, *Science* 311 (Mar. 17, 2006): 1544–46.

5. Mary Jo Feldstein, The cost of conception, *St. Louis Post-Dispatch,* Aug. 6, 2006, p. A1.

6. Lori B. Andrews and Jordan Paradise, Gene patents: the need for bioethics scrutiny and legal challenge, *Yale Journal of Health Policy and Ethics* 5 (2005): 403–12.

7. Stephen Heuser, High tech, biotech clashing on patent bill, *Boston Globe* website, July 19, 2007, available at www.boston.com/business/technology/articles/2007/07/19/high_tech_biotech_clashing_on_patent_bill/?page=1, last visited Aug. 30, 2007.

8. Lori B. Andrews and Jordan Paradise, Gene patents: The need for bioethics scrutiny and legal challenge, *Yale Journal of Health Policy and Ethics* 5 (2005): 403–12.

9. Testimony of Ha T. Tu, Senior Health Researcher, Center for Studying Health System Change, House Committee on Ways and Means, Subcommittee on Health, July 18, 2006.

10. Alex Kuczynski, If beauties multiply, they'll be plain to see, *New York Times,* Dec. 28, 2003, section 4, p. 4.

11. Ramsey Alsarraf, Wayne F. Larrabee Jr., and Calvin Johnson Jr., Cost outcomes of facial plastic surgery, *Archives of Facial Plastic Surgery* 3 (2001): 44–47.

12. Ramez Naam, More than human (New York: Broadway Books, 2005).

13. Peter Temin, Technology, regulation, and market structure in the modern pharmaceutical industry, *Bell Journal of Economics* 10 (1979): 429–46.

14. Ibid.

15. Gregory Stock, Redesigning humans: Our inevitable genetic future (New York: Houghton Mifflin, 2002), p. 186.

16. Jonathan Sandy and Kevin C. Duncan, Does private education increase earnings? *Eastern Economic Journal* 22 (1996): 303–12.

17. *Pierce v. Soc'y of Sisters,* 268 U.S. 510, 535 (1925).

18. The Top of the Class: The complete list of the 1,300 top U.S. schools, avail-

able at www.msnbc.msn.com/id/18757087/site/newsweek/#storyContinued, last visited Sept. 16, 2007.

19. U.S. Department of Education 2006, Comparing private schools and public schools using hierarchical linear modeling (NCES 2006-461), available at http://nces.ed.gov/nationsreportcard/pubs/studies/2006461.asp, last visited Sept. 16, 2007.

20. David Cay Johnston, The gap between rich and poor grows in the United States, *International Herald Tribune,* Mar. 29, 2007, available at www.iht.com/articles/2007/03/29/business/income.4.php, last visited Sept. 14, 2007.

21. G. William Domhoff, Wealth, income, and power, available at http://sociology.ucsc.edu/whorulesamerica/power/wealth.html, last visited Sept. 14, 2007.

22. Elizabeth Warren and Amelia Warren Tyagi, The two-income trap: Why middle-class mothers and fathers are going broke (New York: Basic Books, 2003), emphasis in original.

23. Gary Young, In the U.S., class war still means just one thing: the rich attacking the poor, *The Guardian,* Sept. 3, 2007, available at www.guardian.co.uk/commentisfree/story/0,,2161252,00.html, last visited Sept. 14, 2007.

24. Walter Hamilton, Nation's chief exec enters CEO fray, *Los Angeles Times,* Feb. 1, 2007, p. C1.

25. G. William Domhoff, Wealth, income, and power.

26. Maxwell Mehlman, Wondergenes: Genetic enhancement and the future of society (Bloomington: Indiana University Press 2003), p. 110.

27. Kurt Andersen, A call to arms for populism, before it's too late, http://nymag.com/news/imperialcity/26014/, last visited Sept. 14, 2007.

Chapter 6. Lack of Choice

1. AAP News Release, AAP condemns use of performance-enhancing substances, Apr. 4, 2005, available at www.aap.org/advocacy/releases/aprsubstances.htm, last visited May 30, 2007.

2. J. Habermas, The future of human nature (Cambridge: Polity Press, 2003).

3. *Troxel v. Granville,* 2000. 530 U.S. 57 (Stevens, dissenting).

4. Michael Sandel, The case against perfection, *Atlantic Monthly,* April 2004, p. 57.

5. Ibid.

6. Jeff Alexander, Rare condition gives boy incredible strength, ChicagoTribune.com, May 29, 2007, available at www.chicagotribune.com/news/local/michigan/chi-ap-mi-exchange-musclebo,1,508637.story?coll=chi-newsap_mi-hed, last visited May 30, 2007.

7. Joel Feinberg, Autonomy, sovereignty, and privacy: Moral ideals in the constitution? *Notre Dame Law Review* 58 (1983): 465.

8. Bill McKibben, Enough (New York: Owl Books, 2004), p. 60.

9. Kevin B. O'Reilly, Testing embryos and ethics, *AMA News,* Feb. 26, 2007, p. 9.

10. American Society of Human Genetics and American College of Medical Genetics, Points to consider: Ethical, legal, and psychosocial implications of genetic testing in children and adolescents, *American Journal of Human Genetics* 57 (1995): 1233–41.

11. Andy Miah and Emma Rich, Genetic tests for ability? Talent identification and the value of an open future, *Sport, Education, and Society* 11 (2006): 259–73.

12. Erynn S. Gordon, Heather A Gordish-Dressman, Joseph Devaney, Priscilla Clarkson, Paul Thompson, Paul Gordon, Linda S. Pescatello, Monica J. Hubal, Emidio E. Pistilli, Gary Gianetti, Bethany Kelsey, and Eric P. Hoffman, Nondisease genetic testing: Reporting of muscle SNPs shows effects on self-concept and health orientation scales, *European Journal of Human Genetics* 13 (2005): 1047–54. doi:10.1038/sj.ejhg.5201449; published online June 8, 2005.

13. Julian Savulescu and Bennett Foddy, Comment: Genetic test available for sports performance, *British Journal of Sports Medicine* 39 (2005): 472.

14. Jennifer Alsever, A new competitive sport: Grooming the child athlete, *New York Times,* June 25, 2006, p. BU5.

15. Sparq Training, available at www.sparqtraining.com/ratings/, last visited May 25, 2007.

16. Alsever, A new competitive sport, p. BU5.

17. Savulescu and Foddy, Comment, p. 472.

18. Ibid.

19. Sparq Training, available at www.sparqtraining.com/ratings/.

20. Tamar Lewin, Disability requests reflect change in SAT procedure, *New York Times,* Nov. 8, 2003, p. A10.

21. Pallab Ghosh, Drugs may boost your brain power, BBC News, Apr. 16, 2007, available at http://news.bbc.co.uk/2/hi/health/6558871.stm, last visited Apr. 17, 2007.

22. Shelley Burtt, The proper scope of parental authority: Why we don't owe children an "open future," in Stephen Macedo and Iris Marion Young, eds., *NOMOS XLIV: Child, Family, and State* (New York: New York University Press, 2002), p. 257.

23. Bob Kurson, Sports kids: Pushed too hard? *Chicago Sun-Times,* Oct. 25, 1998, p. 1.

24. *Troxel v. Granville,* 2000. 530 U.S. 57, 65.

25. *Meyer v. Nebraska,* 1923. 262 U.S. 390.

26. *Pierce v. Society of Sisters,* 1925. 268 U.S. 510.

27. *Prince v. Massachusetts,* 1944. 321 U.S. 158.

28. Douglas Diekema, Parental refusals of medical treatment: The harm principle as threshold for state intervention, *Theoretical Medicine* 25 (2004): 243–64.

29. *Parham v. J.R.,* 1979. 442 U.S. 584, 602.

30. *Parham v. J.R.,* 1979. 442 U.S. 584, 603.

31. *In re* Philip B. 1979. 92 Cal App. 3d 796 (Cal. Ct. App.); *Newmark v. Williams,* 1991. 588 A.2d 1108 (Del.); In the matter of Lyle A. 2006. 830 NYS2d 486 (Fam. Ct. N.Y.); *Mueller v. Auker,* 2006. 2007 U.S. Dis. LEXIS 13172 (D. Id. Nov. 28, 2006); and *Hart v. Brown,* 1972. 289 A.2d 386 (Conn. Sup. Ct.).

32. Associated Press, Boy dies of leukemia four years after ruling, *Akron Beacon Journal,* May 23, 2007, p. B3.

33. CNN Presents, Achieving the perfect 10, Aug. 10, 2003, available at http://transcripts.cnn.com/TRANSCRIPTS/0308/10/cp.00.html, last visited Sept. 26, 2007.

34. *Parham v. J.R.,* 1979. 442 U.S. 584, 603.

35. *Wisconsin v. Yoder,* 1972. 406 U.S. 205.

36. *Prince v. Massachusetts,* 1944. 321 U.S. 158.

37. Matter of E.J. 1983. 465 A.2d 374 (DC Ct. App.); *DeMatteo v. DeMatteo,* 2002. 194 Misc. 2d 640 (Sup. Ct. NY); and *In re* Petra, 216 Cal. App. 3d 1163.

38. Associated Press, Vegan couple gets life over baby's death, May 9, 2007, available at http://msnbc.msn.com/id/18574603/, last visited Aug. 22, 2007.

39. *Troxel v. Granville,* 2000. 530 U.S. 57, 65.

40. *In re* Petra, 216 Cal. App. 3d 1163.

41. Douglas S. Diekema, Parental refusals of medical treatment: The harm principle as threshold for state intervention, *Theoretical Medicine* 25 (2004): 243–64.

42. Ohio Rev. Code §2919.22.

43. Diekema, Parental refusals of medical treatment, 243–64.

44. Kenneth A. DeVille and Loretta M. Kopelman, Fetal protection in Wisconsin's revised child abuse law: Right goal, wrong remedy, *Journal of Law, Medicine, and Ethics* 27 (1999): 335.

45. Joel Feinberg, Harm to others (New York: Oxford University Press, 1984).

46. American Academy of Pediatrics, Committee on Bioethics: Religious objections to medical care, *Pediatrics* 99 (1997): 279–81.

47. *In re* Petra, 216 Cal. App. 3d 1163.

48. Arthur Allen, The trouble with ADHD, *Washington Post,* Mar. 18, 2001, p. W8.

49. G. Pascal Zachary, Male order: Boys used to be boys, but do some now see boyhood as a malady? *Wall Street Journal,* May 2, 1997, p. A1.

50. James E. Ryan, The perverse incentives of the No Child Left Behind Act, *NYU Law Review* 79 (2004): 932, 942–43.

51. American Association for the Advancement of Science, Good, better, best: The human quest for enhancement, ed. Mark S. Frankel, available at www.futureguru.com/docs/hesummary.pdf, last visited Oct. 3, 2007.

52. Amy Joice, So much for "personal habits," *Washington Post,* Oct. 15, 2006, p. F1.

53. National Workrights Institute, Lifestyle discrimination in the workplace, available at www.workrights.org/issue_lifestyle/ld_legislative_brief.html, last visited Oct. 3, 2007.

54. U.S. Equal Employment Opportunity Commission, Enforcement guidance: Disability-related inquiries and medical examinations of employees under the Americans with Disabilities Act.

55. U.S. Equal Employment Opportunity Commission, Compliance manual on race and color discrimination, available at www.eeoc.gov/policy/docs/race-color.html, last visited Oct. 4, 2007.

56. U.S. Navy, Performance maintenance during continuous flight operations, a guide for flight surgeons (2000), available at www.globalsecurity.org/military/library/policy/navy/misc/NAVMEDP-6410.pdf, last visited Oct. 3, 2007.

57. Leslie Henry and Lorna Schumann, Inhalation anthrax: Threat, clinical presentation, and treatment, *Journal of the American Academy of Nurse Practitioners* 13 (2001): 164–68.

58. George Annas, Blinded by bioterrorism: Public health and liberty in the 21st century, *Health Matrix* 13 (2003): 33–70.

59. Alexandra Hudson, East German kids bred on steroids, *Rediff India Abroad,* Nov. 1, 2004, available at www.rediff.com/sports/2004/nov/01dope.htm, last visited Oct. 4, 2007.

60. Jere Longman, Just following orders, doctors' orders, *New York Times,* Apr. 22, 2001, section 8, p. 11.

61. Hudson, East German kids.

62. Longman, Just following orders.

63. Ibid.

64. Jordan Bonfante, Dope into gold: Sports officials and the legacy of communism's state-approved abuse of steroids, *Time,* Jan. 19, 1998, p. 46.

65. Andy Coghlan, Casualties of quest for Olympic gold, *New Scientist,* July 20, 1996, p. 44.

66. Bojan Pancevski, German athletes fed steroids and Supertramp, Telegraph online, available at www.telegraph.co.uk/news/main.jhtml?xml=/news/2007/09/23/wsteroids123.xml, last visited Oct. 4, 2007.

67. Mark Starr, Starr gazing: Tarnished gold, *Newsweek,* May 13, 2004.

68. Chris Wood, Ann Walmsley, Shaffin Shariff, Peter Lewis, and Peggy Weddell, The drug busters, *Maclean's,* February 1988, p. 122.

69. Michael Getler, Athlete who fled East Germany cites forced drug use, *Washington Post,* Dec. 29, 1978, p. A1.

70. Ruth R. Faden and Tom L. Beauchamp, A history and theory of informed consent (New York: Oxford University Press, 1986), p. 339.

71. Amateur Athletic Association Newsletter, December 2003, available at www.aafla.org/10ap/SportsLetter14-4/SLhome.html, last visited June 10, 2005.

72. Charles E. Yesalis, Testimony before Subcommittee on Commerce, Trade, and Consumer Protection and Subcommittee on Health, House Energy and Commerce Committee, Mar. 10, 2005.

73. Faden and Beauchamp, A history and theory of informed consent, p. 344, emphasis in original.

74. Jessica W. Berg, Paul S. Appelbaum, Charles W. Lidz, and Lisa S. Parker, Informed consent: Legal theory and clinical practice (New York: Oxford University Press, 2001), p. 68.

75. Robert L. Simon, Good competition and drug-enhanced performance, in William J. Morgan and Klaus V. Meier, eds., Philosophic inquiry in sport, 2nd ed. (Champaign, IL: Human Kinetics, 1995), p. 209.

76. W. M. Brown, Paternalism, drugs, and the nature of sports, in Morgan and Meier, eds., Philosophic inquiry in sport, p. 220.

Chapter 7. Enhancements in Sports

1. Sen. Byron Dorgan, opening statement, Steroid Use in Professional Baseball and Anti-Doping Issues in Amateur Sports: Hearing before Subcommittee on Consumer Affairs, Foreign Commerce and Tourism of the Senate Committee on Commerce, Science, and Transportation, 107th Congress 1, 2002, http://commerce.senate.gov/hearings/hearings0202.htm.

2. Barrie Houlihan, Dying to win (Strasbourg: Council of Europe Publishing, 1999), p. 33, citing J. Puffer, The use of drugs in swimming, *Clinical Sports Medicine* 7 (1986): 77–89.

3. Panayiotis J. Papagelopoulos, Andreas F. Mavrogens, and Panayotis N. Soucacos, Doping in ancient and modern Olympic Games, *Orthopedics* 27 (2004): 1226–31.

4. World Anti-Doping Agency 2005, available at www.wada-ama.org/en/dynamic.ch2?pageCategory_id=20, last visited June 23, 2005.

5. A. J. Higgins, From ancient Greece to modern Athens: 3000 years

of doping in competition horses, *Journal of Veterinary Pharmacology and Therapeutics* 29 (2006): 4–8.

6. David R. Mottram, ed., Drugs in sport, 2nd ed. (London: Routledge, 1996), p. 18.

7. Houlihan, Dying to win, p. 34.

8. Mary Delach Leonard, St. Louis hosts Olympics, *St. Louis Post Dispatch,* Jan. 13, 2004, p. 102.

9. Ivan Waddington, Sport, health, and drugs: A critical sociological perspective (London: Spon, 2000), pp. 114–27.

10. Karen Birchard, Past, present, and future of drug abuse at the Olympics, *The Lancet* 356 (2000): 1008.

11. Some of the following material is based on Maxwell J. Mehlman, Elizabeth Banger, and Matthew Wright, Doping in sports and the use of state power, *St. Louis University Law Review* 50 (2006): 15–73.

12. Higgins, From ancient Greece to modern Athens, 4–8.

13. Waddington, Sport, health, and drugs, pp. 114–27.

14. Ruud Stokvis, Moral entrepreneurship and doping cultures in sport 6 (Amsterdam School for Social Science Research, Working Paper No. 03/04, 2003), available at http://www2.fmg.uva.nl/assr/frdocs/wp/downloads/ASSR-WP0304.pdf, last visited Oct. 10, 2007.

15. International Olympic Committee, Official Bulletin, 1937, available at www.aafla.org/OlympicInformationCenter/OlympicReview/1937/BODEb35/BODEb35b.pdf, last visited Oct. 9, 2007.

16. International Olympic Committee, Official Bulletin, 1938, p. 30, emphasis added.

17. Allen Guttmann, The Olympics: A history of the modern games (Urbana: Illinois University Press, 1992).

18. John Hoberman, Mortal engines: The science of performance and the dehumanization of sport (Caldwell, NJ: Blackburn Press, 2001).

19. Athletes report use of "pep pills," *New York Times,* June 8, 1957, p. 20; and Sports physicians to check on pills, *New York Times,* June 9, 1957, p. 52.

20. G. M. Smith and H. K. Beecher, Amphetamine sulfate and athletic performance, I. Objective effects, *Journal of the American Medical Association* 170 (1959): 542–57.

21. Dane in Rome bike race dies, *New York Times,* Aug. 27, 1960, p. 13.

22. James C. Puffer, Drugs in colleges: To test or not to test, *New York Times,* May 29, 1988, section 8, p. 7.

23. Europack: An education and information guide on sport without doping, available at www.coe.int/T/E/cultural_co-operation/Sport/Doping/eEuropack.asp.

24. Stokvis, Moral entrepreneurship and doping cultures in sport 6.

25. Drugs discovered in cyclist's autopsy, *New York Times,* Aug. 4, 1967,

p. S26; and John L. Hess, Simpson dies in Tour de France, *New York Times,* July 14, 1967, p. 38.

26. John L. Hess, Anti-doping rules threatening Anquetil's bicycle speed mark, *New York Times,* Sept. 29, 1967, p. 70.

27. Waddington, Sport, health, and drugs, pp. 114–27.

28. Michele Verroken, Drug use and abuse in sport, in Mottram, ed., Drugs in sport, pp. 18, 23.

29. Michael A. Hicks, Anti-doping authorities serve as prosecutor, judge and jury: The innocent often pay a high price, *Los Angeles Times,* Dec. 10, 2006, available at www.latimes.com/news/nationworld/nation/la-sp-doping 10dec10,0,2627563,full.story?coll=la-home-headlines, last visited Oct. 10, 2007.

30. John Hoberman, Testosterone dreams (Berkeley: University of California Press, 2005), p. 243.

31. Verroken, Drug use and abuse in sport, pp. 18, 23.

32. Olympian tells of steroid use, *New York Times,* Apr. 21, 1998, p. C5.

33. Verroken, Drug use and abuse in sport, pp. 18, 23.

34. David Galluzzi, The doping crisis in international athletic competition: Lessons from the Chinese doping scandal in women's swimming, *Seton Hall Journal of Sports* 10 (2000): 65–78.

35. Ever faster, ever higher? *The Economist,* U.S. edition, Aug. 7, 2004, special report 1.

36. U.S. Anti-Doping Agency, available at www.usantidoping.org, last visited Oct. 10, 2007.

37. Michael A. Hiltzik, Presumed guilty: Athletes' unbeatable foe, *Los Angeles Times,* Dec. 10, 2006, p. A1.

38. Schmitt Boyer. Does everybody cheat? *Cleveland Plain Dealer,* Feb. 18, 2007, p. A10–11.

39. International Paralympic Committee, Press Release, available at www.paralympic.org/release/Main_Sections_Menu/News/Press_Releases/2004_09_26_a.html, last visited Oct. 10, 2007.

40. Associated Press, Chess: Drug testing has arrived, *New York Times,* Nov. 16, 1999, p. D7.

41. Alwaysclean News, IOC: "Mind" sports must drug test, too, Apr. 16, 2003, available at www.alwaysclean.com/news/atc_news_09.htm, last visited May 30, 2007.

42. Stephen P. Williams, No bridge mix for this crowd, *New York Times,* Feb. 27, 2004, p. F1.

43. Allan H. "Bud" Selig and Robert D. Manfred Jr., The regulation of nutritional supplements in professional sports, *Stanford Law and Policy Review* 15 (2004): 44–46.

44. World Anti-Doping Agency, available at www.wada-ama.org/en/dynamic.ch2?pageCategory.id=264, last visited Oct. 11, 2007.

45. Selig and Manfred, The regulation of nutritional supplements in professional sports.

46. Hiltzik, Presumed guilty, p. A1.

47. Ibid.

48. Michael A. Hiltzik, Cracks in the doping code? *Los Angeles Times,* Jan. 16, 2007, p. D1.

49. Allan H. "Bud" Selig and Robert D. Manfred Jr., The regulation of nutritional supplements in professional sports, 44–46; and Bill Buchalter, Ed Hinton, David Whitley, Andrew Carter, Chris Harry, and Tim Povtak, Super boosters, *Orlando Sentinel* (Florida), Mar. 4, 2007, p. C8.

50. Thomas Banks, Golf to begin drug testing, *Los Angeles Times,* Sept. 21, 2007, p. D8.

51. Schmitt Boyer, Does everybody cheat? *Cleveland Plain Dealer,* Feb. 18, 2007, p. A10–11.

52. Jay Mariotti, No reason to watch if everyone cheats, *Chicago Sun Times,* Aug. 7, 2006, p. 99.

53. George W. Bush, State of the Union Address, Jan. 20, 2004, available at www.whitehouse.gov/news/releases/2004/01/20040120-7.html, last visited June 23, 2005.

54. 38 Stat. 785 (1914); and 41 Stat. 305 (1920).

55. 42 Stat. 596 (1922).

56. Associated Press, Olympics: Marijuana becomes banned substance, *New York Times,* April 28, 1998, p. C5.

57. *Vernonia School District v. Acton,* 1995. 515 U.S. 646.

58. *Board of Education v. Earls,* 2002. 536 U.S. 822.

59. House of Commons Science and Technology Committee Report, Human Enhancement Technologies in Sport, Feb. 22, 2007, p. 26, available at www.publications.parliament.uk/pa/cm200607/cmselect/cmsctech/67/67.pdf, last visited Oct. 13, 2007.

60. Ibid.

61. Michael A. Hiltzik, Anti-doping group to show some leniency, *Los Angeles Times,* Jan. 25, 2007, p. D1.

62. Catherine Carstairs, The wide world of doping: Drug scandals, natural bodies, and the business of sports entertainment, *Addiction Research and Theory* 11 (2003): 263–81, quoting Susan Brownell.

63. WADA, WADA executive committee approves the 2008 prohibited list, available at www.wada-ama.org/en/newsarticle.ch2?articleId=3115475, last visited Oct. 15, 2007.

64. Steve Kelley, Drugs taint today's sports, but we must keep the faith, *Seattle Times,* Oct. 9, 2005, p. C12.

65. Leon Kass, The Wisdom of Repugnance, *New Republic* 2 (1997): 17–26.

66. Charlie Francis, quoted in Charles E. Yesalis, ed., Anabolic Steroids in Sport and Exercise, 2nd ed. (Champaign, IL: Human Kinetics, 2000).

67. Alexandra Hudson, East German kids bred on steroids, *Rediff India Abroad,* Nov. 1, 2004.

68. Hiltzik, Anti-doping rules to show some leniency, p. D1.

69. Quoted in John M. Hoberman, Sport and the technological image of man, in William J. Morgan and Klaus V. Meier, eds., Philosophic inquiry in sport, 2nd ed. (Champaign, IL: Human Kinetics, 1995), p. 202, emphasis added.

70. Editorial: Drugs in sport: A philosophical challenge, *Philosophy* 81 (2006): 559.

71. *Thorpe v. Housing Authority of Durham,* 1967. 386 U.S. 670, 678.

72. 36 U.S.C. §220501.

73. Edward H. Jurith and Mark W. Beddoes, The United States and international response to the problem of doping in sports, *Fordham Intellectual Property, Media and Entertainment Law Journal* 12 (2002): 461–88.

74. Anti-Drug Abuse Act of 1988, Pub. L. No. 100-690, 102 Stat. 4181 (amended 1990).

75. Crime Control Act of 1990, Pub. L. No. 101-647, 104 Stat. 4789 (1990).

76. 21 USCA §812(b)(3).

77. S. Rep. No. 101-433 1990. Steroid Trafficking Act of 1990, S. 1829, 101st Congress, described in Steroids Working Group 2006. U.S. Sentencing Commission Report on Steroids.

78. Athletic Performance-Enhancing Drugs Research and Detection Act 2003. S. 1002, 108th Congress §102.

79. Jack Curry, Four indicted in a steroid scheme that involved top pro athletes, *New York Times,* Feb. 13, 2004, p. A1.

80. George W. Bush, State of the Union Address, Jan. 20, 2004.

81. Steroid Control Act of 2004. Pub. L. 108-358, Oct. 22, 2004, 118 Stat. 1661.

82. 21 U.S.C. §333(h).

83. Restoring Faith in America's Pastime: Evaluating Major League Baseball's Efforts to Eradicate Steroid Use: Hearing before the House Committee on Government Reform, 109th Congress (2005).

84. 150 Congressional Record S3996, 3997–98, 2004 (statement of Sen. McCain).

85. Steroid Use in Sports Part III: Examining the National Basketball Association's Steroid Testing Program: Hearing before the House Committee on Government Reform, 109th Congress (2005); and Steroid Use in Sports Part

II: Examining the National Football League's Policy on Anabolic Steroids and Related Substances, Hearing before the House Committee on Government Reform, 109th Congress (2005).

86. Les Carpenter and Juliet Eilperin, Baseball plan would exile repeat offenders, *Washington Post,* Nov. 16, 2005, p. A1.

87. Jack Curry, To tighten drug tests, teams are secretly monitoring players, *New York Times,* Apr. 1, 2007, section 8, pp. 1, 7.

88. Bill Buchalter et al., Super boosters, p. C8.

89. Hiltzik, Presumed guilty, p. A1.

90. Teri Thompson, Anti-doping head wants government help, *New York Daily News,* May 14, 2007, p. 57.

91. Ibid.

92. Julie Macur, Looking for doping evidence, Italian policy raid Austrians, *New York Times,* Feb. 19, 2006, available at www.nytimes.com/2006/02/19/sports/olympics/19drug.html, last visited Oct. 19, 2007.

93. Associated Press, Austrian coach who fled in mental hospital, MSNBC, Feb. 26, 2006, available at www.msnbc.msn.com/id/11446789/from/RSS/, last visited Oct. 19, 2007.

94. Jason Cohen, Rick Collins, Jack Darkes, and Dan Gwartney, A league of their own: Demographics, motivations, and patterns of use of 1,955 male adult nonmedical anabolic steroids users in the United States, *Journal of International Society of Sports Nutrition* (2007), available at www.eurekaalert.org/pub_releases/2007-10/bc-tr100907.php, last visited Oct. 10, 2007.

Chapter 8. The Lessons from Sports

1. World Anti-Doping Agency, Athletes Passport, April 2004, available at www.wada-ama.org/rtecontent/document/April_04.pdf, last visited June 10, 2005.

2. Francis Fukuyama and Franco Furger, Beyond bioethics: A proposal for modernizing the regulation of human biotechnologies (Washington, D.C.: Paul H. Nitze School of Advanced International Studies, 2007).

3. John Robertson, Genetic selection of offspring characteristics, *Boston University Law Review* 76 (1996): 421, 479.

4. Ronald M. Green, Parental autonomy and the obligation not to harm one's child genetically, *Journal of Law, Medicine, and Ethics* 25 (1997): 5–15.

5. *Lifchez v. Hartigan,* 1990. 735 F. Supp. 1361 (N.D. Ill.), *aff'd,* 914 F.2d 260 (7th Cir. 1990), *cert. denied,* 498 U.S. 1069 (1991).

6. *Cameron v. Board of Education of Hillsboro,* 1991. 795 F. Supp. 228 (S.D. Ohio).

7. Robert Pear, Fertility clinics face crackdown, *New York Times,* Oct. 26, 1992, p. A15; and 42 U.S.C. §263a-1-263a-7.

8. Human Fertilization and Embryology Authority Code of Practice,

G-12-3-2, available at http://cop.hfea.gov.uk/cop/pdf/COP.pdf, last visited Oct. 22, 2007.

9. Allan H. "Bud" Selig and Robert D. Manfred Jr., The regulation of nutritional supplements in professional sports, *Stanford Law and Policy Review* 15 (2004): 44–46.

10. Jack Curry, To tighten drug tests, teams are secretly monitoring players, *New York Times*, Apr. 1, 2007, section 8, pp. 1, 7.

11. Michael A. Hiltzik, Presumed guilty: Athletes' unbeatable foe, *Los Angeles Times*, Dec. 10, 2006, p. A1.

12. House of Commons Science and Technology Committee, Human Enhancement Technologies in Sport (advance copy), Feb. 22, 2007, p. 30.

13. Ibid., p. 41.

14. Liz Brody, Easy drugs online, *Glamour*, Apr. 2000, p. 102.

15. Ibid.

16. Steve P. Callandrio, Cash for kidneys? Utilizing incentives to end America's organ shortage, *George Mason Law Review* 13 (2004): 69–133.

17. Cosmetic Surgery and Healthcare Holidays Abroad, available at www.cosmeticsurgeryholidays.com, last visited Oct. 27, 2007.

18. Treatment Abroad, available at www.treatmentabroad.net/cosmetic-abroad, last visited Oct. 27, 2007.

19. Council of Europe, Convention on human rights and biomedicine, Art. 13 (European Treaty Series No. 164).

20. Denver Summit of the Eight, communique of June 22, 1997, available at www.g7.utoronto.ca/summit/1997denver/g8final.htm, last visited Oct. 26, 2008.

21. Council of Europe, Convention on human rights and biomedicine, additional protocol on the prohibition of human cloning (European Treaty Series No. 164); and European Parliament, 2000, Resolution on human cloning (85-0719, 0751, and 0764/2000).

22. George J. Annas, Lori B. Andrews, and Rosario M. Isasit, Protecting the endangered human: Toward an international treaty prohibiting cloning and inheritable alterations, *American Journal of Law and Medicine* 28 (2002): 151–78.

23. HUGO, Ethics committee statement on cloning, *Eubios Journal of Asian and International Bioethics* 9 (1999): 70.

24. 50 U.S.C.A. §1701(b).

25. Adam Smith, A high price to pay: The costs of the U.S. economic sanctions policy and the need for process-oriented reform, *UCLA Journal of International Law and Foreign Affairs* 4 (1999–2000): 325–76.

26. American Association for the Advancement of Science, 2006, Good, better, best: The human quest for enhancement, ed. Mark S. Frankel, avail-

able atwww.futureguru.com/docs/hesummary.pdf, last visited Oct. 3, 2007.

27. U.S. Congress, Office of Technology Assessment, Human gene therapy: A background paper (OTA-BP-BA-32) (Washington, D.C.: Government Printing Office, 1984).

28. Transplant News, Japan bans Seed from setting up cloning research center, Jan. 15, 1999, available at www.allbusiness.com/health-care-social-assistance/ambulatory-health-services/151398-1.html, last visited Nov. 3, 2007.

29. Jane Barrett, Doctor vows cloning effort will proceed, *Philadelphia Inquirer,* Aug. 7, 2001, p. A2.

30. Tracy Wilkins, Italy bars fertility aid to older women, gays, *Los Angeles Times,* Dec. 12, 2003, p. A1; and Reuters, Italian lawmakers enact rules that limit reproductive rights, *New York Times,* Dec. 12, 2003, p. A16.

31. How to build your own atomic bomb, available at http://students.fct.unl.pt/users/osv/bomb.htm, last visited Oct. 31, 2007.

32. James Ridgeway, Al Qaeda duped? *Village Voice,* Nov. 16, 2001, available at www.villagevoice.com/news/0147,ridgeway2,30078,6.html, last visited Nov. 3, 2007.

33. William J. Broad, U.S. web archive is said to reveal a nuclear primer, *New York Times,* Nov. 3, 2006, available at www.newyorktimes.com/2006/11/03/world/middleeast/03documents.html, last visited Nov. 3, 2007.

34. Jorge Chabat, Mexico's war on drugs: No margin for maneuver, *Annals of the American Academy of Political and Social Science* 582 (2002): 134–48.

35. Congressional Research Service, Mexico's drug cartels: Report for Congress, available at www.fas.org/sgp/crs/row/RL34215.pdf, last visited Oct. 31, 2007.

36. *Haig v. Agree,* 1981. 453 U.S. 280.

37. Carla K. Johnson, CDC quarantine officers ever on watch, *USA Today,* July 14, 2007, available at www.usatoday.com/news/health/2007-07-14-2008900088_x.htm, last visited Nov. 5, 2007.

38. U.S. Department of Homeland Security, Form I-693: Medical examination of aliens seeking adjustment of status, available at www.uscis.gov/files/form/I-693.pdf, last visited Nov. 5, 2007.

39. 18 U.S.C. §2251–57.

40. *U.S. v. Harvey,* 1993. 2 F.3d 1318 (3d Cir.).

41. 31 U.S.C.A. §5314.

42. 31 U.S.C.A. §5316.

43. 26 U.S.C.A. §7206(1).

44. Personal communication from Lori Andrews.

45. U.S. Anti-Doping Agency, available at www.usantidoping.org/what/stats/quarterly.aspx, last visited Oct. 26, 2007.

46. Richard Willing, DNA lag leaves potential for crime, *USA Today*, Sept. 4, 2007, p. 8A, 1A.

47. Johnson, CDC quarantine officers ever on watch.

48. Charles E. Yesalis, Testimony before Subcommittee on Commerce, Trade, and Consumer Protection and Subcommittee on Health, House Energy and Commerce Committee, Mar. 10, 2005.

49. Centers for Disease Control and Prevention, National Center for Health Statistics 2004 data, available at www.cdc.gov/nchs/fastats/druguse.htm, last visited Oct. 27, 2007.

50. Charles E. Yesalis, Testimony before Subcommittee on Commerce, Trade, and Consumer Protection and Subcommittee on Health, House Energy and Commerce Committee, Mar. 10, 2005.

51. Columbia Pictures, 1997.

52. National Cancer Institute, Simian Virus 40 and Human Cancer: Questions and Answers, available at www.cancer.gov/newscenter/sv40, last visited Nov. 16, 2007.

53. Paul Berg et al., Potential biohazards of recombinant DNA molecules, *Science* 185 (1974): 303.

54. Alan Lightman, The discoveries (New York: Pantheon Books, 2005).

55. HUGO Ethics Committee, Statement on cloning, *Eubios Journal of Asian and International Bioethics* 9 (1999): 70.

56. World Medical Association, available at www.wma.net/e/policy/c7.htm, last visited Nov. 17, 2007.

57. Michael A. Grodin, George J. Annas, and Leonard H. Glantz, Medicine and human rights: A proposal for international action, *Hastings Center Report* 23 (1993): 8–12.

58. Lightman, The Discoveries.

59. AMA Council on Ethical and Judicial Affairs, *Archives of Family Medicine* 3 (1994): 633–42.

60. AMA Council on Ethical and Judicial Affairs, Current Opinion E2.11: Gene Therapy, 2004.

61. AMA, The AMA policy system, available at www.ama-assn.org/ama1/pub/upload/mm/450/amapolicysystem0306.pdf, last visited Nov. 19, 2007.

62. Emile Durkheim, Professional ethics and civic morals, trans. Cornelia Brookfield (New York: Routledge, 1957).

63. White House, Fact Sheet: President Bush's Stem Cell Research Policy, available at www.whitehouse.gov/news/releases/2006/07/20060719-6.html, last visited Nov. 19, 2007.

64. California Institute for Regenerative Medicine, available at www.cirm.ca.gov/, last visited Nov. 19, 2007.

65. Ron Bailey, Do we really need the feds? Funding stem cell research

without Uncle Sam, available at www.reason.com/news/show/34993.html, last visited Nov. 19, 2007.

66. Robert C. Black, Monkeywrenching the justice system? *UMKC Law Review* 66 (1997): 11–40.

67. Joan W. Howarth, Adventures in heteronormativity: The straight line from Liberace to Lawrence, *Nevada Law Journal* (Fall 2004): 260–83.

68. Robert E. Rodes Jr., On law and chastity, *Notre Dame Law Review* 76 (2001): 643–79.

Chapter 9. The War on Enhancements

1. NIH, Recombinant DNA research, request for public comment on "points to consider in the design and submission of human somatic-cell gene therapy protocols." 50 *Federal Register* 2940 (Jan. 22, 1985).

2. AMA Council on Ethical and Judicial Affairs. 1994. Current Opinion EB2.11: Gene Therapy.

3. AMA Council on Ethical and Judicial Affairs, *Archives of Family Medicine* 3 (1994): 633–42.

4. Courtney S. Campbell, Biotechnology and the fear of Frankenstein, *Cambridge Quarterly of Healthcare Ethics* 12 (2003): 342–52.

5. Willard Gaylin, The Frankenstein factor, *New England Journal of Medicine* 297 (1977): 665–67.

6. Jon W. Gordon, Genetic enhancement in humans, *Science* 283 (1999): 2023–24.

7. Centers for Disease Control and Prevention, Preliminary 2005 fertility clinic success rates and national summary, available at www.cdc.gov/ART/index.htm, last visited Nov. 30, 2007.

8. William Hermann, DEA steroid probe widens across valley, *Arizona Republic*, July 24, 2007, p. 1.

9. C. Swanson, L. Gaines, and B. Gore, Police officer use of anabolic steroids, *FBI Law Enforcement Bulletin* 60 (1991): 19–23.

10. Stephen Hudak, Steroids: A threat to police officers "a larger problem than people think," *Cleveland Plain Dealer*, July 25, 2003, p. B1.

11. Duff Wilson, Aging: Disease or business opportunity? *New York Times*, Apr. 15, 2007, section 3, p. 1.

12. Available at www.antiagingquackery.com/illegal/doctorsandclinics.html, last visited Dec. 2, 2007.

13. Liu Hau, Dena M. Bravata, Ingram Olkin, Smita Nayak, Alan M. Garber, and Andrew R. Hoffman, Systematic review: The safety and efficacy of growth hormone in the healthy elderly, *Annals of Internal Medicine* 146 (2007): 104–24.

14. Stanley D. Silverman, Letter to Dr. Thomas Perls, Oct. 4, 2004, avail-

able at www.bumc.bu.edu/www/BUSM/Cen/images/oct_2004.pdf, last visited Dec. 2, 2007.

15. Available at www.antiagingquackery.com, last visited Dec. 2, 2007.

16. Ibid.

17. Brian Fitzgerald, Longevity researcher Thomas Perls: Study proves growth hormone injections are harmful, *B.U. Bridge,* Jan. 10, 2003, available at www.bu.edu/bridge/archive/2003/01-10/longevity.htm, last visited Dec. 2, 2007.

18. Blair Tindall, Better playing through chemistry, *New York Times,* Oct. 24, 2004, section 2, p. 1.

19. William J. Robbins, Congress gets Nixon's bill to curb drug abuses, *New York Times,* July 16, 1969, p. 1.

20. Alex Baenninger, Jorge Alberto Coasta e Silva, Ian Hindmarch, Hans-Jurgen Moeller, and Karl Rickels, Good chemistry: The life and legacy of Valium inventor Leo Sternbach (New York: McGraw-Hill, 2004).

21. M. K. Shear, C. Greeno, J. Kang, D. Ludewig, E. Frank, H.A. Swartz, and M. Hanekamp, Diagnosis of nonpsychotic patients in community clinics, *American Journal of Psychiatry* 157 (2000): 581–87.

22. Baenninger et al., Good chemistry.

23. Michael Tackett, Scientologist campaign shakes drug firm, advertising industry, *Chicago Tribune,* June 30, 1991, p. 17.

24. Paula Span, The man behind the bitter pill debate: Lawyer Leonard Finz presses the case against Eli Lilly and Prozac, *Washington Post,* Aug. 14, 1991, p. C1.

25. Eric G. Wilson, In praise of melancholy, *Chronicle of Higher Education,* Jan. 18, 2008, available at http://chronicle.com/temp/reprint.php?id=t5wqrs9hpxt70zjz3bv348pqg1hcxz0r, last visited Feb. 25, 2008.

26. WADA 2008 Monitoring program, available at www.wada-ama.org/rtecontent/document/Monitoring_Program_2008_En.pdf, last visited Dec. 10, 2007.

27. National Collegiate Athletic Association, http://www1.ncaa.org/membership/ed_outreach/health-safety/drug_testing/banned_drug_classes.pdf, last visited Dec, 10, 2007.

28. NCAA Drug Testing Information, available at www.stockton.edu/ospreys/ATDrugTesting.htm, last visited Dec. 10, 2007.

29. Michael Mason, Energy drinks may feed reliance on caffeine, *Cleveland Plain Dealer,* Dec. 23, 2006, p. E6.

30. Ibid.

31. Ibid.

32. Medical News Today, French ban on Red Bull (drink) upheld by European court, Feb. 8, 2004, available at www.medicalnewstoday.com/articles/5753.php, last visited Dec. 10, 2007.

33. Red Bull, available at www.redbullusa.com/en/ProductPage.FAQS/htmlProductPage.action?faqIndex=5, last visited Dec. 10, 2007.

34. Tara Parker-Pope, Soda makers to disclose caffeine content on labels, *Wall Street Journal,* Feb. 27, 2007, p. D1.

35. Kaye Spector, Shaker stirred up over coffee; caffeine caution prompts grumbles, *Cleveland Plain Dealer,* Feb. 9, 2006, p. B1.

36. Tom Feran, Readers are flush with toilet tales, *Cleveland Plain Dealer,* Feb. 28, 2006, p. E1.

Chapter 10. Promoting Safety, Efficacy, and Informed Decisionmaking

1. John Buescher, Spiritualism, Dictionary of Unitarian Universalist biography, available at www.uua.org/uuhs/duub/articles/spiritualism.html, last visited Dec. 27, 2007.

2. Susan Gilbert, Medical fakes and frauds (New York: Chelsea House, 1989).

3. James Harvey Young, The medical messiahs: A social history of health quackery in twentieth-century America (Princeton, NJ: Princeton University Press, 1974).

4. Maxwell J. Mehlman, Robert H. Binstock, Eric T. Juengst, Roselle S. Ponsaran, and Peter J. Whitehouse, Anti-aging medicine: can consumers be better protected? *Gerontologist* 44 (2004): 304–10 (references omitted).

5. C. W. Nevius, Radio station sued in water stunt death, *San Francisco Chronicle,* Jan. 26, 2007, p. B12.

6. 21 CFR §§312.80, 314.610.

7. Sharona Hoffman, The use of placebos in clinical trials: Responsible research or unethical practice? *Connecticut Law Review* 33 (2001): 449–501.

8. *Warner-Lambert Co. v. Heckler,* 1986. 787 F.2d 147 (3rd Cir.).

9. Baruch A. Brody, Ethical issues in drug testing, approval, and pricing: The clot-dissolving drugs (New York: Oxford University Press, 1995).

10. Anita Bernstein and Joseph Bernstein, An informal prescription for prescription drug regulation, *Buffalo Law Review* 54 (2006): 569–618.

11. FDA Modernization Act of 1997, Pub. L. 105-115, 111 Stat. 2296, §114.

12. Botox Prescribing Information, available at www.botoxcosmetic.com/resources/pi.aspx, last visited Dec. 31, 2007.

13. Carol Lewis, Botox cosmetic: A look at looking good, U.S. Food and Drug Administration, FDA Consumer magazine, July-August 2002, available at www.fda.gov/fdac/features/2002/402_botox.html, last visited Dec. 31, 2007.

14. S. R. Ahmad, Adverse drug event monitoring at the Food and Drug Administration, *Journal of General Internal Medicine* 18 (2003): 57–60; and J. Lazarou, B. H. Pomeranz, and P. N. Corey, Incidence of adverse drug events

in hospitalized patients: A meta-analysis of prospective studies, *JAMA* 279 (1998): 1200–1205.

15. 21 U.S.C. §321(ff)(1).

16. Life Source Nutrition, available at www.lifesource4life.com/hgh.html, last visited Jan. 2, 2008.

17. 21 U.S.C. §350b; and 21 U.S.C. §355(d).

18. U.S. General Accounting Office, Health products for seniors: "Anti-aging" products pose potential for physical and economic harm (GAO-01-1129), (Washington, D.C.: U.S. Government Printing Office, 2001).

19. Dietary Supplement and Nonprescription Drug Consumer Protection Act 2006, Public Law 109-462, 120 Stat. 3471.

20. Allan H. "Bud" Selig and Robert D. Manfred Jr., The regulation of nutritional supplements in professional sports, *Stanford Law and Policy Review* 15 (2004): 35–59.

21. U.S. Food and Drug Administration, Statement of policy for regulating biotechnology products, 49 *Federal Register* 50 (1984): 878; and U.S. Food and Drug Administration, Application of current statutory authorities to human somatic cell therapy products and gene therapy products, 58 Federal Register 53 (1993): 248.

22. 21 U.S.C. §321(g).

23. 21 C.F.R. §600.3(h), emphasis added.

24. Gail H. Javitt and Kathy Hudson, Regulating (for the benefit of) future persons: A different perspective on the FDA's jurisdiction to regulate human reproductive cloning, *Utah Law Review* 2003: 1201–29.

25. Ibid.

26. Richard A. Merrill, Human tissues and reproductive cloning: New technologies challenge FDA, *Houston Journal of Law and Policy* 3 (2002): 1–82.

27. Ibid.

28. Erik Parens and Eric Juengst, Editorial: Crossing the germ line, *Science* 292 (2001): 397.

29. Gail H. Javitt and Kathy Hudson, Regulating (for the benefit of) future persons, 1201–29.

30. American College of Medical Genetics, ACMG statement on direct-to-consumer genetic testing, available at www.acmg.net/resources/policies/Direct_Consumer_Testing.pdf, last visited Jan. 8, 2008.

31. Available at www.gtldna.com/dnatests.html, last visited Jan. 8, 2007.

32. Andrew Pollack, The wide, wild world of genetic testing, *New York Times*, Sept. 12, 2006, p. G4.

33. John E. Wennberg, Which rate is right? *New England Journal of Medicine* 314 (1986): 310–11.

34. E. Haavi Morreim, A dose of our own medicine: Alternative medicine, conventional medicine, and the standards of science, *Journal of Law, Medicine and Ethics* 31 (2003): 222–35.

35. David A. Hyman and Charles Silver, The poor state of health care quality in the U.S.: Is malpractice liability part of the problem or part of the solution? *Cornell Law Review* 90 (2005): 893–993.

36. John Carey, Medical guesswork, *Business Week*, May 29, 2006, pp. 72–79.

37. Neil A. Holtzman and Michael S. Watson, Final report of the Task Force on Genetic Testing, available at www.genome.gov/10001733, last visited Jan. 8, 2008.

38. Janet L. Dolgin, Debating conflicts: Medicine, commerce, and contrasting ethical orders, *Hofstra Law Review* 35 (2006): 705–35; Marcia Angell, The truth about the drug companies: How do they deceive us and what to do about it? (New York: Random House, 2004); Jerome P. Kassirer, On the take: How medicine's complicity with big business can endanger your health (New York: Oxford University Press, 2005); and David Blumenthal, Nancyanne Causino, Eric Campbell, and Karen Seashore Louis, Relationships between academic institutions and industry in the life sciences: an industry survey, *New England Journal of Medicine* 334 (1996): 368–74.

39. Eric G. Campbell, Russell L. Gruen, James Mountford, Lawrence G. Miller, Paul D. Cleary, and David Blumenthal, A national survey of physician-industry relationships, *New England Journal of Medicine* 356 (2007): 1742–50.

40. Melissa Healy, Sold on drugs, wooing the gatekeeper, *Los Angeles Times*, Aug. 6, 2007, p. F3.

41. Ford Fessendon and Christopher Drew, Bottom line in mind, doctors sell ephedra, *New York Times*, Mar. 31, 2003, p. A8.

42. E. Haavi Morreim, Medical research litigation and malpractice tort doctrines: Courts on a learning curve, *Houston Journal of Health Law and Policy* 4 (2003): 1–86.

43. *Pegram v. Herdrich*, 2000. 530 U.S. 211.

44. American College of Medical Genetics, ACMG statement on direct-to-consumer genetic testing.

45. AMA Council on Ethical and Judicial Affairs, *Archives of Family Medicine* 3 (1994): 633–42; and AMA Council on Ethical and Judicial Affairs. Current Opinion E2.11: Gene Therapy.

46. Mark S. Frankel and Audrey R. Chapman, Human inheritable genetic modifications: Assessing scientific, ethical, religious, and policy issues, available at www.aaas.org/spp/sfrl/projects/germline/report.pdf, last visited Jan. 9, 2008.

47. American Academy of Pediatrics, Policy statement: Use of performance-enhancing drugs, *Pediatrics* 115 (2005): 1103–6.

48. Federal Trade Commission, FTC targets bogus anti-aging claims for pills and sprays promising human growth hormone benefits, available at www.ftc.gov/opa/2005/06/greatamerican.shtm, last visited Jan. 10, 2008; and Federal Trade Commission, Marketers of Bloussant breast enhancement product to stop making false and unsubstantiated claims, available at www.ftc.gov/opa/2003/07/wellquest.shtm, last visited Jan. 10, 2008.

49. Federal Trade Commission, Marketers of Bloussant breast enhancement product to stop making false and unsubstantiated claims.

50. Howard Beales, Prepared statement of the Federal Trade Commission before the U.S. Senate Special Committee on Aging, Swindlers, hucksters and snake oil salesmen: The hype and hope of marketing anti-aging products to seniors, available at www.quackwatch.com/01QuackeryRelatedTopics/Hearing/ftc.html, last visited Jan. 10, 2008.

51. Dan Horn, Ex-Berkeley exec: Male-enhancement ads a lie, *Cincinnati Enquirer,* Jan. 16, 2008, p. 1A.

52. James Nash, Cap on lawsuit damages upheld: Right to jury trial does not rule out $350,000 limit, *Columbus Dispatch,* Dec. 28, 2007, p. 1A.

53. *Neotonus, Inc. v. AMA,* 2007. 2007 U.S. Dist. LEXIS 56656 (N.D. Ga.).

54. Peter D. Jacobson and Stefanie A. Doebler, We were all sold a bill of goods: Litigating the science of breast cancer treatment, *Wayne State Law Review* 52 (2006): 43–112.

55. 42 USC §1395y(a)(1)(A); and 42 USC §1395y(10).

56. Comprehensive Major Medical Health Care Certificate, Case Western Reserve University (Medical Mutual of Ohio), 1997.

57. David C. Radley, Stan N. Finkelstein, and Randall S. Stafford, Off-label prescribing among office-based physicians, *Archives of Internal Medicine* 166 (2006): 1021–26.

58. A. Elizabeth Blackwell and James M. Beck, Drug manufacturers' First Amendment right to advertise and promote their products for off-label use: Avoiding a pyrrhic victory, *Food and Drug Law Journal* 58 (2003): 439–62; and David M. Smolin, Nontherapeutic research with children: The virtues and vices of legal uncertainty, *Cumberland Law Review* 33 (2002–2003): 621–44.

59. Cephalon, Inc. Investor Overview, 2007, available at www.corporateir.net/ireye/ir_site.zhtml?ticker=CEPH&script=2100, last visited Nov. 12, 2003.

60. U.S. Department of Justice, Press Release: Warner-Lambert to pay $430 million to resolve criminal and civil health care liability relating to off-label promotion, 2004, available at www.usdoj.gov/usao/ma/presspage/May2004/Warner-Lambert-globalsettlemnt.htm, last visited May 24, 2004.

61. Anita Bernstein and Joseph Bernstein, An information prescription for drug regulation, *Buffalo Law Review* (2006): 569–618.

62. Rebecca S. Eisenberg, The role of the FDA in innovation policy, *Michigan Telecommunications and Technology Law Review* 13 (2007): 345–88.

63. Catherine T. Struve, The FDA and the tort system: Postmarketing surveillance, compensation, and the role of litigation, *Yale Journal of Health Policy, Law and Ethics* 5 (2005): 587–669; and Daniel R. Cahoy, Medical product information and the transparency paradox, *Indiana Law Journal* 82 (2007): 623–71.

64. Roselie A. Bright, Strategy for surveillance of adverse drug events, *Food and Drug Law Journal* 62 (2007): 605–15.

65. Struve, FDA and the tort system.

66. Oregon Health Services Commission, Prioritization of health services: A report to the governor and the legislature (1993).

67. 35 U.S.C. §287.

68. H. A. Slagter, L. L. Greischar, and A.D. Francis et al., Mental training affects distribution of limited brain resources, *Public Library of Science Biology* 5 (2007), available at doi:10.1371/journal.pbio.0050138, last visited Jan. 11, 2008.

69. Maxwell J. Mehlman, Robert H. Binstock, Eric T. Juengst, Roselle S. Ponsaran, and Peter J. Whitehouse, Anti-aging medicine: Can consumers be better protected? *Gerontologist* 44 (2004): 304–10.

70. S. Jay Olshansky, Leonard Hayflick, and Bruce A. Carnes, No truth to the fountain of youth, *Scientific American* 286 (2002): 92–95.

71. Mark A. Hall, Law, medicine, and trust, *Stanford Law Review* 55 (2002): 463–527.

72. AMA Council on Ethical and Judicial Affairs, Current Opinion E8.20: Invalid medical treatment.

Chapter 11. Protecting the Vulnerable

1. Daniel Callahan, The vulnerability of the human condition, in Peter Kemp, Jacob Rendtorff, and Niels Mattsson Johansen, eds., Bioethics and biolaw, volume II: Four ethical principles (Copenhagen: Rhodos International Science and Art Publishers; and Centre for Ethics and Law in Nature and Society, 2000), pp. 115–22.

2. Michael H. Kottow, The vulnerable and the susceptible, *Bioethics* 17 (2003): 460–71.

3. 45 C.F.R. §46.111(a)(3).

4. Erika Blacksher and John R. Stone, Introduction to "vulnerability" issues of theretical [*sic*] medicine and bioethics, *Theoretical Medicine and Bioethics* 23 (2002): 421–24.

5. David C. Thomasma, The vulnerability of the sick, *Bioethics Forum*

16 (2000): 5–12; and Patricia Backlar, Human subjects research, ethics, research on vulnerable populations, in Thomas H. Murray and Maxwell J. Mehlman, eds., Encyclopedia of ethical, legal, and policy issues in biotechnology 2:641–51 (New York: John Wiley and Sons, 2000).

6. Jim Vertuno, High school steroid testing plan moves forward in Texas, *USA Today,* Jan. 10, 2008, available at www.usatoday.com/sports/2008-01-10-3430990485_x.htm, last visited Jan. 30, 2008; and Gary Sharrer, Vendor chosen for drug testing in high schools, *Houston Chronicle,* Jan. 22, 2008, available at www.chron.com/disp/story.mpl/sports/5474634.html, last visited Jan. 30, 2008.

7. CNN, Bill bans teens from tanning booths, available at www.cnn.com/2004/HEALTH/05/21/tanning.ban.ap/index.html, last visited May 21, 2004.

8. *Feres v. United States,* 1950. 340 U.S. 135.

9. *Gonzalez v. U.S. Air Force,* 2004. 88 Fed. Appx. 371 (10th Cir.) (unpublished opinion).

10. Edith Starzyk, Bill would prohibit paddling in Ohio schools, *Cleveland Plain Dealer,* Jan. 29, 2008, p. A1.

11. *Ingraham v. Wright,* 1977. 430 U.S. 651.

12. John B. Breaux and Orrin G. Hatch, Confronting elder abuse, neglect, and exploitation: The need for elder justice legislation, *Elder Law Journal* 11 (2003): 207–71.

13. Harry Brighouse and Adam Swift, Parents' rights and the value of the family, *Ethics* 117 (2006): 80–108.

14. Kenneth A. DeVille and Loretta M. Kopelman, Fetal protection in Wisconsin's revised child abuse law: Right goal, wrong remedy, *Journal of Law, Medicine, and Ethics* 27 (1999): 335.

15. Personal communication from Sigmund Loland, Norwegian University of Sports, May 16, 2007.

Chapter 12. Access and Inequality

1. Internal Revenue Service, Publication 502, 2007, available at www.irs.gov/publications/p502/index.html, last visited Feb. 5, 2008.

2. Fritz Allhoff, Germ-line genetic enhancement and Rawlsian primary goods, *Kennedy Institute of Ethics Journal* 15 (2005): 36–59.

3. Office of Technology Assessment, Evaluation of the Oregon Medicaid proposal (Washington, D.C.: Government Printing Office, 1992).

4. John Rawls, A theory of justice (Cambridge, MA: Belknap Press of Harvard University Press, 1971); Norman Daniels, Just health care: Studies in philosophy and health policy (Cambridge, MA: Cambridge University Press, 1985); and Daniel W. Brock and Norman Daniels, Ethical founda-

tions of the Clinton administration's proposed health care system, *JAMA* 271 (1994): 1189–96.

5. Amy Goldstein, U.S. tells states to cover Viagra prescriptions under Medicaid, *Washington Post,* July 3, 1998, p. A21.

6. CMS says states should not cover impotence drugs for sex offenders, *BNA Health Law Reporter* 14 (2005): 755.

7. Alison Keith, The economics of Viagra, *Health Affairs* (March-April 2000): 147–57.

8. Maxwell Mehlman, Wondergenes: Genetic enhancement and the future of society (Bloomington: Indiana University Press, 2003).

9. Patricia Reaney, Surgery in Prague, Czech Republic: Plastic surgery lottery shocks UK, XtraMSN, Oct. 1, 2007, available at http://xrtramsn.co.nz/lifestyles/0,,12607-6970416,00.html, last visited Jan. 24, 2007.

10. Congressional Budget Office, Prices for brand-name drugs under selected federal programs, 2005, available at www.cbo.gov/ftpdocs/64xx/doc6481/06-16-PrescriptDrug.pdf, last visited Feb. 9, 2008.

11. Bradley Graham, Anthrax vaccine firm in trouble: Pentagon's inoculation program supplier near bankruptcy, *Washington Post,* July 1, 1999, p. A27.

12. Guy Gugliotta, Pentagon's missteps stalled new vaccines, *Washington Post,* Apr. 12, 2002, p. A13.

Chapter 13. Abominations

1. Julian Savulescu, Human-animal transgenesis and chimeras might be an expression of our humanity, *American Journal of Bioethics* 3 (2003): 22–25; and Andy Miah, Genetically modified athletes: Biomedical ethics, gene doping, and sport (London: Routledge, 2004).

2. Elliot Marshall, Legal fight over patents on life, *Science*NOW, 1999, available at http://sciencenow.sciencemag.org/cgi/content/full/1999/617/3, last visited Feb. 22, 2008.

3. George J. Annas, Lori B. Andrews, and Rosario M. Isasi, Protecting the endangered human: Toward an international treaty prohibiting cloning and inheritable alterations, *American Journal of Law and Medicine* 28 (2003): 151–78.

4. Burke K. Zimmerman, Human germ-line therapy: The case for its development and use, *Journal of Medicine and Philosophy* (1991): 593–612.

5. Stephen Holden, Film review: Kinkiness and piercing, branding and flogging, *New York Times,* Dec. 11, 1998, p. E1.

Chapter 14. Research on Enhancement

1. National Commission for the Protection of Human Subjects of Biomedical and Behavioral Research, The Belmont report: Ethical principles

and guidelines for the protection of human subjects of research, 1979, available at www.hhs.gov/ohrp/humansubjects/guidance/belmont.htm, last visited Oct. 2, 2008. See also 46 CFR 46.111(a)(2); 21 CFR 312.42 (b)(i); and 45 CFR 46.120(a).

2. 45 C.F.R. 46.116(a)

3. Subparts B, C, and D of the HHS guidelines.

4. 45 C.F.R. 46.111(b).

5. Anne Wood, Christine Grady, and Ezekiel J. Emanuel, Regional ethics organizations for protection of human research participants, *Nature Medicine* 10 (2004): 1283–88.

6. B. R. Furrow, T. L. Greaney, S. H. Johnson et al., Bioethics: Health care law and ethics, 5th ed. (St. Paul, MN: Thomson/West, 2004), p. 446.

7. B. Barrett, R. Brown, M. Mundt et al., Using benefit harm tradeoffs to establish sufficiently important difference: The case of the common cold, *Medical Decision Making* 25 (2005): 53.

8. N. Agar, Liberal eugenics: In defence of human enhancement (Malden, MA: Blackwell, 2004), pp. 167–68.

9. Anjan Chatterjee, Cosmetic neurology: the controversy over enhancing movement, mentation, and mood, *Neurology* 63 (2004): 968–74.

10. President's Council on Bioethics. Beyond therapy: Biotechnology and the pursuit of happiness (Washington, D.C.: President's Council on Bioethics, 2003), p. 306.

11. F. Bokhari, R. Mayes, and R. M. Scheffler, An analysis of the significant variation in psychostimulant use across the U.S., *Pharmacoepidemiology and Drug Safety* 14 (2005): 267–75.

12. L. G. Martin, R. F. Schoeni, V. A. Freedman et al., Feeling better? Trends in general health status, *The Journal of Gerontology. Series B, Psychological Sciences and Social Sciences* 62 (2007): S11–21.

13. 45 C.F.R. §46.111.

14. 45 C.F.R. §46.111(b).

15. 45 C.F.R. §46.204(b).

16. 45 C.F.R. §46.204(e).

17. 45 C.F.R. §§46.304-46.306.

18. Ian Urbina, Panel suggests using inmates in drug trials, *New York Times,* Aug. 13, 2006, available at www.newyorktimes.com/2006/08/13/us/13inmates.html, last visited Feb. 16, 2008.

19. Institute of Medicine, National Academy of Sciences, Ethical considerations for research involving prisoners (Washington, D.C.: National Academies Press, 2006).

20. Office of Human Subjects Protections, National Institutes of Health, IRB guidebook, available at www.hhs.gov/ohrp/irb/irb_guidebook.htm, last visited Feb. 20, 2008.

21. Ibid.

22. Amateur Athletic Association Newsletter, December 2003, available at www.aafla.org/10ap/SportsLetter14-4/SLhome.html, accessed June 10, 2005. As the newsletter explains, some critics deride the survey as unscientific.

23. Benjamin A. Alman, Naweed Razal, and W. Douglas Biggar, Steroid treatment and the development of scoliosis in males with Duchenne muscular dystrophy, *Journal of Bone and Joint Surgery* 86 (2004): 519–24.

24. Dena S. Davis, Medical research with college athletes: Some ethical issues, *IRB* (July-August 1998): 10–11.

25. WADA, available at www.wada-ama.org/en/dynamic.ch2?pageCategory.id=291, last visited Feb. 18, 2008.

26. Greg Bishop, Steroids issue offers no room in the middle, *Seattle Times*, Oct. 11, 2005, p. D7.

27. 45 CFR §46.111(a)(3).

28. National Commission for the Protection of Human Subjects of Biomedical and Behavioral Research, The Belmont report, 1979.

29. U.S. General Accounting Office, Human experimentation: An overview on Cold War era programs, Testimony of Assistant Comptroller General Frank C. Conahan before the Legislation and National Security Subcommittee, House Committee on Government Operations, Sept. 28, 1994, available at http://archive.gao.gov/t2pbat2/152601.pdf, last visited Feb. 18, 2008.

30. U.S. Congress, Report of the Senate Committee on Veterans' Affairs: Is military research hazardous to veterans' health? Lessons spanning half a century. 103d Congress 2d Sess. Dec. 8, 1994 (S. Prt. 103-97), available at www.gulfweb.org/bigdoc/rockrep.cfm#hallucinogens, last visited Feb. 18, 2008.

31. John McManus, Sumeru G. Mehta, Annette R. McClinton, Robert A. De Lorenzo, and Toney W. Baskin, Informed consent and ethical issues in military medical research, *Academic Emergency Medicine* 12 (2005): 1120–27.

32. David Dishneau, Church role in germ-warfare research debated, *Houston Chronicle*, Oct. 31, 1998, p. 8.

33. Ann LoLordo, Project Whitecoat: Human testing done with care, *Baltimore Sun*, Apr. 3, 1994, p. 1E.

34. Mark D. Somerson, Church blessed germ experiments: Army's biological warfare research used Seventh-Day Adventist volunteers, *Columbus Dispatch*, Nov. 8, 2001, p. 1A.

35. 32 CFR §§219.101ff.

36. 10 U.S.C. §980; and 21 CFR §50.24.

37. Keri D. Brown, Comment: An ethical obligation to our servicemembers: Meaningful benefits for informed consent violations, *S. Texas Law Review* 47 (2006): 919–47.

38. 10 U.S.C. §1107.

39. U.S. Army, Human Research Protection Office, Institutional policies and procedures, VI.B.2 (Possibility of coercion or undue influence), 2005, available at https://mrmc-www.army.mil/docs/rcq/HRPO_Policies_Procedures.pdf, last visited Feb. 18, 2008.

40. U.S. Army, Office of the Surgeon General. Reg. 15-2 I/11/89, 1989, available at https://mrmc-www.army.mil/docs/rcq/otsg15-2.pdf, last visited Feb. 18, 2008.

41. John McManus, Sumeru G. Mehta, Annette R. McClinton, Robert A. De Lorenzo, and Toney W. Baskin, Informed consent and ethical issues in military medical research, *Academic Emergency Medicine* 12 (2005): 1120–27.

42. F. X. Castellanos and J. L. Rapoport, Effects of caffeine on development and behavior in infancy and childhood: A review of the published literature, *Food and Chemical Toxicology* 40 (2002): 1235–42.

43. Thomas H. Murray, The worth of a child (Los Angeles: UCLA Press, 1996), quoting Paul Ramsey, The patient as person (New Haven: Yale University Press, 1970).

44. 45 CFR §46.102(i).

45. U.S. National Commission for the Protection of Human Subjects of Biomedical and Behavioral Research, Research involving children: Report and recommendations (Bethesda, MD, 1977); and M. J. Field and Richard E. Behrman, Institute of Medicine (U.S.), Committee on Clinical Research Involving Children, Ethical conduct of clinical research involving children (Washington, D.C.: National Academies Press, 2004).

46. Carol A. Tauer, The NIH trials of growth hormone for short stature, *IRB* 16 (1994): 1–9.

47. S. Shah, A. Whittle, Benjamin Wilfond, G. Gensler, and D. Wendler, How do institutional review boards apply the federal risk and benefit standards for pediatric research? *JAMA* 291 (2004): 476–82.

48. 45 CFR §46.407.

49. Personal communication from Ori Lev, Franklin G. Miller, and Ezekiel J. Emanuel, Jan. 3, 2008.

50. *Grimes v. Kennedy Krieger Inst., Inc.*, 2001. 782 A.2d 807 (Md. Ct. App.).

51. National Commission for the Protection of Human Subjects of Biomedical and Behavioral Research, The Belmont report, 1979.

52. Sharona Hoffman, The use of placebos in clinical trials: Responsible research or unethical practice? *Connecticut Law Review* 33 (2001): 449–501.

53. Recombinant DNA Advisory Committee, Points to Consider in the Design and Submission of Protocols for the Transfer of Recombinant DNA Molecules into One or More Human Research Participants (Points to Consider), Appendix M, 1985, available at http://www4.od.nih.gov/oba/rac/guidelines_02/Appendix_M.htm, last visited Aug. 17, 2007.

Index